VINCENNES UNIVERSITY LIBRARY

Practicing Yoga as Resistance

Bringing together a diverse chorus of voices and experiences in the pursuit of collective bodily, emotional, and spiritual liberation, *Practicing Yoga as Resistance* examines yoga as it is experienced across the Western cultural landscape through an intersectional, feminist lens.

Naming the systems of oppression that permeate our lived experiences, this collection and its contributors shine a light on the ways yoga practice is intertwined with these systems while offering insight into how people challenge and creatively subvert, mitigate, and reframe them through their efforts.

From the disciplines of yoga studies, embodiment studies, women's and gender studies, performance studies, educational studies, social sciences, and social justice, the self-identified women, queer, BIPOC, and White allies represented in this book present an interdisciplinary tapestry of scholarship that serves to add depth to a growing assemblage of yoga literature for the 21st century.

Cara Hagan is an assistant professor and scholar of dance studies at Appalachian State University. Hagan founded and facilitates the Boone, North Carolina-based organization, Small and Mighty Acts (SAMA). She is an interdisciplinary artist working at the intersections of movement, digital space, words, contemplative practice, and community.

Routledge Research in Race and Ethnicity

Ethnic Subjectivity in Intergenerational Memory Narratives
Politics of the Untold,
Mónika Fodor

Cool Britannia and Multi-Ethnic Britain
Uncorking the Champagne Supernova
Jason Arday

Translocational Belongings
Intersectional Dilemmas and Social Inequalities
Floya Anthias

Diasporas, Weddings and Trajectories of Ethnicity
Terence Heng

Black Families and Recession in the United States
The Enduring Impact of the Great Recession of 2007–2009
Dorothy Smith-Ruiz and Albert M. Kopak

Practicing Yoga as Resistance
Voices of Color in Search of Freedom
Edited by Cara Hagan

For a full list of titles in this series, please visit https://www.routledge.com/sociology/series/RRRE

Practicing Yoga as Resistance

Voices of Color in Search of Freedom

Edited by Cara Hagan

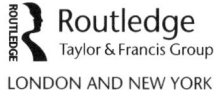

LONDON AND NEW YORK

First published 2021
by Routledge
2 Park Square, Milton Park, Abingdon, Oxon OX14 4RN

and by Routledge
52 Vanderbilt Avenue, New York, NY 10017

Routledge is an imprint of the Taylor & Francis Group, an informa business

© 2021 selection and editorial matter, Cara Hagan; individual chapters, the contributors

The right of Cara Hagan to be identified as the author of the editorial material, and of the authors for their individual chapters, has been asserted in accordance with sections 77 and 78 of the Copyright, Designs and Patents Act 1988.

All rights reserved. No part of this book may be reprinted or reproduced or utilised in any form or by any electronic, mechanical, or other means, now known or hereafter invented, including photocopying and recording, or in any information storage or retrieval system, without permission in writing from the publishers.

Trademark notice: Product or corporate names may be trademarks or registered trademarks, and are used only for identification and explanation without intent to infringe.

British Library Cataloguing-in-Publication Data
A catalogue record for this book is available from the British Library

Library of Congress Cataloging-in-Publication Data
Names: Hagan, Cara, editor.
Title: Practicing yoga as resistance: voices of color in search of freedom/ edited by Cara Hagan.
Description: Abingdon, Oxon; New York, NY: Routledge, 2021. | Series: Routledge research in race and ethnicity; 38 | Includes bibliographical references and index.
Identifiers: LCCN 2020049577 (print) | LCCN 2020049578 (ebook) | ISBN 9780367470524 (hardback) | ISBN 9781003033073 (ebook)
Subjects: LCSH: Hatha yoga–Social aspects–United States. | Minorities–United States–Social conditions. | Feminism–United States. | Oppression (Psychology) | Resistance (Philosophy) | United States–Race relations.
Classification: LCC RA781.7 .P733 2021 (print) | LCC RA781.7 (ebook) | DDC 613.7/046–dc23
LC record available at https://lccn.loc.gov/2020049577
LC ebook record available at https://lccn.loc.gov/2020049578

ISBN: 978-0-367-47052-4 (hbk)
ISBN: 978-0-367-75390-0 (pbk)
ISBN: 978-1-003-03307-3 (ebk)

Typeset in Times New Roman
by Deanta Global Publishing Services, Chennai, India

Contents

List of figures	viii
List of tables	x
List of contributors	xi
Foreword	xix
Preface: An introduction	xxi
Acknowledgement	xxv

PART I
Invitations   1

1 Essential questions for inner and outer liberation   3
  CARA HAGAN

2 Towards a White spiritual antiracism   17
  JARDANA PEACOCK

PART II
Yoga, Self, and Community   25

3 Embodied radical healing through the collective: A Black Lotus autoethnography   27
  DOMINIQUE A. MALEBRANCHE

4 Reclaiming spaces, reshaping practices: Yoga for building community and nurturing families of color   38
  AMY ARGENAL AND MONISHA BAJAJ

5 The city of radical love: A Philly story of oppression, resistance, and healing   49
  SHEENA SOOD AND MARI MORALES-WILLIAMS

6 Body science of survivorship: Mapping the
   neurological impacts of interlocking systems of oppression and
   co-designing equitable solutions through movement and breath   66
   MORGAN VANDERPOOL

7 Pedagogy of movement: Yoga in migrant projects from a race
   and class perspective   82
   FIRDOSE MOONDA

8 White hygiene, White womanhood, and wellness in the United
   States   109
   RUMYA S. PUTCHA

9 Incomplete: Impeding the settler colonial project through Yoga
   for Black Lives   118
   STEPHANIE D. HICKS

10 Hozho Yoga: Indigenous movements illuminating human and
   more-than-human interconnections   133
   TRIA BLU WAKPA

11 Yoga asana and the performance of gender
   in American exercise   157
   CARA HAGAN

12 Embodying liminality through yoga: An autoethnography
   exploring the spaces between   175
   SANAZ YAGHMAI

PART III
Yoga in Educational Spaces   201

13 Yoga, engaged pedagogy, and the process of *becoming:*
   Explorations of a socially just yoga intervention   203
   KIMBERLY NAO

14 White teachers, Brown yoga: Teacher candidates
   learning yoga   219
   ERIN ADAMS, SOHYUN AN, JILLIAN FORD, AND SANJUANA RODRIGUEZ

15 Trials and transformations: Ruminations of a community
   college yoga teacher   238
   SHYAMALA MOORTY

16 Situating girls of color in K–12 yoga research: Reflections and
   results from studying an after school yoga program for at-risk
   youth   255
   MICHELE TRACY BERGER

17 Yoga and arts: Positive disruptors in the school to
   prison pipeline   273
   SUZANA PLAISANT MCCALLEY

18 Tending communities: Yoga as an integrative, collaborative,
   and transformative practice   291
   NARIN HASSAN

   Index   305

Figures

1.1	Consider This: A Read-In for 21st Century Literacies	12
1.2	The Author, in an advertisement photo for one of the Essential Questions workshops	13
4.1	Family yoga post and image	43
4.2	Laxman and Prashad in a pose during class	45
4.3	Laxman and both his children in a pose during class	46
7.1	Timeline of data collection	87
7.2	Ourmala participant demographics – nationality	89
7.3	Ourmala participant demographics – race	90
7.4	Ourmala participant demographics – religion	90
7.5	OMPowerment participant demographics – nationality	91
7.6	OMPowerment participant demographics – race	91
7.7	Ourmala and OMPowerment – participant race demographics	92
7.8	Ourmala and OMPowerment – teacher and assistant teacher race demographics	92
8.1	Promotional photographs of Marilyn Monroe, 1948	111
8.2	Ruth St. Denis performing in brownface in Yogi (1911) and Nautch (1908) debuted in Vienna. Courtesy New York Public Library	112
8.3	Brillo advertisement, 1968	113
9.1	Musical theater actress Akilah Sailers has provided live music for YBL classes	122
10.1	Haley Laughter, in Warrior Three, transforming into a soaring eagle with white tailfeathers	134
10.2	Laughter connecting her palms and feet with the earth in Downward Facing Dog	140
10.3	After flipping her Downward Facing Dog, Laughter lifts and arcs her left arm, gesturing to the more-than-humans surrounding her	141
10.4	In Eagle Pose, Laughter's wrapping of her arms and legs resemble bean tendrils climbing corn stalks	144

10.5	In Garland Pose, Laughter's hands in prayer at the crown of her head suggest an eagle feather and her Diné/Native identity	147
10.6	Laughter appears like a plant in upside-down Garland Pose	149
10.7	Laughter "opening her heart" in Dancer's Pose	150
10.8	Laughter realizing one of her visions by teaching yoga to Native people in a Hogan	152
11.1	Clipping from "The Women's Page" of the *Mercury* newspaper, 1935	162
11.2	Madonna performs "Vogue" on her "Re-Invention tour in 2004. Getty Images	165
11.3	The Naked Athena, Portland, Oregon, 2020	167
11.4	Ardhanarishvara	170
15.1	"I did Down-guard facing dog." (Student Journal, 2012)	240
15.2	"I practiced Worrier Pose." (Student Journal, 2012)	242
15.3	"Is feeling this good illegal?" (Student journal, Fall 2015)	245
15.4	"When I do Dark Vader I feel more calm and end my day great." (Student Journal, Spring 2013)	250
15.5	A forest of Tree Poses, photo taken with permission of West LA Yoga students	252
17.1	Photo by Suzy McCalley	276
17.2	Photo by Christine Bloomfeld	281
17.3	Rameka Warren, photo by Christine Bloomfeld	283

Tables

16.1	Mindful Attention Awareness Scale (1)	262
16.2	Mindful Attention Awareness Scale (2)	262
16.3	Mindful Attention Awareness Scale (3)	262
16.4	Mindful Attention Awareness Scale (4)	263
16.5	Difficulties in Emotional Regulation Scale (1)	264
16.6	Difficulties in Emotional Regulation Scale (2)	264
16.7	Difficulties in Emotional Regulation Scale (3)	265
16.8	Difficulties in Emotional Regulation Scale (4)	265
16.9	Depression Anxiety Stress Scale (1)	266
16.10	Depression Anxiety Stress Scale (2)	266
16.11	Depression Anxiety Stress Scale (3)	266
16.12	Depression Anxiety Stress Scale (4)	267

Contributors

Erin Adams is Assistant Professor at Kennesaw State University in Kennesaw, Georgia where she teaches courses in elementary social studies methods, classroom community building and teacher leadership. Dr. Adams is interested in the teaching and rhetoric of economics education. Her work has been published in several edited volumes and social studies education journals.

Sohyun An is an associate professor of social studies education at Kennesaw State University. She received B.S. and M.S. degrees in social studies education from Seoul National University in South Korea, and a Ph.D. degree in Curriculum and Instruction from the University of Wisconsin-Madison. Since 2009, she has been teaching and researching in the field of social studies education. Her work is informed by scholarship on AsianCrit, critical race theory, critical pedagogy, and global citizenship. As a critical race scholar, elementary social studies teacher educator, and immigrant mother of Asian American children, she studies, teaches, and parents with a hope for anti-racist, anti-oppressive school and society for all children. Some of her works are published in journals namely, *Journal of Curriculum Studies*, *Theory and Research in Social Education*, *Journal of Social Studies Research*, and *Social Studies Research and Practice*. Her current project is a critical race parenting research in which she, as a parent-researcher, seeks to learn from her child-participants regarding how Asian American children make sense of and respond to race/ism and White supremacy in school and society.

Amy Argenal completed her doctorate in International and Multicultural Education at the University of San Francisco, where she also received her master's in the same area of study. She received her second master's in Human Rights from Mahidol University in Thailand, where she continued to partner with human rights activists in South East Asia, through her doctorate research focusing on human rights activism in Myanmar. She has published on critical service learning and presented at various conferences on teaching race, power and privilege. She is also an adjunct faculty at the University of San Francisco, teaching courses in the School of Education Human Rights Education program, the Critical Diversity Studies program and the Masters in Migration Studies.

Monisha Bajaj is Professor of International and Multicultural Education at the University of San Francisco. She is also a Visiting Professor at Nelson Mandela University – Chair, Critical Studies in Higher Education Transformation in South Africa. Dr. Bajaj is the editor and author of six books, including, most recently, *Human Rights Education: Theory, Research, Praxis* (University of Pennsylvania Press, 2017), as well as numerous articles. She has also developed curriculum – particularly related to peace education, human rights, anti-bullying efforts, and sustainability – for non-profit organizations and inter-governmental organizations, such as UNICEF and UNESCO. In 2015, she received the Ella Baker/Septima Clark Human Rights Award (2015) from Division B of the American Educational Research Association (AERA).

Michele Tracy Berger is Associate Professor in the Department of Women's and Gender Studies at the University of North Carolina-Chapel Hill. She is the author and co-editor of several books, including *Workable Sisterhood: The Political Journey of Stigmatized Women with HIV/AIDS* (2004); *The Intersectional Approach: Transforming the Academy Through Race, Class and Gender* (2009); and *Transforming Scholarship: Why Women's and Gender Studies Students Are Changing Themselves and the World* (2011, 2014).

Her research, teaching, and practice all focus on intersectional approaches to studying areas of inequality, especially racial and gender health disparities. This work spans the fields of public health, sociology, and women's and gender studies. Her recent work is focused on the health and wellness practices of Black women and girls. "Black Women's Health: Paths to Wellness for Mothers and Daughters" will be published in 2021 by New York University Press. Since 2014, she has been a co-investigator with Keval Kaur Khalsa researching yoga and mindfulness interventions with at-risk elementary and middle school children through Duke University's Bass Connections: Mindfulness in Human Development project.

Tria Blu Wakpa is an Assistant Professor of Dance Studies in the World Arts and Cultures/Dance Department at UC Los Angeles. She received a Ph.D. and M.A. from the Department of Ethnic Studies at UC Berkeley and an M.F.A. in Creative Writing from San Diego State University. She is a scholar and practitioner of Indigenous dance, North American Hand Talk (Indigenous sign language), martial arts, and yoga, and performs and publishes her poetry in a variety of venues. For her scholarly and creative writing, she has received major fellowships from the Ford Foundation, the Fulbright Program, the UC President's Postdoctoral Program, and the Hellman Fellows Fund. Her book project, *Settler Colonial and Decolonial Choreographies: Native American Embodiment in Educational and Carceral Contexts*, theorizes how and why the U.S. has attempted to manage Native mobilities, and conversely, how Native bodies and movement forms (dance, basketball, boxing, gardening, theater, and yoga) have carried, generated, and transmitted knowledge in educational and carceral institutions on Lakota lands in what is often referred to as South Dakota. A co-founder and Co-Editor-in-Chief of *Race and Yoga*, the first peer-reviewed journal in the emerging field of Critical Yoga Studies, Dr. Blu Wakpa has also served as a guest editor for special issue journals that feature writing by people who are imprisoned. She has taught a wide range of interdisciplinary and community-engaged classes at public, private, tribal, and carceral institutions. She is married to Dr. Makha Blu Wakpa and the mother of their two children.

Jillian Ford (she/they) is an associate professor of social studies education at Kennesaw State University where she teaches about education for liberation through courses in educational research methods and embodied learning. She draws on Black feminist, womanist, and abolitionist theory to inform her teaching, research, and community engagement. Her work has appeared in numerous journals and edited volumes.

Narin Hassan is Associate Professor in the School of Literature, Media, and Communication (LMC) at Georgia Tech. Her research and teaching interests include Victorian literature and culture, gender and postcolonial studies, and histories of medicine. Her book, *Diagnosing Empire: Women, Medical Knowledge and Colonial Mobility* (Ashgate, 2011), traces the rise of the woman doctor within the context of empire. Her research surveys a range of materials, including Victorian women's travel writing and fiction, 19th-century medical manuals, health guides, and botanical images to examine notions of embodiment, mobility, and colonialism. She is currently researching yoga and 19th-century physical culture in relation to gender, medicine, and globalization. Along with her interests in the gendered and colonial histories of yoga, Narin has begun to incorporate practices of yoga and mindfulness within the academic classroom and plans to research the intersections of theory and practice within cultures of both academia and yoga. She has been teaching yoga for 15 years, and opened a studio in Atlanta in 2018.

Stephanie Hicks is a Lecturer at the Program on Intergroup Relations at the University of Michigan, and a faculty affiliate of the Institute for Research on Women and Gender at U-M. A scholar in educational policy studies, her teaching and research foci include diversity, equity and inclusion policy in higher education, intergroup dialogue and social justice education. A Chicago native, Hicks received a dissertation grant from the Institute for Research on Race and Public Policy at the University of Illinois at Chicago, and was named a Diversifying Higher Education Faculty Fellow by the Illinois Board of Higher Education. Her work has been published in the *National Political Science Review* and the *Black History Bulletin*, and is featured in the book *Discussing Democracy: A Primer on Dialogue and Deliberation in Higher Education*. Hicks is also a yoga teacher, and in 2016, began *Yoga for Black Lives*, a series of donation-based yoga classes to support Chicago organizations resisting state violence against Black people.

Dominique A. Malebranche is a licensed psychologist and Assistant Professor in the Division of Counseling and Psychology, at Lesley University. Her intersectional experiences as a first-generation Haitian-American offers her a critical lens to center her teaching, practice, and scholarship in liberatory and trauma-informed approaches. Dr. Malebranche's work has a strong commitment to dismantling relational and structural violence through the study of oppression, trauma, culture and the practice of embodied healing justice. As a Harvard Medical School Teaching Affiliate at the Center for Mindfulness and Compassion, and former postdoctoral fellow at the internationally known Trauma Center at JRI in Brookline, MA, she specializes in the treatment and assessment of psychological traumatic stress and mind-body interventions. In addition to her university appointment, self-identified activist-practitioner-scholar, Dr. Malebranche provides multicultural and trauma-informed consultation services in local and global clinical, organizational, and community settings. As a 500-hr certified yoga teacher (Vinyasa and Trauma Center Trauma Sensitive Yoga), she also values and encourages multiple ways of knowing, practices meditation and embodiment, teaches trauma-informed yoga, and participates in radical healing justice community with Black Lotus Collective in occupied Wôpanâak traditional territory (Boston, MA).

Suzana Plaisant McCalley is a Brazilian American singer, songwriter, musician, playwright, poet, screenwriter, and actor. Suzy is also an award-winning artist and community leader. Her play "Little Bird in The Night" has been produced in North Carolina and Off Broadway in New York City. Recently she starred in "Gem," a feature film that premiered in London and Tokyo. Her original music album "Into the Flame" is available on Spotify and iTunes.

Suzana holds a Masters of Fine Arts in Interdisciplinary Arts from Goddard College, Vermont. Suzana received her Bachelor of Arts in Philosophy from the University of Texas at Austin. Her main areas of research involve critical cultural art, theory, and pedagogy; specifically, how yoga, mindfulness, and the arts can heal and empower communities and contribute to social change. Suzy is the Founder and Owner of the Breathing Room, a yoga, arts, and wellness center in Winston Salem, North Carolina. She also founded and serves as Executive Director of Breathing Access 501c3, that brings yoga and arts education to underserved schools and communities. Suzana received her 500hr Yoga Instructor Certification at the Asheville Yoga Center and is a Yoga Alliance Continuing Education Provider. She is also a certified trauma-informed yoga practitioner, a certified Reiki Master, EFT Practitioner and Personal Development Coach with 12 years of experience helping clients achieve results. As a Speaker, Facilitator, and Educator, Suzana has worked with health care systems, school systems, universities, mental health and correctional facilities, corporations, and non-profit organizations to promote positive cultural shifts in the areas of creativity, stress management, innovation, diversity, inclusion, and equity.

Firdose Moonda is a researcher, yoga teacher, and sports writer based in Cape Town, South Africa. She holds a Masters Degree in the Traditions of Yoga and Meditation from the School of Oriental and African Studies, a 500-Hour Yoga Alliance Accredited Teacher Training and works as the South African correspondent for ESPNcricinfo. Her areas of interest include: post-colonial theory, social history, the history of the body, the development of cultural wellbeing practices, race theory, critical pedagogy, and sound as a technology of healing and community. She is undertaking doctoral research which investigates historical developments of yoga across the Indian Ocean and through the Indian diaspora. Her aim is to develop a decolonized yogic pedagogy, rooted in the epistemologies of the South, in order to create and promote an inclusive and accessible form of yoga. Firdose runs her own yoga company, Souldier Yoga, which seeks to use yoga as a form of social activism. She teaches yoga history and philosophy on yoga teacher trainings, offers ad hoc courses which explore different aspects of yoga theory and has founded the yoga program for refugees at the Scalabrini Centre in Cape Town. A longer version of her essay was used as her dissertation for completion of her M.A.

Shyamala Moorty has taught yoga, dance, and Pilates at various community colleges in Southern CA for over 10 years. She is dedicated to sharing the growth, healing, and self-actualization that is possible through each of these forms. In addition to teaching, Shyamala is a founding member of the Post Natyam Collective, a transnational, web-based coalition of dance artists whose work triangulates between art-making, activism, and theory; and the Dancing Storytellers who create South Asian inspired performances for the whole family. Shyamala also has worked with TeAda Productions as an ensemble member, director, producer, and facilitator of self-expression and healing through the arts for various groups including people of colour, survivors of domestic violence, and gender non-conforming individuals. Shyamala's yoga background includes teacher training with Yoga Works (200hr), Kava Yoga (300hr), and specialty training in restorative and wall strap modalities. She also has Pilates mat training from BASI, and an MFA in choreography from UCLA. Shyamala currently teaches hatha yoga, restorative yoga and "healthy back" wall strap classes at KAVA Yoga, where she lives in Long Beach, CA. For more information visit her website at www.shyamalamoorty.com.

Mari Morales-Williams, originally from East Harlem and the Bronx, has been a social justice educator for the past 15 years, with a particular focus on holistic leadership development for Black and Brown female identified youth. A former Social Studies teacher, advisor, and administrator of El Centro de Estudiantes, she is the founding director of T.U.F.F. Girls, a youth organization focused on wellness, political education, and restorative justice skill building. As an internationalist, yogi, organizer, and prison abolitionist, she is committed to teaching young people how to lead with their heart, and how to fight for and create more liberated worlds. She holds a Masters and Ph.D.

in Urban Education from Temple University. She is currently integrating her passion for transformative justice and food/land sovereignty as a farmer at Life Do Grow Farm in North Philadelphia.

Kimberly Nao is an Associate Professor of Education at Mount Saint Mary's University where she is the Director of the Instructional Leadership and Teacher Induction Programs. Throughout her 25 years in the field of education, she has valued holistic, experiential, and transformative pedagogical practices as a professor, student advocate, and former English teacher. Her areas of research include critical pedagogy, language and voice, and most recently yoga in schools. She currently teaches courses on linguistics, language diversity, and professional development and facilitates workshops and trainings on diversity, equity, and inclusion with a focus on the intersection of race, gender, and sexuality. As a consultant for Peace Pros LA, she has trained university faculty and staff, K–12 educators, police officers, counselors and parents with the goal of breaking down toxic gender norms that can lead to discrimination and violence. As a certified kundalini yoga instructor, Kimberly has studied yoga philosophy and practices in the U.S. and at the Kaivalyadhama Institute and the Swami Vivekananda Yoga Anusandhana (SVYASA) in India. She researches yoga as a new pedagogical frontier and as a tool for personal and social transformation.

Jardana Peacock (they/them) is the author of *Practice Showing Up: A Guidebook for White People Working for Racial Justice*. Their work and essays have been featured in YES! Magazine, Elephant Journal, Decolonizing Yoga, Avatar Review, Mother, Feminist Wire, and more. They facilitate white ancestral healing and antiracism retreats across the U.S. They are a 500-hour certified yoga teacher and are committed to bringing their practice into movements for change and antiracism into spiritual communities. They have helped to found seven social justice organizations including Liberation School South, a healing and spirituality school for changemakers and Showing Up for Racial Justice (SURJ). Jardana has worked as a cultural organizer at the Highlander Research and Education Center and the Anne Braden Institute for Social Justice Research. They often travel to other worlds through their imagination, and prefer to be barefoot. They are happiest by water, in the mountains or desert, and playing in the sun with their kids. Jardana lives in Louisville, KY and serves as Director of Development and Communications at PeoplesHub.

Rumya S. Putcha is an assistant professor in Hugh Hodgson School of Music and the Institute for Women's Studies. Her research interests center on post-Enlightenment, colonial, and anti-colonial thought, particularly around constructs of citizenship, race, gender, sexuality, the body, and the law. Professor Putcha received her Ph.D. from the University of Chicago in 2011 and her first book, *Mythical Courtesan | Modern Wife: Performance, Transnationalism, Praxis*, develops a transnational feminist approach to South Asian performance cultures. Her second book project, *Namaste Nation: Orientalism and Yoga in the 21st Century*, extends her work on South Asian and South Asian American performance cultures to critical analyses of capitalist yoga practices within legal and affective discourses of body, race, wellness, and citizenship.

Sanjuana C. Rodriguez is an Assistant Professor of Reading Education in the Elementary and Early Childhood Department at Kennesaw State University. Sanjuana is the co-director for the Academy for Language and Literacy in the Bagwell College of Educational at Kennesaw State University. Her research interests include the early literacy development of culturally and linguistically diverse students, early writing development, literacy development of students who are emergent bilinguals, and Latinx children's literature. She has published in journals such as *Journal of Language and Literacy Education*, *Race Ethnicity and Education*, and *Journal of Children's Literature*.

Sheena Sood (she/her) is a Philly-based activist, educator, and healing justice visionary of South Asian descent. Sheena earned her Ph.D. in Sociology at Temple University. As a sociologist, Sheena's scholarship explores topics of race and ethnicity, immigration, political solidarity, social movements, and critical yoga studies. Recently, Sheena has brought a geopolitical focus to her research by examining the ethical implications of yoga's integration in military, policing, and corporate mindfulness programs around the world. Using India, the U.S. and Israel (occupied Palestine) as case studies, Sheena explores how regimes that advance ethnonationalist and neoliberal agendas weaponize yoga to sanitize their public images.

As a certified advanced yoga practitioner and South Asian American from an upper-caste family, Sheena brings a complicated legacy to the work of decolonizing yoga. She curates *healing justice* offerings through frameworks that simultaneously recognize yoga's oppressive layers and its liberatory potential. Rather than propagate narratives that glorify yoga's ancient past, Sheena envisions a futuristic yoga that centers collective freedom and embodied political action. In her yoga programs, Sheena encourages herself and others to envision how yoga can be purposed toward a liberatory spirituality that centers all of humanity, all living beings, and Mother Earth.

Finally, Sheena is grateful to call Philly home and to be in relationship with the incredible organizers of the Campaign to Bring Mumia Home, The MOVE Organization, and grassroots collectives that work to prioritize social justice by abolishing the carceral state and freeing all political prisoners.

Morgan Vanderpool is a genderqueer/non-binary, clinical social worker and movement facilitator, based in the unceded territory of the Puyallup tribe in Tacoma, WA. They focus their life's practice on the em-bodied and em-brained restoration and resolution of complex trauma – i.e. the survivorship of interlocking systems of oppression.

Morgan is committed to leveraging their survivorship, and their access to protection within systems of oppression, to instigate and co-create equitable access to the knowledge and practices necessary to restore nervous systems, to effectively, and collectively, engage in trauma-sensitive and anti-oppressive systems change. Morgan collaborates cross linguistically (Spanish/English) and in a multiculturally adept and anti-colonialistic way, to cultivate trauma sensitive practice communities along the west coast of North America, and throughout Latin America, and the Caribbean, and Spanish speaking communities worldwide.

Sanaz Yaghmai is a Trauma-Informed Coach and birthworker. Formerly a psychologist, she has worked in the mental health field for over a decade. Her personal experience of trauma recovery through yoga, empowerment coaching, and therapy redirected her career. Today, she is the founder of the Alchemy Of Trauma, a Trauma-Informed practice centred around coaching, yoga, and resilience-building services. Sanaz combines the tools of embodiment and psychology with the ancient healing art form of yoga, supporting clients towards awakening their innate resilience and self-healing abilities.

Foreword

By Dianne Bondy

What is Freedom? In the true sense of the word, freedom can be described as a state of being. To be free requires the absence of coercion and restraint. In some parts of the world, freedom is a right that many vehemently uphold, while in others, freedom is a privilege reserved only for a select few. Here in the West, freedom is fluid. *Who gets to be free, and why?* What resources are at our disposal in our quest for personal freedom? Are those resources restricted by the color of our skin, sexual identity, socio-economic status, and gender?

As I read through this incredible anthology, I am struck by how it illuminates our individual and collective struggle for freedom from the restrictive powers in our society that so clearly target those of us living on the margins of mainstream culture. Racism, capitalism, sexism, and ableism are insidious and ubiquitous strongholds that, if left unexamined, threaten to inhibit our potentiality for greater evolution.

If we wish to embrace a radical view of our future, one in which freedom is accessible to *every*body, we must first be able to envision ourselves as valuable players in this quest for freedom. This anthology brings attention to, and calls into focus, all the barriers that people of color experience when it comes to finding and participating in the healing practices that hold the keys to freedom – both internally and within the greater landscape of our shared society. Our community wants to heal from the trauma of our past, while also strengthening our collective voice in the war against ongoing oppression.

Representation matters. It's the touchstone of equity. It links together all parts of our existence and reinforces that we all belong. Representation is the path to radical healing and the cornerstone in our quest for freedom. It's how we break down the biases and oppressive structures that govern our culture and politics. Diversity gives us a broader and more balanced view of what it means to be human; it gives us a collective understanding of our shared humanity. Together we achieve justice and evolve society as a whole. When we join together, when we can envision our black skin, our differently abled-bodies, our non-binary selves as *free*, that is when the radical healing begins.

It is my belief that mind-body practices, like yoga, provide us with invaluable tools in our search for liberation. Yoga, after all, is a practice created by Brown people, for Brown people. Its aim, from inception, has always been the attainment of liberation – *moksha*. The intentionality behind the yoga practice is to lift the veil of ignorance so that we can see our innate connection to Spirit, and the oneness of all beings.

When I started practising yoga nearly 50 years ago, there were no expensive yoga studios, branded mats, or trendy clothing. Yoga was a practice of self-study, movement, and connection to our Source. Since then, yoga moved more fully into the mainstream capitalist culture where it became commodified. It became cool and trendy. Now yoga was something to aspire to. As a fat Black woman, I no longer felt like I belonged. I felt displaced, unseen, and uninvited to a practice that had been a part of me for my whole life, a practice that was created by people who suffered the same kinds of oppression as I had. It was then that yoga changed for me. It was now something tangible that didn't belong to me because I was fat and Black. I watched as the overarching systems of White supremacy and capitalism changed my beloved practice into something exclusive and White. The western world of yoga taught me yoga as a function of beauty. My new narrative of yoga: White, young, thin, able-bodied, straight, and cis-gender.

When I noticed this shift toward the wilful exclusion of voices of color and the need to center whiteness, I decided to push back. In my study of the Bhagavad Gita, I learned it was my sacred duty – my Dharma if you will – to seek justice and yoga for all of us. It was time to teach dominant culture that people of color and people at the margins are not props within the practice. We should not be reduced to educating White people on why equity and representation matter.

Practicing Yoga as Resistance: Voices of Color in Search of Freedom is a collection of lived truths, experiences, and research that exposes the power biases, cultural conditioning, and discrimination that has impacted on our collective psyche. These stories demonstrate how yoga can strengthen, uplift, and empower, underestimated and underrepresented communities. This work illuminates how spiritual practices can change lives and the trajectory of our collective consciousness as well as profoundly heal communities of color through action, self-actualization, and unity. The lived experiences shared in this book demonstrate that all communities are worthy and valuable and that yoga belongs to all of us. Yoga is a practice of the many, not the few. Everyone is welcome on the mat regardless of race, sexual identity, gender, size, ability, or age. By witnessing the experiences of others, we learn how to uplift our communities and rewrite our own narratives.

Now, more than ever, we get to decide how the world sees us. We get to define who belongs and who doesn't. We get to stand in our power and our truth, creating a different narrative: one where we all belong, we all deserve freedom, and where diversity is what makes this life so beautiful.

Preface
An introduction

By Cara Hagan

Yoga has become ubiquitous with lifestyle culture in the West and people can't get enough. Whether it's because Western culture can't seem to do away with being over-busy, or because people are obsessed with finding ways to achieve physical beauty, or because it's seen as exotic, or because yoga means big money for an industry that shows no signs of slowing down anytime soon, yoga has captured the imagination of the masses. It is in part because of its mass appeal that yoga has taken on a variety of manifestations that continually expand the pool of those who consider themselves to be practitioners and enthusiasts. These days, you can practice a variety of yoga styles found in gyms and studios, in addition to niche yoga classes, like goat yoga, happy hour yoga (which includes wine, of course!), and "Broga," a type of yoga that specifically caters to male yogis in a society where women practitioners and instructors vastly outnumber their male counterparts. For many people, the studios, parks, community centers, university campuses, and make-shift yoga spaces where yoga can be found represent important facets of their communities. People come together to learn, to practice, and to grow in their bodies, minds, and spirits. But for others, these spaces represent sites of judgment, trauma, oppression – barriers to healing and growth. They represent a wilful unawareness of the entities and systems that hinder one's ability to give full attention to the body and the breath, withdraw from the senses, concentrate on the infinite, and pursue bliss or enlightenment. Practically, the ability to simply arrive in one of these spaces is fraught with financial, locational, and cultural realities that mean access is not universal.

To begin to talk about the popularity of yoga, its uses among various communities and trends in the yoga ecosystem in the West, is important to name the ways yoga arrived here. The story of yoga's import to the West is one that includes a back-and-forth exchange of ideas and practices via a history of settler-colonialism, nationalism, transnationalism, capitalism, and a fascination by the West with Eastern spirituality and philosophy. These histories and their consequences are taken up with more detail in the chapters collected for this volume. Subsequent to the efforts of personalities like Swami Vivekananda, Tirumalai Krishnamacharya, Indra Devi, K. Pattabhi Jois, B.K.S. Iyengar, and Bikram Choudhury to popularize yoga among westerners, the proliferation of yoga in the United States, Europe, and Canada has been part and parcel of an ongoing settler-colonial project such that yoga spaces across the West are engaged in the othering and oppression of people of color, people with disabilities, fat people, and queer people. Further, the perpetuation of yoga as a means of quelling physical and cultural characteristics and ways of being that are disruptive to the status quo are par for the course in yoga spaces and in the dissemination of Western yogic practice. The more than $16 billion yoga industry perpetuates a clear socio-economic divide between those who can afford to practice formally and those who cannot, continually creating the conditions for homogenous representation and authority in yoga.

As yoga scholars and practitioners of the 21st century are beginning to more forcefully name the disparities that exist in these spaces, women and queer people of color, in particular, are excavating the racist, sexist, ableist histories of yoga as they existed prior to its import to the West and since. Additionally, they are both participating in and reporting about how their communities have historically cultivated, and continue to find creative ways of utilizing the practices and teachings of yoga to work toward anti-oppression efforts and collective liberation.

Practicing Yoga as Resistance: Voices of Color in Search of Freedom is one such resource that explores the complexities of race, gender, and social justice in Western yogic practice through the voices of women and queer-identified yoga studies scholars, educators, and practitioners of color, along with a small handful of White allies. Through an intersectional feminist lens, the cohort unpacks histories of oppression in a variety of contexts while confronting the ways institutionalized and capitalism-driven discrimination in yoga negatively affects marginalized people. With contributors from a variety of racial and ethnic backgrounds, the work grapples with philosophies and practices that are specific to these communities and acknowledge the ways that White supremacy affects different communities in distinct ways.

Therefore, the essays found in this collection exist in three realms: invitations; yoga, self, and community; and yoga in educational spaces. For the purposes of this volume, community spaces are ones defined as existing separate from institutional bodies such as K-12 schools, colleges and universities, and prisons. They include neighborhoods, studios, community centers and gatherings, and other communal spaces. Institutional spaces include those listed above that community spaces are not – spaces dependent on imposed structures of institutionalized and capitalist hierarchies deemed necessary for the operation and survival of these spaces. More specific to this volume, the educational institutions where yoga has become more commonplace in recent years are of interest as the politics of race, gender, and class therein collide with the holistic aims of yoga practice. Autoethnography, case studies, and empirical research act as the vehicles for the exploration of the topics in this volume, with each mode of exploration contributing to a multifaceted, embodied experience.

Thus, this collection opens with two invitations: the first, by Cara Hagan, invites readers to consider the role of the Western yoga community in reinforcing oppressive systems and offers tools for individuals to excavate their own participation in systems of oppression on the road to collective liberation. This piece also demonstrates the need for POC-specific spaces, a topic which is considered in more detail in subsequent chapters. Jardana Peacock's *Towards a White spiritual anti-racism* addresses White readers specifically by inviting them to interrogate spiritual bypassing while offering a framework to begin the work of dismantling systems of oppression in yoga spaces and society at large.

As readers encounter the work of other authors in the collection, a dynamic tapestry of social, political, and cultural discourse emerges that elucidates the diversity with which yoga is experienced, though not always made visible. Several of the chapters here explore the "politicized healing and the revolutionary potential" of yoga through the stories of specific civic movements including MOVE Philadelphia and the Black Lives Matter movement by authors Sheena Sood and Mari Morales-Williams, and Stephanie Hicks, respectively. Other pieces in this vein explore the experiences of displaced people through the work of Sanaz Yaghmai and Firdose Moonda, who grapple with the complexities of geo-political affairs, White saviorism, and power dynamics within refugee communities.

The role of family and shared learning spaces on the path to collective liberation through popular education and community-supported initiatives are discussed by several authors in addition. Amy Argenal and Monisha Bajaj present a model of family yoga practice and community care through their piece, *Reclaiming spaces, reshaping practices: Yoga for building community and nurturing families of color*. Dominique A. Malebranche explores the importance of embodied knowledge in the role of collective restoration in her piece, *Embodied radical healing through the collective: A Black Lotus autoethnography*. Narin Hassan demonstrates how she uses yoga to build bridges between the two seemingly disparate communities of the academy and the city of Atlanta, Georgia in her work, *Tending communities: Yoga as an integrative, collaborative, and transformative practice*. Bringing together the body, nature, and indigenous philosophy, Tria Blu Wakpa explains the way yoga discourse often leaves out indigenous voices, while it continues to grow in popularity among indigenous people in her essay, *Hozho Yoga: Indigenous movements illuminating human and more-than-human interconnections*. In their work, Morgan Vanderpool explains the mind-body science of oppression and offers insights on how to engage in a practice that acknowledges and honors generational trauma.

And although this volume deals most expressly with race, gender plays an important role in this discourse. Both Rumya S. Putcha and Cara Hagan explore the racialized and gendered dynamics of beauty and fitness in their chapters on women's wellness culture. While Hagan's essay surveys philosophical and medical trends concerning the care of women's bodies dating back to the 19th century, Putcha's work utilizes over ten years of ethnographic work in yoga studios in the United States to discuss the ways yoga maintains what she calls, "White hygiene." Both essays demonstrate how notions of White womanhood in western society are harmful to those who do not fit the trope of a thin, able-bodied, White, wealthy, female, lifestyle enthusiast.

More essays take readers on a journey through our educational system from elementary school, through high school and the collegiate experience. Author Michele Tracey Berger discusses a study on the effects of yoga on the mental health of middle school girls of color in an after school program in her chapter, while Suzy McCalley looks at the school to prison pipeline through her work teaching yoga in title-one elementary schools and prisons in central North Carolina. Kimberly Nao presents a series of short case studies on individuals from a high school practicing yoga as part of a freshman seminar experience. Shamala Moorty offers her own series of case studies on the experiences of students taking yoga as part of their community college courses in West LA. Inviting us into the world of the academy as it trains future teachers, co-authors and educators to pre-service teachers Erin Adams, Sohyun An, Jillian Ford, and Sanjuana Rodriguez discuss how perceptions of yoga's use in classroom settings leads to yoga being employed as a tool of bodily control, instead of a liberatory one.

As a whole, this collection addresses the need for increased awareness in the yoga community, in activist spaces, and in educational spaces around nuanced issues of race and systemic oppression. For yoga studies specifically, this anthology offers another important resource among a growing panorama of literature helping people to understand the complexities of yoga as both a personal and cultural practice. As the world at large grapples with these issues under increasingly volatile circumstances, I hope that this book can offer readers solidarity, along with knowledge and tools to imagine a more just existence in the world.

In closing, I would like to thank all of the contributors who so graciously offered to create works for this collection. Through our time working on this book, I have learned much about each of their particular expertise, valuable gifts, and passion for both the practice of yoga and its social, political, and cultural contexts. I am grateful to our publisher, who saw the value of this work and has worked hard to bring it to you in this form. Finally, I am grateful to you, dear readers, for your interest in the topics surveyed in this book, and for uplifting our voices every time you open it to read.

Acknowledgement

As seekers of and workers for liberation, we acknowledge the injustice of forced displacement and the erasure of languages and customs attributed to the tribes whose ancestral lands we occupy. We employ the power of our words to amplify the urgent need for the repatriation of sacred lands to disenfranchised peoples across the United States and the world.

Part I

Invitations

Chapter 1

Essential questions for inner and outer liberation

Cara Hagan

An exposition of personal experience is useful in that it provides an accessible entryway into larger conversations. In a conversation about yoga, where it is easy to spiral into philosophical territory, personal experience helps to keep the conversation grounded in an embodied realm. In this essay, I impart my personal journey to arriving at a set of questions I hope you'll consider deeply in your own yoga practice, and as you move through this volume. Too, it is my hope that this piece is an opening to a larger conversation about the need for healing spaces full of people who are more aware of the ways oppression and discrimination effect some of the people who may show up in those spaces, and those people who may choose not to show up at all because they do not feel welcome or understood. As a Black woman living in America, I am familiar with the reticence communal yoga practice can provoke and the desire and express need for yoga spaces for people of color. Marching along my own journey in yoga practice and philosophy, I have found that regular reevaluation has served me in shedding unhelpful patterns and making important breakthroughs. These breakthroughs most often bloom from the seed of a question. In the spirit of inspiring open and honest dialogue, I present this piece to you in the form of a letter. I begin this letter with questions. At the climax of the piece, I propose a set of questions which have become my most important touchstones both in yoga and in life. Finally, I end the piece with questions for the future. Let's begin:

Dear Reader,
    What do we do with collective trauma? What do we do with collective fear? How do we transform a culture of panic into a culture of understanding? More specifically, how do we cultivate and maintain an ethos of peace? To answer these questions and to begin to move into a place of actionable outcomes, it is important to ask exactly what *peace* includes. I imagine the way one describes peace is different from person to person, but I also imagine each definition has something to do with ease, and with the ability to live without environmental, personal, interpersonal and institutional obstacles or burdens. For me, peace requires freedom from oppression, as oppression in my opinion – forms of oppression imposed by both outer forces and inner struggle – is the biggest

barrier to freedom. As ever, it seems that the world is at odds with how to balance the roles of peace and power in our societies, and it remains up to us to determine how we will proceed toward a future with which contemporary generations, and generations yet to come, can live.

Like many, results of the 2016 presidential election sent me reeling.[1] The idea that our country had willfully chosen racism, xenophobia, misogyny, contempt for the poor and working class, disregard for collective education and collective well-being among other social ills as the new order, sickened me. It rendered me fearful for what the future held. The most alarming events in the year following the inauguration included the rise of an emboldened White supremacist movement (Blow, 2017), a year of gun violence and police brutality with numbers of incidents and victims on par with the previous two years (Sullivan et al., 2017), attempts at dismantling public education and healthcare (Green, 2017a and b, Pear et al., 2017), imposed barriers to refuge for people in need of safe places to live (Shear and Cooper, 2017), and attempts to further damage an already ailing earth (Popovich and Schlossberg, 2017). Fast forward to 2020, and the confluence of the Coronavirus pandemic and renewed attention to the murders of innocent Black and Brown people by police and White vigilantism has created a dystopian world we could never have imagined. While not all of the events of the past four years can be attributed directly to the general election results, it can be argued that the presidential election and the minutia surrounding the installation of the Trump administration created an environment where the oppression of marginalized people and wide-spread ignorance have become socially and politically acceptable.

In the year leading up to, and directly following the election in my small, Southern, Appalachian town, I observed a multitude of reactions: panic, sadness, paralysis, apathy, and for some, a kind of giddy excitement that people could finally express sentiments about the world that may have been previously considered objectionable, at least on the surface, by accepted social norms. On the campus where I work, several White students took to the sidewalks at night, writing racist messages in chalk for our students of color to find in the mornings. For our undocumented students, messages encouraging them to "go home," were particularly disconcerting. Several minority students experienced repeated incidents of verbal harassment on campus and expressed feelings of unsafety (Cole, 2017 Hayes, 2016). A pick-up truck, with the muffler sawed off and a large Confederate flag flying off of the back hitch, would speed down our small main street each day, as if to remind everyone what the new America was going to be like and to challenge anyone brave enough to dispute it. On televisions in bars and restaurants across the region, Fox News claimed to predict a revitalized American society where order would be restored and the American dream could be repaired (Manning, 2017, Smith, 2020). As one of a small community of people of color at my institution and in my town, I felt isolated, afraid, and wondered how any response I could muster would help to ease the impact of these events, both nationally and right at home, much less make any real change. A longtime community-engaged artist and activist, I was no stranger to action. And though I realized that the events of 2016 and 2017 were just more knots in a long string of injustices our country has experienced, the anxiety they produced felt uncontrollable. And what do I do when it feels like I can't get a grasp on a dizzying world?

> I gather people. I make place. I make art. And I step onto my mat.
> Except, this time, I could not get on my mat.

At the same time I found myself fretful about the direction and future of American society, I found myself disillusioned with the yoga community. As a Black woman who has been practicing yoga for over fifteen years in the United States, this was certainly not the first time I've felt cynicism toward the yoga community. This time though, the sting of what felt like abandonment by that community left me deflated and unmotivated to practice. Like the times I had become disillusioned in the past, I found the violence and discrimination I saw and experienced out in the world repackaged for me under the guise of spirituality, in spaces that claimed to offer refuge from those very injustices. I found yoga teachers who problematized bodies of color, disguising such discussions as anatomy lessons.[2] I found fellow yogis uninterested in the ways my experiences as a Black woman informed my experiences on the mat. I experienced out-and-out discouragement from speaking about race, gender, and class in yoga spaces. And, I encountered White yogis who claimed that the election and the events that followed were karmic events, and that the only victims of the events were those who victimized themselves. Already feeling the pressure of needing to dialogue about the role of contemplative practice in times of sociopolitical turbulence with other practitioners of color – people who could better identify with my concerns and experiences – I was compelled to begin a project entitled, *Mindfulness and Resistance*, in the spring of 2016. It began as a series of interviews, and a survey I sent out on social media, with the intention to write an article. However, the *real* intention, a deeper intention I hadn't even admitted to myself going into the project, was to find a community. As soon as I began conducting the interviews, with such teachers, inspirers, and change-makers like Jassamyn Stanley, Dr. Chelsea Jackson Roberts, Jana Long, Hillary Lopes, and more, I realized that the project was going to grow to be more than an article. Ultimately, that initiative grew into this book and the community of writers who have shared their talents with us. In the spirit of wanting to be energetically engaged in resistance to mounting injustice and wanting to feel less isolated in my home community, in October 2016, I started a grass-roots organizing group in my town called, *Small and Mighty Acts (SAMA)*. SAMA is a space where anyone who wants to find creative ways of being involved in community building, activism, and local politics can gather to pitch ideas, learn collective organizing strategies, and be inspired to participate in civic life from a place of power (Hagan, 2016). Built on the philosophy of *Creative Social Stewardship,* - "a method of community engagement, which invites citizens to tap into their whimsical, radical, colorful, innovative selves to foster and preserve inclusive, emotionally sustainable community environments that combat social stigma, discrimination and systemic oppression through outward creative expression" (Hagan, 2016) – SAMA represents an approach to activism through community care.

Despite what felt like enlivening developments, I still found it difficult to practice with any regularity. I realized that if I had any hope of returning to my practice and to the yoga community – and not in a superficial way – I had to start digging. I had to ask questions that both scrutinized and challenged my reticence, and my relationship to the practice and the community around it. I had to confront the reasons why the confluence of the election, my experience of the fallout from that, and my perceived abandonment by the yoga community had left me averse to being deep in my practice, and therefore, deep in myself.

The line of inquiry that emerged from this realization changed my practice, and it changed the ways I show up to what I consider my ongoing call to resistance in the face of injustice. Finally, the experience offered me a repeatable methodology to share with others who wish to creatively engage yogic practice as a platform for inner and outer liberation.

Instead of sitting down for a series of long, probing meditations I assumed would be wholly uncomfortable and counterproductive, I thought it best to begin with my body. Throughout the year of 2016 and the first half of 2017, I experienced incredible physical discomfort, marked by migraines, regular bouts of vertigo, muscle weakness, digestive trouble, lower back pain, swelling in my right Achilles tendon, swelling in my left knee, and tension throughout my shoulders, neck and jaw. It was a year-and-a-half riddled with insomnia from an inability to shut my mind off. I spent more time in a doctor's office between 2016 and 2017 than I had in the ten years prior. My initial reaction to the physical sensations I was experiencing was to get rid of them, however necessary, however possible. Interestingly enough, after several visits to specialists and a battery of tests, the doctors found nothing inherently wrong with my body. They could not medicate me. *Yes*, they did find some allergies of which I was previously unaware, but those were mitigated easily enough. And *yes*, I was officially diagnosed with migraines, but other than that, everyone told me I was one of the healthiest individuals they had ever met. Many of the doctors suggested I try stress-reduction, or relaxation techniques. When I left their care, I was left with those uncomfortable sensations and no answers as to how to address them. I felt trapped.

I began to imagine my life as never feeling "normal," again. I began to devise ways to work around my ailments, tricks and strategies to mentally override my body's signals, and not let on to others that I didn't feel well. One day though, I cracked. "I can't do this anymore," I said to myself in the bathroom mirror. I needed to get free.

"What does liberation look like?" I asked myself. "What does it feel like? What does liberation move like?"

My question, I found, was not just about physical discomfort. It was about the oppression I was experiencing in the world around me and within my own body.

It was about *collective liberation*. A series of yoga poses may work to alleviate the discomfort in my body (and any body) temporarily, but I surmised that if I wanted to truly experience liberation I needed to look closely at mechanisms of oppression and how they permeate our bodies and our minds. I needed to interrogate my relationship to oppression and how that oppression may be affecting me physically. Just after New Year's, 2017, I went to my mat for the first time in months. With the intention to move through the physical sensations I was feeling, my sociopolitical anxieties, and to lean into how they were interconnected, I moved through a series of slow asana, holding each pose for several breaths. I lingered in poses I found to be uncomfortable, for one reason or another, barring actual danger to my joints and muscles. Simple forward folds felt suffocating. Backbends, which had been longtime favorites of mine, felt strained. I explored the ways I confronted difficulty and discomfort – which I discovered, was by pursing my lips and muscling through. This was the way I observed myself moving out in the world, too. When confronted with racist or misogynist comments by White and/or male students and colleagues, I gritted my teeth, smiled, and offered tempered responses. When I read the news each day and sat with the participants of *Small and Mighty Acts* in our meetings thereafter, I put aside my own anxieties to make space for theirs. When students of color came to me in fear, needing refuge and advice,[3] I swallowed my own fear and held theirs. When I continued to feel the pangs of injustice rippling throughout the yoga community, instead of speaking out, I distanced myself.

"How do I participate in my own oppression?" I asked myself. "How do I participate in the oppression of others?" After several practices, moving through poses slowly, gauging my physical and emotional responses to the poses, it seemed natural that these questions arose next. I couldn't just move about them, though. I felt the urge to write. One morning, I picked up my notebook and began to free write. I wrote, and wrote, and wrote. When I stopped, I read through what I had written and circled a phrase. I turned over a new page, and began to write about that phrase. And write, and write. Once more, I stopped, circled a phrase, and wrote. I circled one more phrase. Each time, I wrote, I wrote a little faster, for a shorter amount of time. I call this exercise, "*Three Leagues Deep*,"[4] and it is one of my favorite ways to get to the bottom of things. When I got to the bottom of this particular day's writing though, I was dismayed to read my final response. It wasn't particularly profound, and it went against the ways I worked to show up, or rather, be *perceived* to show up, in the world.

"I'll have what you're having: I'll eat whatever you serve me."
"I'll eat whatever you serve me?!" I mused.

I had to admit that I had been eating a lot of other people's stuff. I was taking on their fears, their anxieties, their needs, and not attending to my own. I was internalizing racism, misogyny, and my dissatisfaction with the yoga community and other communities and spaces I frequented for work, art, activism, and socializing. I was working hard to make myself agreeable to others, presenting myself as capable, independent, safe, supportive, and when it suited those around me, invisible. So, I sat down on my cushion and I decided to meditate…with my final response from the Three Leagues Deep exercise, as my mantra. As I repeated the phrase in my head, it felt and tasted icky. I sensed my attachment to comfort, familiarity and safety, even though that comfort was unproductive, even though it had been hurtful to me, and possibly hurtful to others. I began to sense all the ways I participate in my own oppression for the sake of making others feel comfortable, safe, competent, or taken care of, and how that participation often sets the stage for the oppression of others through insensitive expectations and maintenance of the status quo. I sensed the ways the tension and discomfort in my emotional body were connected to the tension and discomfort in my physical body. Though I became frustrated and my mind began to wander, it felt important to keep going; to move through what was my mind resisting a deep dive into the core of my experience. Regaining my focus, the feeling and meaning of the words began to change.

> *"I'll have what you're having: I'll eat whatever you serve me."*
> *"I'll eat whatever you serve me."*
> *"I'll eat whatever you serve me."*

I began to feel the words, "I'll have what you're having," as a call to part with my attachment to comfort and familiarity. Originally, I interpreted those words to represent the ways I made space for others to feel comfortable and to uphold the status quo. Now, the words meant that I could choose to feel into the space of the suffering of others and relinquish comfort for action informed by a deeper connection to my (and all of our) trauma. It was a call to practice more fully the principle of Aparigraha (non-possessiveness) as a path to practicing Satya (truthfulness) and Ahimsa (non-violence). (Satchidananda, 2012)

I began to envision my eating as a form of resistance. I can eat something, as a way of transforming it, instead of holding on to it and allowing it to make me ill, physically, emotionally, or socially. I can eat whole institutions, systems of tyranny, I can eat fear, and I can transform those into actionable steps toward peace. I can choose how I assimilate turmoil. I can choose how much I take on for the sake of others, and how much of my energy is spent fostering my own freedom. I can choose not to eat, if I'm not hungry.

Following my asana, writing, and meditation experiences, I wanted to begin to share some of my discoveries with others as a way of moving into my reframed relationship to resistance and my desire to more strategically destabilize systems of oppression and to decenter fear.

Naturally, more questions came in this next stage of development. "How do I keep my intellectual and spiritual growth sacred? How do I keep the intellectual and spiritual growth of my community sacred?" Yoga compels us to hold our spiritual and intellectual growth sacred most notably through Svadhyaya, or self-study. My experiences in returning to my practice thus far had felt like the kind of inquiry that could be described as Svadhyaya, and I wanted to take that study further by sharing it. Distilling my experience into a transmittable package, I now had a concrete series of questions, what I call my *Five Essential Questions*. They are:

1. What does liberation look like?
2. How do I participate in my own oppression?
3. How do I participate in the oppression of others?
4. How do I hold my intellectual and spiritual growth sacred?
5. How do I hold the intellectual and spiritual growth of my community sacred?

In February 2017, I was invited to present at the Embodied Learning Summit at Duke University. The title of the Summit was *Bring it to the Mat: Yoga, Mindfulness and Racial Justice* (Embodied Learning Summit, 2017). The proposal for my presentation was entitled, *Mindfulness and Resistance: the Body as Chronicle*. Originally, I envisioned it to be an exploration through asana and meditation, of our relationship to implicit bias within the yoga community, through the lens of my work interviewing women and non-binary people of color on the intersections of contemplative practice and resistance. Of course, after reconsidering my relationship to oppression and resistance, I felt I had to regroup and present on my recent personal experiences. In that first iteration of that work, I explained my disillusionment with the yoga community to a diverse group of practitioners and educators. It was a short (fifty minutes) but rich session where we were able to walk through some of the steps I had walked through in my personal work. We began with a free writing exercise, exploring the question, "Where does resistance live in my body?" We discussed our answers in small groups, then entered into a short, very simple asana practice where we focused on areas of comfort and discomfort. We followed with an exercise where participants witnessed each other in positions that they considered uncomfortable during that short practice (they were instructed not to go into any positions that were dangerous or counter indicated), and provided feedback as to what they saw and what feelings that experience cultivated. They reflected on the difference between what it was like to be a witness, and what it was like to be witnessed. To conclude our session, I presented a short "unburdening" meditation, meant to help participants release any residual tension from our experiences together. I presented my Five Essential Questions as fodder for the participants to take away with them. My intention for this short workshop was to heighten awareness around our inner resistance, with the purpose of working to show up more fully to the resistance of our time; to look at our relationships to bias especially, and to explore our own relationships to oppression. While we did not do the mantra meditation as I had in my own work, this beginning offered me a platform on which to build the practice as a facilitator.

As I continued to live the questions in my own life, it was important for me to explore the questions not only in yoga spaces, but in non-yoga spaces that lent themselves to contemplative work. In March of 2017, I was invited to the Boone Universalist Unitarian Church (BUUF, 2020) to speak on racial discrimination. During my address to the fifty-or-so mostly White attendees, I presented the five questions and invited the congregation to join me in an activity. I passed around small cards and envelopes. I invited each participant to choose one question to ponder, to write a response down on a card and put it in an envelope. I requested that they do so without putting their names on the cards, so responses would remain anonymous. When everyone had put their cards in their envelopes, I asked them to walk around the room and pass the envelopes several times. When passing concluded, I asked everyone to open the envelopes they received, to read the responses, and to have a conversation with someone next to them about what they read. To my surprise, many responded to the two questions I assumed people would avoid: "How do I participate in my own oppression?" and, "How do I participate in the oppression of others?"

Some of the responses to the question, "How do I participate in my own oppression" included:

- "My role in my own oppression is to question my ability to speak openly. I hold onto guilt."
- "My role in my own oppression is my constant thinking that others must always come before myself."

Responses to the question, "How do I participate in the oppression of others" included:

- "My role in other's oppression is COMPLACENCY."
- "My oppression of others is in discounting or discrediting contributions of others because of who they are."
- "My role in oppression of others is nothing short of participating within the system that keeps humans separate, in order to gain for themselves."

Responses to the questions, "How do I hold my intellectual and spiritual growth sacred," and "How do I hold the intellectual and spiritual growth of my community sacred" included:

- "I hold my creative/intellectual growth by encouraging the curiosity of learning in children and learning from them."
- "I advocate for the growth of my community by sharing knowledge about learning and ecocentrism (not a human-centered society)."
- "I advocate for the growth of my community by organizing events open to multiple generations."

Finally, a response to the question, "What does liberation look like," was this:

- "Liberation looks like equality – of expression, of education, of religious and sexual expression, IT LOOKS LIKE JUSTICE."

We concluded with a short, large-group discussion where we talked about ways we could continue to explore these questions for ourselves, and how we could take actionable steps to embody our inner work.

Continuing my exploration of these questions outside of yoga spaces, I set up a booth in the library of my university as part of *Consider This: A Read-In for 21st Century Literacies*. The read-in was an offering of Small and Mighty Acts, and included a series of mini-events like, a panel discussion with representatives from the Prison Books Collective (Prison Books, 2020) about the intersections of literacy and justice, readings and discussions of works like Octavia Butler's *Parable* series, and a protest songwriting workshop.

In the rotunda of the library, where there is ample foot traffic as students pass through en route to classes and to the multiple levels of the library, I set up a table with my typewriter, a basket of quotes related to my Five Essential Questions, and the questions themselves, which were written on cards that hung from string stretched across two pylons. I intended the strings to act as a sort of "analog conversation thread." As students passed, I invited them to choose a quote from the basket and have mini-conversations with me. I made a record of each conversation through an ongoing roll of typewriter paper, and asked each student to leave a small token of our conversation on the analog conversation thread. Engaging over the course of four hours with quotes on liberation, oppression, collective fear, trauma, intellectual freedom, the power of literacy, and spirituality carefully curated by me, the students surprised and delighted me with their insights. On my paper roll I typed observations like:

> *"Marissa comes to join me – a dance minor whom I've not had in class yet. Her quote by Bertrand Russell talks about collective fear. She connects her experience as a Jewish woman to the experiences of those who are Muslim in our country right now. She says 'education' is the antidote to collective fear. She puts that one word on the conversation line above."*

I converse with forty students in total, from a variety of majors and backgrounds. By the end of my time, my analog conversation thread is full of comments like, "If you haven't changed your mind lately, how can you be sure you still have one?" And, "Don't be afraid to do the right thing, even if it's different from what everyone else is doing." And, "What are you really afraid of?"

In July of 2017, I was finally able to offer a full-length *Mindfulness and Resistance: The Body as Chronicle* workshop. The workshop was donation-based – all donations went to the Immigrant Justice Committee of the Watauga

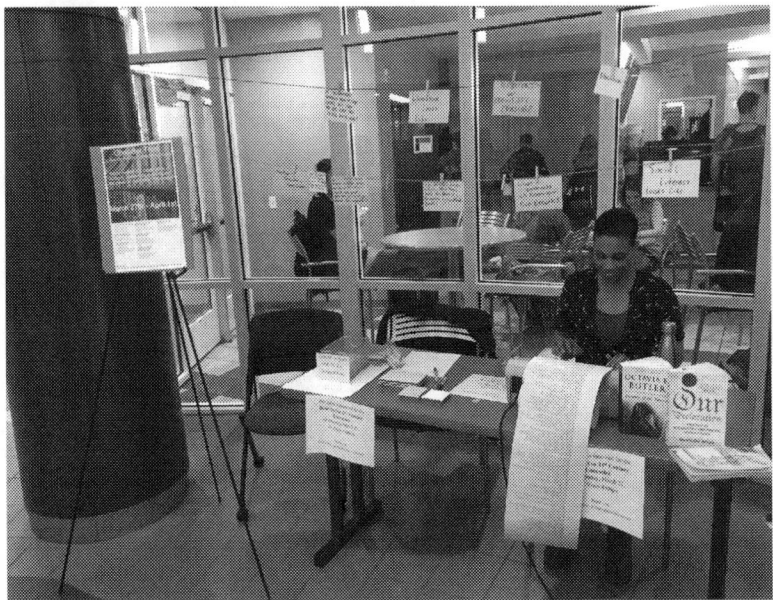

Figure 1.1 Consider This: A Read-In for 21st Century Literacies.

County NAACP[5] – and was hosted by SAMA and a local yoga studio. It was here that I was able to include insights from everything that had happened between my initial explorations in January 2017 and the events of that spring. The workshop was attended by sixteen people between the ages of twenty-one and seventy. There were three White men and five women of color among the rest of the group of White women. The workshop began as the workshop did at the Embodied Learning Summit, with a discussion and writing exercise on where resistance lives in the body. We followed with an asana practice that lasted an hour and fifteen minutes, where I was able to present questions about how we respond to challenges and discomfort while we are in movement. We followed the asana practice with the witnessing exercise[6] I presented at the Embodied Learning Summit, followed by a more robust post-activity reflection that included both written response and verbal discussion. To our group discussion, I offered the notion that the ways we saw our partners during our witnessing exercise, and what we felt as we were being witnessed has "everything to do with how we view ourselves, each other, and the world; both consciously and subconsciously." Finally, we did my Three Leagues Deep exercise. Each participant chose one of the Five Essential Questions on which to reflect. I led them through the three iterations of their exploration, each time, giving them less time to write.

When I told them that we would be using their final responses from the exercise as mantra for meditation, I was met with surprise and curiosity. During the meditation itself, several participants had visceral experiences, visible through physical responses like fidgeting and tears rolling down the cheeks. After bringing everyone out of the meditation, we had the chance to discuss the experience. Why had several of the participants had such emotional responses to the work? In discussion, participants pointed out that confronting inner resistance and our relationships to oppression is hard work. They said that often in yoga classes, they aren't asked to explore as deeply as this experience invited them to do. One participant who had a particularly emotional response to the work, a twenty-two-year-old Black woman, spoke with me in an interview, and wrote to me after the event. She said that as a woman of color in yoga spaces, she generally feels ignored. "I wasn't sure I wanted to show up when I saw who was going to be in the room. My previous experience has showed me that these people are going to ignore me. I'm glad that wasn't the case." She cited finding an unexpected connection with her witnessing activity partner (a White woman, twenty years her senior), and that although doing the deep emotional work required of each new experience in the workshop was awkward among a group of strangers, "it was necessary." The biggest takeaway from the workshop for her though, was the mantra meditation: "I want to be liberated to the point where I can love those who have wronged me."

In 2018, I had a handful of opportunities to present the work in people-of-color only spaces and spaces for trauma-informed communities. I presented at the American Dance Festival Studios in Durham, North Carolina for an intimate

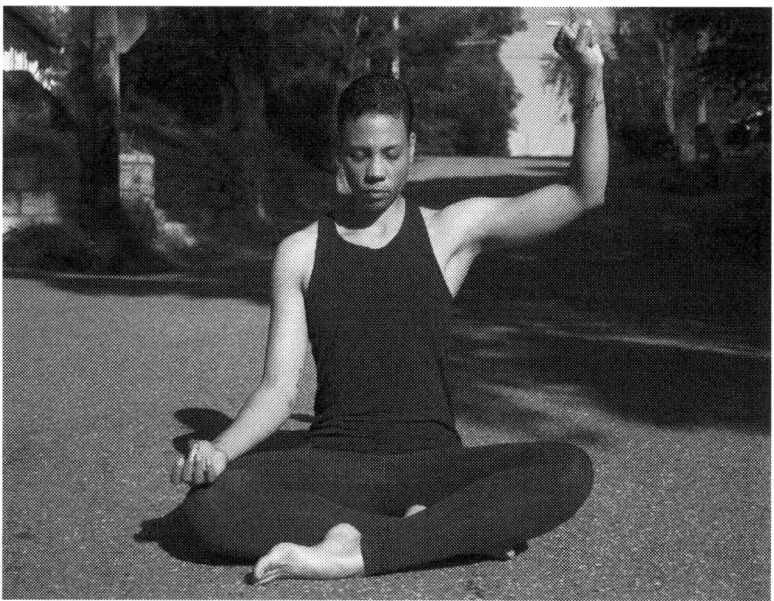

Figure 1.2 The Author, in an advertisement photo for one of the Essential Questions workshops.

group of five people where for the first time, the ratio of people of color in the room (three) was greater than the ratio of White people in the room (two). At this workshop, we raised $100 for Alerta Migratoria, a North Carolina based immigrant advocacy organization. I presented a workshop for women of color through Amplify and Activate, a Charlotte, North Carolina-based yoga and social justice organization run by Black women, at the CTZNWell Summit in the fall of 2018 and in Leicester, England as part of programming for Light Seekers, another social justice based organization.

As 2019 began, I became pregnant with my daughter, who was born in December that year. Hence, I took a hiatus from traveling and giving workshops. 2020 and the COVID-19 pandemic came and implored all of us to practice stillness. This has been an interesting time to continue to live the Five Essential Questions and their corresponding actions in the world.

One piece of insight I am taking away from the experience of the past few years is that the path to inner and outer liberation and the mitigation of oppression are long, and winding journeys. Even so, I can say that I am able now to check in with myself to discern whether or not I am attending to my own freedom, while working to attend to the freedom of others. I have used the work with the Five Essential Questions both in my own yoga practice, the timbre of which has become malleable, yet steady, and out in the world as touchstones to decide whether an activity or endeavor aligns with my commitment to liberatory self-care, decentering fear and dismantling the status quo. In some situations, I've successfully parted with comfort – my own, and the comfort of others – to speak out against words, actions and systems that affect us all, in ways that I would not have felt comfortable speaking out before. I must admit though, that this is a work in progress. My relationship with the yoga community remains precarious: I'm still critical, but I'm more willing to engage and speak to those criticisms than to walk away. Now, the work is more salient than ever, as I make space for the new shape of my life with my family and contend with the realities of the pandemic and the continued injustice people of color face in the United States. The trauma of these events will unfold for years to come, for all of us, in different ways.

As a parting thought, I wish to recognize how we are all at different stages in our development. As an invitation to consider how you wish to proceed, I offer these questions as a springboard: When history looks back on this time, how do you want to remember your response? As you look to the future, what kind of world are you imagining?

All the best to you, Dear Reader.
-Cara

Notes

1 The American Psychological Association reports that levels of stress across America rose markedly between August 2016 and January 2017 (Bethune, 2017).

2 For years in the yoga community, I've heard talk about "lordosis," or an anterior tilt of the pelvis. This is often described as a structural issue that needs to be addressed to avoid back injury. In a workshop, the instructor was explaining that the psoas, which is tight in many people due to sitting causes lordosis, which creates more possibility for low-back injury. They then posited that some people have thicker psoas muscles than others, with Black people having the thickest psoas, therefore, the most instances of lordosis. In a room of White students, this explanation (with no sources to bring forward to support the claims) perpetuated the idea that we must "fix" bodies of color. However, studies since the 1980s have disputed the structural inferiority of Black and Brown bodies. One study of women in 1989 showed that while the *perceived* amount of lordosis between White and Black women is different due to varying amounts of gluteal muscle tissue, *actual* amounts of lordosis are similar. A 1998 study on psoas thickness in young men found that the psoas of Black men are often thicker than those of White men, but that there were no indicators that this thickness causes a disproportionate amount of injuries.
3 Several studies have demonstrated how female professors are expected by students and fellow faculty, to do more emotional labor than their male counterparts (El-Ayali et al., 2018). Further, faculty of color are often expected to do emotional labor through diversity work – diversity work, which is also meant to support them (Matthew, 2016).
4 Three Leagues Deep is a misnomer! Fathoms go deep, leagues go wide. In any case, I hope the exercise brings people expansiveness and depth of all kinds. I digress.
5 Now the Immigrant Justice Coalition, it is a stand-alone group as the NAACP in Watagua County dissolved.
6 Again, this is where participants are partnered and the observe each other moving through discomfort in asana. Following the witnessing, partners report back to each other what they saw. They also reflect on what it is like to witness and to be witnessed.

Works Cited

Bethune, Sophie. "Many Americans Stressed about Future of Our Nation, New APA Stress in America™ Survey Reveals." *American Psychology Association*, February 2017. https://www.apa.org/news/press/releases/2017/02/stressed-nation.

Blow, Charles M. "Trump, Proxy of Racism." *The New York Times*, November 30, 2017. https://www.nytimes.com/2017/11/30/opinion/trump-racism-white-supremacy.html.

BUUF, 2020. http://www.buuf.net/.

Cole, Mia. "Appalachian State Students of Color Become Target of Harassment after Racist Chalkings on Campus." *Fresh U*, September 2017. http://www.freshu.io/mia-renee-cole/appalachian-state-students-of-color-target-of-harassment-after-chalkings.

ElAlayli, Amani, Ashley A. Hansen-Brown, and Michelle Ceynar. "Dancing Backwards in High Heels: Female Professors Experience More Work Demands and Special Favor Requests, Particularly from Academically Entitled Students." *Sex Roles* 79, no. 3–4 (2018): 136–50. doi: 10.1007/s11199-017-0872-6.

Embodied Learning Summit, 2017. https://embodiedlearning.weebly.com/.

Green, Erica L. "DeVos Delays Rule on Racial Disparities in Special Education." *The New York Times*, December 15, 2017a. https://www.nytimes.com/2017/12/15/us/politics/devos-obama-special-education-racial-disparities.html.

Green, Erica L. "To Understand Betsy DeVos's Educational Views, View Her Education." *The New York Times*, June 10, 2017b. https://www.nytimes.com/2017/06/10/us/politics/betsy-devos-private-schools-choice.html.

Hagan, Cara. *Symposium for Creative Social Stewardship*, 2016. https://socialstewardship.weebly.com/.

Hayes, Megan. "Chalk Talk: App State Board of Trustees Passes Unanimous Resolution Aimed at Inclusiveness." *Blowing Rock News*, October 5, 2016. https://blowingrocknews.com/chalking-appalachian-university-trustees/.

Manning, Richard. "Trump's Budget Really Could Make America Great Again. Will Congress Allow Him to Do It?" *FOX News Network*, May 22, 2017. https://www.foxnews.com/opinion/trumps-budget-really-could-make-america-great-again-will-congress-allow-him-to-do-it.

Matthew, Patricia A. "What Is Faculty Diversity Worth to a University?" *Atlantic Media Company*, November 23, 2016. https://www.theatlantic.com/education/archive/2016/11/what-is-faculty-diversity-worth-to-a-university/508334/.

Pear, Robert, Maggie Haberman, and Reed Abelson. "Trump to Scrap Critical Health Care Subsidies, Hitting Obamacare Again." *The New York Times*, October 12, 2017. https://www.nytimes.com/2017/10/12/us/politics/trump-obamacare-executive-order-health-insurance.html.

Popovich, Nadja, and Tatiana Schlossberg. "23 Environmental Rules Rolled Back in Trump's First 100 Days." *The New York Times*, May 2, 2017. https://www.nytimes.com/interactive/2017/05/02/climate/environmental-rules-reversed-trump-100-days.html.

Prison Books Collective, March 14, 2020. http://prisonbooks.info/.

Satchidananda, Swami. *The Yoga Sūtras of Patañjali*. Buckingham, VA: Integral Yoga Publications, 2012.

Shear, Michael D., and Helen Cooper. "Trump Bars Refugees and Citizens of 7 Muslim Countries." *The New York Times*, January 28, 2017. https://www.nytimes.com/2017/01/27/us/politics/trump-syrian-refugees.html.

"Small and Mighty Acts." smallandmightyacts.org, 2016. http://smallandmightyacts.org/.

Smith, Samantha. "Most Say American Dream Is within Reach for Them." *Pew Research Center*, May 30, 2020. https://www.pewresearch.org/fact-tank/2017/10/31/most-think-the-american-dream-is-within-reach-for-them/.

Sullivan, John, Reis Thebault, Julie Tate, and Jennifer Jenkins. "Number of Fatal Shootings by Police Is Nearly Identical to Last Year." *WP Company*, July 1, 2017. https://www.washingtonpost.com/investigations/number-of-fatal-shootings-by-police-is-nearly-identical-to-last-year/2017/07/01/98726cc6-5b5f-11e7-9fc6-c7ef4bc58d13_story.html?utm_term=.d8b84ae081cd.

Chapter 2

Towards a White spiritual antiracism

Jardana Peacock

If spirit, god(dess), the creator, Allah, love is in all of us then why do systems of oppression exist? Where is the god in White supremacy, sexism, homophobia, classism, and ableism?

I asked this question to a council of elders from a range of spiritual backgrounds in the fall of 2007 at the Bioneers conference. Patricia St. Onge, an indigenous activist based in Oakland, California and White eco-spiritual Buddhist Joanna Macy's responses continue to inform me:

> "We are all related. However. Because we have brokenness in the world, our authentic selves get veiled. We've stopped trusting what's inside of us. The spiritual work of our time is to lift up the veils." – Patricia St. Onge, Mokawk.

> "Our capacity to choose is great. This exquisite choice is sacred to me. When we show up, through our practice, we respond to our future and our ancestors and our present with grace." – Joanna Macy, Buddhist.

Onge and Macy's words touch on two vital components for White people to consider in our journeys as spiritual practitioners. Interconnection is implicit in our world, however systems of oppression, racism, and internalized supremacy and oppression have severed us from feeling our interconnection. Macy emphasizes that we have a *choice* to show up, for White people this means we have a *choice* to interrupt centuries of power and domination. Zenju Earthlyn Manuel's wisdom in *The Way of Tenderness* is also valuable. She states:

> Although systemic oppression does not feed us (quite the contrary), we need not be smothered by it. We can use it to awaken. (Manuel, 2015)

I suggest that White people's spirituality must include antiracism if we are to actualize self and collective liberation. Embodying antiracism as White people is both spiritual and ancestral work.

White people are racist

The practice of antiracism was introduced to me by activist Anne Braden, a White Kentuckian who purchased a home for a Black couple, the Wades, in Louisville, Kentucky in 1954 (Braden, 1999). At the time it was illegal for Black people to own homes. The house was bombed and she was tried for sedition, along with her husband Carl Braden. As articulated in Sheena Sood and Mari Morales-Williams's essay, *The City of Radical Love: A Philly Story of Oppression, Resistance, and Healing* (Sood and Morales-Williams, 2020), these scare tactics by the state were sanctioned across the U.S. as a way to suppress and oppress radical thought and action in the 50s and 60s – and still today although less overt at times. Anne and Carl Braden embodied a White antiracism that challenged state violence and for that they were jailed.

Anne became a mentor to me in her last year of life. She openly talked about whiteness whereas most other people taught me to ignore it. She asked me to examine my thoughts and actions through the prism of my whiteness, my biases, and my privilege. She encouraged me to confront the internal and external realities of White supremacy. Anne stated that all White people are racist. This was a hard truth to admit. "I'm not racist," I thought. I am a good person. I had Black friends and Black romantic partners throughout my life. Anne stated that being racist had nothing to do with good intent and everything to do with our inherent power and racial prejudice. Whiteness is constructed to protect White people in a positionality of privilege. This makes it challenging to understand or know when our words, actions, and subconscious harm People of Color and uphold systems of oppression.

As White people we are born into feeling and enacting supremacy; we inherit privilege because we are born White (Braden, 2005). Through my mentorship with Anne, I came to understand that as White people we are taught anti-Blackness from an early age. We *are* racist and we have to do everything possible to reverse this truth by dismantling a significant portion of the messages we've grown up believing, including the more subtle ones from the culture of White supremacy that values perfectionism, individualism, power, and control. There is a choice that White people are granted because we are White. Anne asked me and her other students to consider: how are we using our bodies and life for racial justice? I've since considered living my life answering the question: is my whiteness a bridge or does it divide myself from others –especially Black people and People Of Color?

Antiracism is spiritual work

Following my introduction to Anne Braden, my antiracism journey continued to unfold through the guidance of a powerful multiracial social justice community in Louisville, Kentucky (Peacock, 2018). At the same time my activism began to deepen, my spiritual practices did as well. While Anne did not call antiracism a spiritual practice, understanding whiteness is key to White people's healing and spiritual work. Understanding whiteness and dismantling racism is both painful and liberating. This is in essence what spirituality holds us in as humans, a journey towards living into our best selves, an ability to hold complexity and a commitment to continual growth and reflection which informs our external actions. Antiracism is similar. White antiracism asks us to examine the truth of our thoughts and actions, to locate the ways we've been indoctrinated to believe in our superiority and to toss those ideologies out in exchange for living more honestly into our values of interconnection and equity.

However, as I entered more deeply into spiritual communities, it became clear that systems of oppression are alive there too. At the start of a new training or class, spiritual teachers often began by saying, "You are here for a reason. You are chosen to be on a path for the enlightened." Even now when I look around the yoga studio, or the Buddhist temple, I see others like me – White people. If only those present are on a path towards enlightenment, where is everyone else? The yoga and meditation spaces I began to frequent looked vastly different than the multiracial alliances that informed my activist life.

In a seminal yoga text, Patanjali's Yoga Sutras, yoga is defined as liberation (Satchidananda, 1990). Liberation is connected to more than an individual experience. We exist in the world with others and when others suffer, we suffer. I came to understand that yoga is ahimsa, or nonviolence. Nonviolence isn't a passive practice and yet most Western teachings of yoga focus on the inner work without linking it to the outer actions needed to create a better world. On the other hand, many activist communities focus on the outer injustices without tending to the inner work. Both communities miss the link about how self and collective liberation is inner and outer work which returns us to righteous interconnection and equanimity.

The practice I have studied most in-depth, Tantra yoga, focuses on the energetic body. Pandit Rajmani Tigunait, a spiritual teacher and cultural bearer of the Sri Vidya Tantra tradition states: "Sri Vidya is based on a philosophy that tells us our body, mind, senses, and the universe are designed on exactly the same pattern: anything that exists in the universe exists in our body, and anything that exists in our body exists in the universe" (Tigunait, 2017). Tantra Hatha asana practice focuses on enhancing the health of the spine and thus your life, whether that is addressing a psychosomatic pain in the hip or knee or a deep-seated fear.

Some of the hidden fears I uncovered through my practice are how I hid inside of roles and identities that protected me from pain, for example hiding behind White privilege – which acts as a bubble to protect and divide me from others. If I remain disconnected, I am "safe." I began to use the tools of Tantra yoga towards a deeper examination of how oppression and supremacy exist inside of myself and inside of the world. With the development of this inner work, I found myself able to speak up with more courage when my family made racist remarks at the dinner table, or when activist communities committed to social justice outwardly but would cut each other down inside groups.

In my activist life, along with many others – I began to interrupt the breakneck speed of meetings, campaign schedules, and coalition strategy sessions – to attend to building a culture of care: taking time to enjoy food with each other, pausing for moments throughout meetings to check in with each other or share in breath and meditation together. We found that this enhanced our bonds with each other and our activism moved from a more rooted place of care and love. I learned the healing balm of silence, contemplative spaces, embodied movement, and a reconnection to the ways that our minds, bodies, and hearts respond to the trauma of oppression. Through Tantra practices, I came into a more compassionate and loving antiracism. I began to create more meaningful relationships across race and with other White people. I showed up to hard interpersonal conversations where I had enacted harm despite my best intentions. The healing work of meditation, yoga, breath, and silence aided our campaigns and activist projects. My activist community became more focused, less stressed, and moved more from a relational foundation.

Antiracism is as much a journey inward as it is outwards and through it I have learned to love myself and other White people (Peacock and Germaine Strickland 2017). The practices of yoga and meditation show me a mirror around how I am going into the pain of oppression or how I am avoiding it. I discovered in my meditation practice that when I avoid pain, I'm not breathing and not connected to my body. When I am confronting the pain of whiteness and oppression, I come into my body and I am better able to show up to the harm I create and the truth about the harm of my ancestors. White supremacy tears us from belonging. White supremacy separates us. Breathing brings us back to the truth of our collective humanity.

Spiritual bypassing

Unfortunately, the deeper healing work yoga was created to facilitate, as I've described above, is often glazed over in Western yoga teaching (Williams, Owens, and Syedullah, 2016 and Johnson, 2020). Instead it was antiracism that grounded me in the liberatory intentions of yoga. I question the purpose of many Western yoga and healing spaces, which have supported me in many ways but also continually fail to apply anti-oppression values. These spaces serve as an escape for White people. These spaces foster a way for White people to avoid the truth of the oppression we uphold inside and out or what is otherwise known as spiritual bypassing. I recognize that if I do not make visible the ways whiteness contributes to oppression, I will never be able to adequately dismantle it. To face myself, to face my whiteness is to begin to heal and go deeper into my spiritual understanding of living on this earth in this moment in time. As White people, as White spiritual practitioners, we can no longer separate ourselves from the truth demons of our history and present.

The purpose of practice is to strengthen our resilience as we enter into conversation with the truth. White privilege aids in spiritual bypassing and hinders our ability to shift and change internal and external hate and violence. This brings me to a sunny room in Boone, North Carolina when my former White yoga teacher boldly named Trump as an igniter of a much-needed revolution. "The election of Donald Trump was predestined. It is America's karma. Trump is igniting a revolution. He is God too, " she stated. The room was made up of mostly liberal White women, from working-class and middle-class backgrounds from the southern United States. There were a few social justice organizers in the circle, including one Black woman.

In her statement, the White yoga teacher ignored the truths about the inequity experienced across race, class, and gender. She invisiblized her own whiteness and failed to lift up a history of resistance from Black and Brown people to injustice. These are the ways that our privilege protects us from feeling havoc and trauma that the inhumane policies of the U.S.A. continue to enact. This is how whiteness functions in many yoga and spiritual spaces. Our White bodies and assertions are rarely questioned. Our White bodies do not know the fear of dropping our kids at the bus stop under a looming threat of ICE, as immigrant neighbors of mine experience in Louisville, Kentucky. Whiteness protects us from these realities. Whiteness keeps us relatively safe but it also keeps us disconnected.

That afternoon, I spoke up and asked her to go deeper into an understanding of intergenerational trauma, power, and privilege. Others joined in and we had a healthy discussion. Part of the spiritual work of antiracism is the ability to give up "being right;" in yoga practice that is what people often refer to as the ego. While I definitely felt like I was right in that moment, the teacher and I continued to grapple throughout our relationship around what it means to be in a White body teaching practices that are not from our own lineages. We wrestled together around how those practices are political and why our language matters.

Zenju Earthlyn Manuel wrote, "Whatever we see and hear in regard to race, sexuality and gender has been learned. That doesn't mean we should disengage from dialogue, however. To the contrary, it means we must engage in it more honestly so that we can unearth our ancestral and karmic tendencies and reclaim our ancient, lost kinship with one another" (Manuel, 2015). Although the yoga teacher and I were never able to come to a mutual understanding, a lot of growth happened for both of us as we dived into these tensions around whiteness, trauma, power, and privilege in the context of a spiritual community. We must continue to interrupt White privilege, power, and supremacy in our spiritual spaces.

Antiracism as a path towards interconnection

What we seek most as human beings and as spiritual practitioners is connection and belonging. Our interconnection is intimate and messy, it is uncomfortable and difficult but worthy and liberating to attend to. Interconnection requires self and collective examination. As Zenju reminds, "We are all one" (Manuel, 2015). This is what yoga serves to teach us, this is how spiritual practice supports us in embodying collective liberation. Being in the mess is one of White folks' greatest challenges. However, we cannot realize interconnection until we confront the messiness of oppression.

White people are set up in our culture to value competition over connection, individualism over interconnection, insolation over community. Examining and dismantling racism as a White person is a pathway through White privilege and supremacy and towards actualizing interconnection and healing. This messiness is necessary to understand and act upon if we are to create different ways of being and relating.

The spiritual revolution White folks need to be a part of is one of antiracism and decolonization. We must step through the looking glasses of privilege and into a place of reimagination. adrienne maree brown states that we are caught inside a White man's imagination (brown, 2017). Whiteness limits what is possible, suggesting that there must be those who have and those who do not, that Black men, women, and trans and queer folks are disposable, that the pandemic of missing indigenous women can continue without policy shifts or action by the general population. As spiritual practitioners we often assume spirituality will be enough but the truth is Black and Brown folks are dying in our inaction. I believe this can change.

If spiritual practice isn't positively transforming society, then we need to change our understanding and embodiment of our spiritual practices. Perhaps it is not that "more people need to meditate" but rather that those who do need to enact their meditation out loud and help create a world where people are treated with dignity and respect. Instead, we must move forward a radical imagination (Kelley, 2003) of what's possible when we move together: neighborhood mutual care networks, a solidarity economy, freedom for all people, a world where everyone has enough.

Interconnection isn't an ideal that White people can realize without first doing the deep internal work of changing, reprogramming, and understanding whiteness and how it contributes to the violence of our world. When we understand this, then we begin to live into an antiracism which builds a different world in which our whiteness isn't violence but rather solidarity. Racism is a disease of the heart and body. In order to shift that, we have to embody what we value every day and show up in some way that aligns our actions with values of liberation. A White spiritual antiracism comes into conversation, heals, and strives to interrupt our ancestral lineages of violence and power.

We were born into this moment, on this planet, for a reason. Our work in this lifetime as White people is to confront oppression and unroot it at its core. Our lives are answers to our ancestors' questions and dreams (Burns-Jones and Dendy-Green, 2019). For White people, this means reconciling the deep wounds of genocide, slavery, and the violence of our ancestors. Spiritual practice is a bridge toward liberation but without a commitment to antiracism it will never be enough.

Works cited

Bioneers Conference, 2007. https://bioneers.org.

Braden, Anne. *The Wall Between*. Knoxville: University of Tennessee Press, 1999.

Braden, Anne. "Finding the Other America." *Fellowship of Reconciliation*, January/February, 2005. http://www.november.org/BottomsUp/reading/america.html.

brown, adrienne maree. *Emergent Strategy: Shaping Change, Changing Worlds*. Chico: AK Press, 2017.

Burns-Jones, Amber and Sara Dendy-Green. "Personal Correspondence." *Liberation School South*, 2019. https://www.liberationschoolsouth.org.

Johnson, Michelle Cassandra. *Skill in Action: Radicalizing Your Yoga Practice to Create a Just World*. Boulder: Radical Transformation Media, Shambhala Publications, 2020.

Kelley, Robin D. G. *Freedom Dreams: The Black Radical Imagination*. Beacon Hill: Beacon Press, 2003.

Manuel, Zenju Earthlyn. *The Way of Tenderness, Awakening Through Race, Sexuality and Gender*. Somerville: Wisdom Publications, 2015.

Peacock, Jardana. *Practice Showing Up: A Guidebook for White People Working for Racial Justice*. Lexington: Create Space, 2018.

Peacock, Jardana and Kelly Germaine Strickland. "Ancestral Healing for White Anti-Racist Folks." *Irresistible Podcast*, 2017. https://podcasts.apple.com/us/podcast/14-ancestral-healing-for-anti-racist-white-folks-jardana/id1308078502?i=1000401043475.

Satchidananda, Sri Swami. *The Yoga Sutras of Patanjali*. Buckingham: Integral Yoga, 1990.

Sood, Sheena and Mari Morales-Williams. "The City of Radical Love: A Philly Story of Oppression, Resistance, and Healing." In *Practicing Yoga as Resistance: Voices of Color in Search of Freedom*. Edited by Cara Hagan. Abington: Routledge, 2021.

Tigunait, Pandit Rajmani. "Foundations of Sri Vidya Tantra." *Himalayan Institute*, 2017. https://www.himalayaninstitute.org/series/foundations-sri-vidya-tantra/.

Williams, Rev. angel Kyodo, Owens, Lama Rod and Jasmine Syedullah. *Radical Dharma, Talking Race, Love and Liberation*. Berkeley: North Atlantic Books, 2016.

Part II

Yoga, Self, and Community

Chapter 3

Embodied radical healing through the collective
A Black Lotus autoethnography

Dominique A. Malebranche

I met asana before I knew yoga.

I was introduced through an asana practice at a small-town studio, while studying for my PhD in counseling psychology. I was drawn to the title "community" class, that was a third of the price of their regular weekly classes. Upon arrival, I mentally noted being the only person of color in the room, and was not met with community, but instead with mixed feelings. My background in dance informed my participation; I engaged with the yoga flow like I was learning choreography for the first time. However, there were no counts, no drum and bass, and no "boom-kats", just breath, sweat, and ambient music.

Fast-forward a few years, my continued asana practice later reflected my resonance with dance. I always yearned for the high of embodied expression, without words, language, and cognitive understanding. A blissful break from the default analytical self. Over time and through cultural exploration, the practice of yoga allowed me to be in my body. The beat of my own pulse was the drumming that I needed to find flow, guided by the organic rhythm of Haitian blood that danced through me. My body created the choreography. Dancing on the mat, with contemplative intention; it was a spiritual dance. A spiritual dance connected to a cultural rhythm of movement and energy, not inherently connected to a particular aesthetic, though I mindfully practiced in my embodiment as a Black woman.

However, that first afternoon, I was focused and determined to get the choreography and spent most of the time in my own head evaluating my progress and trying to physically mimic those around me. The class ended with an Om and chant, "shanti, shanti, shanti; that means peace…". My eyes shot open, as I anxiously surveyed the room at everyone else who seemed secure in their practice. My heartbeat became more pronounced, as I wondered what I had just participated in; in that moment, the fear of sacrilege was present. I came alone and left alone, experiencing no sense of community and ignorant to the real meaning of yoga in practice.

All too often, people of color are introduced to yoga under similar circumstances, or perhaps avoid the practice all together because of such experiences. Some individuals experience further marginalization in yoga classes, which create barriers for certain communities to access the transformative qualities of the practice. This chapter outlines a brief context of Western yoga and its historical and contemporary connections to trauma dynamics that reflect roots of systemic oppression and relational disconnection from the original intentions of cultural and spiritual liberation. It continues to contextualize the cultural embodied knowledge, lived experiences of a Black Haitian-American female-bodied author, through contemplative radical healing. Before concluding with a discussion of considerations for culturally and politically contextualized embodied yoga, the chapter offers a complementary approach to Westernized asana practice through the exploration of yoga philosophy in a contemplative healing justice community: Black Lotus Collective.

Cultural (dis)embodiment in Western yoga

> We grieve to stay in touch with what is…We cannot afford to dissociate from this moment, to become numb or distracted for prolonged periods – we owe it to the seven generations before us and the seven generations ahead of us.
> – @Flordelotonegra, Black Lotus Collective

Western yoga, in its current state, engenders links to larger historical and contemporary traumatic forces such as colonization, oppression, and structural racism. Its early history is situated in European imperialism in India where yoga was intentionally outlawed under British occupation and colonization in the late 1700s (Singleton, 2010). Dalit peoples and Hatha yogis were further marginalized and the West's influence in India reinforced a physical culture of the spiritual practice. Presently, various parts of India continue to experience broken lineages and ancient traditions lost, which leave a lasting impact on collective identity (Barkataki, 2017). Meanwhile in the West, Euro-American ideas of India have been reified in its import to the United States. Appropriated elements of Indian spirituality were reintroduced with yoga through decontextualized trinkets of Hindi sculptures, displayed phrases of "Om," "Namaste," and other Sanskrit terms, while seemingly erasing yoga's representation of practitioners and teachers of color. Yoga's origination of ancient spiritual practice, to be translated from Sanskrit as "yoking," or unifying mind, body, and spirit (Bryant, 2015), has since been secularized and (mis)appropriated in the West as a capitalist endeavor.

This history has transferred its impact of colonial power to contemporary isolating dynamics of cultural trauma. American sociologists describe cultural trauma as occurring when "members of a collectivity feel they have been subjected to a horrendous event that leaves indelible marks upon their group consciousness, marking their memories forever and changing their future identity in fundamental and irrevocable ways" (Alexander et al., 2004, p. 1). Scholars have begun to document the experience of imperial trauma, its enduring intergenerational impacts, and ongoing oppression as fundamentally altering the health and well-being of people of color (see Akbar, 2017; Brave Heart, 2000; DeGruy, 2017; Yehuda et al., 2001). Cultural appropriation of yoga, as defined by the "taking, marketing, and exotification of cultural practices from historically oppressed populations" (Deshpande, 2019, p. 3) shows up in two forms of cultural trauma in the United States: commodification and cultural erasure.

Mainstream yoga in the West, predominately represented by thin, White, upper-middle-class, able-bodied, cis-women, lends itself to fostering a false sense of community in the form of emphasizing elite access through the exoticized representations of asanas, or postures, as yoga. The commercialization of yoga, often illustrated as core power and exercise routines in exclusive attire, contributes to the privatization of yoga, which further appropriates a devotional practice once free of cost for thousands of years to now being marketed and sold (Deshpande, 2019). That said, the cost of Western yoga classes can be prohibitive for low to middle-income individuals, often excluding communities of color and creating barriers for historically marginalized individuals and immigrants to whom the practices inherently belong (Gandhi & Wolff, 2017).

Practices in today's Western yoga culture also invisibilize Brown and Black people, who were the original creators and practitioners, and instead center White ableist cisheteropatriarchy and a neoliberal embodiment of health. Though there has been a shift to address this gap, the invisible oppression further implicates the impact of racism and colonialism to describe the role of power in yoga's import and its legacies of imperialism (Putcha, 2019). Yoga teacher and decolonizing yoga activist, Susanna Barkataki, describes feeling "dehumanized" by the erasure of her culture being "stripped of its meaning" and noted, "To be colonized is to become a stranger in your own land. As a desi, this is the feeling I get in most Westernized yoga spaces today" (2017). The early construction of Whiteness, that included European assimilation to establishing roots in the US, may have also been a carried source of cultural trauma that contributed to the dominant society rapidly seeking practices such as yoga. As a result, the decolonizing movement urges a critical deepening of practice that returns yoga to its liberatory roots that can center cultural embodied knowledge.

Eight limbs for radical healing

> Breathing in, I acknowledge the harm I have caused myself and others while in my learning process. Breathing out, I offer curiosity, tenderness and accountability.
> – Flowerthief, co-founder of Black Lotus Collective

Although Western science has begun to evaluate the psychological and physiological "benefits" of yoga as asana practice, it is the "healing" philosophy of the ancient yogic practices that should be further emphasized in efforts toward liberation. *Patanjali's Yoga Sutras* discuss the classical philosophy that engages the eight limbs of yoga to guide mastery of mind and emotions and offer spiritual wisdom (Bryant, 2009). The philosophy includes ethical and social restraints (*yamas*), observances (*niyamas*), postures (*asanas*), breath control (*pranayama*), withdrawal of the senses (*pratyahara*), concentration (*dharana*), meditation (*dhyana*), absorption into the Divine or enlightenment (*samadhi*). In these eight limbs for liberation, he begins with ethics and emphasizes breathing, meditation, and concentration practices as critical embodiments of yoga. These practices aim to unite individual consciousness with universal consciousness and can be understood as offering practice for the potential for both personal and collective liberation.

In order to (re)orient our practices toward liberation for all beings, we have to first engage the experiences of those who have been historically traumatized by ongoing oppressive structures, then re-envision those structures. Researchers have referred to this approach as radical healing, grounded in a love ethic that involves addressing the individual, focusing on interpersonal relationships and communities, and transforming root issues of harm in systems (Ginwright, 2015). A radical healing framework also centers "being able to sit in a dialectic and exist in both spaces of resisting oppression and moving toward freedom" (French et al., 2019, p. 11). The reclamation of the embodied ethics of yoga can be a path for the global majority and historically marginalized to both resist and reclaim liberation.

Indigenous researcher and scholar-activist, Michael Yellow Bird, reminds us of the possibility of collective liberation through community emancipation from hegemony, also understood as the essence of decolonization, which includes pulling away and rebuilding (Gray et al., 2008). Given the historical and cultural trauma narratives for people of color and other marginalized groups, personal liberation is bound in the collective. Modern asana practice alone in Western yoga spaces fails to connect to a deeper level of liberation that reflects the need to consider a cultural context to address internalized oppression, as well as nourish the yogic practice. The following offers a response to root causes of harm in Western yoga spaces and explores supportive structures for marginalized individuals and communities in the context of a contemplative healing justice collective.

Embodied yoga ethics in community: Black Lotus Collective

> You are held, you are seen, you are loved, your life matters.
> – Juliana Santoyo, co-founder of Black Lotus Collective

As I have since deepened my yoga practice in this embodiment, I have found that I have to feed my yoga "soul offerings" by identifying what nourishes my spirit – spaciousness, community, collective healing, and collective visibility, to name a few. Collective visibility is the practice of seeing others and being seen, at the heart level in loving presence and at a cultural level in acknowledgment of sociopolitical impact. The quote above was initially presented to me at my first community sit in our closing meditation; it is in the way of being that *Black Lotus Collective* embodies yoga and offers soul nourishment for radical healing.

Black Lotus Collective (BLC), originally organized around the *Radical Dharma* (Kyodo Williams, Owens & Syedullah, 2016) community conversations, is a model for personal and social liberation in contemplative spaces. BLC is a QTBIPOC healing justice and liberation community practicing in colonized Wôpanâak (Wampanoag) traditional territory, also known as Greater Boston Area, that centers marginalized experiences in healing endeavors through meditation, transformative justice, future-building art, and embodiment practices. Developed in 2016, it responded to historical and ongoing oppression and trauma perpetuated by institutions of power and the state, as well as to address the erasure of marginalized identities within contemplative spaces (Gathers, Jones, Martin, Santoyo & Santoyo, 2018). The Collective engages healing through liberation and ancestral work, cultural, Indigenous and ancestral practices, meditation, as well as accountability processes with one another that address cultural trauma by challenging dominant notions of White supremacy and its byproducts of systemic and internalized oppression. BLC practice aligns with the radical healing framework that asserts a focus on building critical consciousness, promoting cultural authenticity and self-knowledge, as well as providing hope, emotional and social support, and connecting with strength and resistance (French et al., 2019). The relational way of being within this community fosters an ethical practice of yoga and yogic philosophy that enhances asana practice. Though not explicitly stated, BLC engages yogic thought at the intrapersonal, interpersonal, and community level through the ethical precepts of the sutra's yamas and niyamas.

Yamas in community

The yamas, translated as "social restraints," can be seen as vows and practices of self-discipline (Adele, 2009). Restraint is expressed in the following forms – nonviolence (*ahimsa*), truthfulness (*satya*), non-stealing (*asteya*), non-excess (*brahmacharya*), non-possessiveness (*aparigraha*). Ahimsa, satya, and brahmacharya are explored in the context of BLC.

Ahimsa, nonviolence or non-harming, has been described as the force unleashed when the desire to harm is eradicated. However, it is not meant to suggest the absence of violence but also 'love in action' that can be practiced through deeds, thoughts, and words. The practice of accountability and addressing harm is fundamental to the Collective, and a pillar of yogic ethical principles. In community, these healing tenets of ahimsa are informed by centering identities and dismantling systems of oppression of hierarchy. Restorative practice and circle processes are used to minimize harmful dynamics with one another and in the community. The founders strive to redistribute power by flattening hierarchical structures as an active process in contemplative sits, community events, and relational engagements. Leadership is shared, participation is diverse, and engagement is voluntary.

The notion of internalized oppression is consistently addressed through the accountability process. We use each other as a mirror for deconstructing systems of oppression in our language, behaviors, and ways of relating to our own and each other's emotions. As a result, individuals can find agency in their sense of power to disrupt oppressive internalizations, reclaim cultural integrity, and further understand and affirm lived experiences in their embodiment. Oftentimes, self-love and acceptance are conditioned out of individuals who embody nondominant positions within society. The active practice of ahimsa in relationships offers a felt sense of dignity and affirmation in one's humanity.

The cultivation of self-compassion in practice is also used to engage the principle of ahimsa. Contemplative practices are contextualized in the lived experiences that center those navigating interpersonal and systemic oppression. Holding space for mixed emotions and honoring compassionate responses for external circumstances are also reflected in the meditation practices. In practice, we are guided to sit with our "body as home, the universe" and in doing so, noticing "how one is governing the hierarchy inside of self; which emotions do and do not get space; which get prioritized and which get seen and heard." Through acknowledging how the external systems of oppressive hierarchy impact lived experiences, individuals are offered space to recognize how these systems become reinforced in one's personal experience. The intent to dismantle external systems of oppression through collective practice is just as critical as disrupting internal systems of oppression for personal transformation. To consider new structures and ways of operating, we are called to address how we are governing our own "universe."

Truthfulness, or satya, is practiced through right speech and self-expression without causing harm to others in community. BLC provides and encourages freedom to show up as one's true self, in full expression. Whether it be in a traditional Western yoga studio, or within the greater social context, marginalized communities with a history of cultural trauma are often silenced, invisibilized, and tokenized. Individuals learn that it may be unsafe to authentically present themselves. While strategies, like code switching, have been reinforced for survival in navigating normative spaces, they fragment identities of individuals and therefore communities. Community practice is linked to prioritizing accountability for authentic presence. Restorative justice practices, informed by indigenous traditions, provide a structure of utilizing a talking piece to share authentic stories and insights born from contemplative and embodied practice in the present moment. Often the experience of resonance is alive in the room through a spectrum of collective experiences from joy to grief. It is in these collective practices that we can learn how to be truthful to ourselves and to be lovingly witnessed at the same time.

I was assisting in a weekend intensive trauma treatment workshop that included long hours of supporting a community in healing, managing trauma dynamics in participants, and witnessing and participating in theatrical dramas of previous traumatic experiences. I was in need of engaging the lightness of my own spirit and needed to leave the workshop to do so. At the end of the day, participants went off to bed and I left to be in community with BLC.

That night, BLC was hosting an event titled, S.O.O.P. (Stories of Our People). Community members were invited to bring one ingredient for a communal soup, a story or wisdom to share, or just their being for presence. I brought my being. At a community soup kitchen, focused on social enterprising to support the physical, economic, and social well-being of the community, we all savored music, song, stories of our names, struggles, and joys. Stunned from my intensive work, I allowed myself to absorb the energy and resonate with the heightening vibrations of the group. I became re-energized in the divinity of my relationships in the Collective and the divine experience of being together and coming alive through stories that connected us to our roots. I grew keenly aware of the sacredness of culture, community, and collective catharsis. Following the community share that blessed the meal, the soup was simmered and spiced to feed the entire room. There was just enough – just enough laughter, just enough tears, just enough "Say That!", and just enough food to satisfy. We might as well have called it "soup joumou¹," because in that moment I felt like we were celebrating freedom.

Driving back to the workshop that evening, I was full. I had just enough to satisfy my own spiritual hunger, and in that satisfaction, I was grounded in centeredness and the experience of sacred collective liberation that affirmed rootedness and balance for the remainder of the weekend.

The spirit of brahmacharya, non-excess, was resonating throughout my experience. Broader interpretations of brahmacharya can be understood as a practice of moderating and conserving energy. It requires being aware of one's behaviors, as they change in the moment, and preventing dissipation of one's energy through the misuse of the senses. In the above example, the collective energy assisted in moderating the individual energy with a soulful and cultural offering.

Niyamas in community

Niyamas, translated as active "observances," include purity (*saucha*), contentment (*santosha*), self-discipline (*tapas*), self-study (*svadhyaya*), and surrender (*ishvara pranidhana*) (Adele, 2009). These niyama tenets emphasize the ways in which we treat ourselves and interact with others. Saucha, tapas, and svadhyaya are further discussed through BLC community practices.

Music has long been a form of medicine to purify the spirit of collectivist cultures across the globe. During a monthly sit, we were invited into meditation practice through the sounds of a saxophone played by a community member. They framed it with discussion of the growing reality of burdens for marginalized communities, including the increase of ecological grief due to the impact of climate crises, and we sat in movement and flow, tension and conflict, resistance and release, all illustrated through sound. Lodged emotions moved through the body supported by the melody as it offered clarity and the opportunity to awaken energy within us. Only through the deep rhythms and contemplation could our community move into the authentic experience of carried burdens of responsibility as future ancestors. The cleansing of negativity and weight resonated throughout the day, as I continued to experience the visceral quality of the purification process.

Saucha invites us to purify our bodies through mental, emotional, and physical practices, as well as purifying the relationships and world around us. Using the practice to declutter the mind and emotional space has been essential to community healing. As people of color with intersectional identities, such as queerness and disability, there is a burden to carry in the simple practices of navigating work, academic, and life spaces. What individuals and community experience in microaggression, bias, and discrimination is paralleled to the experiences of structural violence noted within larger society. However, attending a BLC sit and preparing for meditation are consistent acts of moving into ease and working to make space to hold our heaviness with compassion.

Prior to the sound meditation, BLC engaged in a year-long exploration of identifying the emotional, physical, and spiritual responses that are necessary for practicing right effort of personal and collective liberation as conscious ancestors-in-training. Self-discipline in monthly gatherings included contemplative practice that was oriented around restoring the oppressed spirit and activating cultural resiliency and integrity. One of these practices focused on the human connection to the ecological system and invited the community into an embodied exercise to illustrate the past and future perspectives in regard to the current needs and long-lasting impacts of climate crises and eco-grief. The invitation was a demonstration of tapas, and a call to "burn non-supportive habits" in our daily lives for the sake of future rewards to the next several generations (Adele, 2009, p. 135). Tapas is about doing the work. Sitting with a balance of grief and responsibility, the practice of self-discipline in our current embodiment became critical for the healing of current selves and our past and future lineage.

Overall, these intentional gatherings facilitate the practices of svadhyaya, self-study. The response to "who am I" can become convoluted underneath the many labels forced without consent by the broader society. By engaging in the process of learning who we are in our true identities as divinely free, and unlearning the compounded layers of oppression and internalization, the community engages in a collective evolution of growing the witness. Each meditation and embodiment practice encourages the understanding of multiple layers of self, and the context in which self operates and functions.

Cultural healing and the future of yoga in context

> If you really want to disrupt the system, start reclaiming your body.
> – Lama Rod Owens, Buddhist activist, author, and spiritual teacher

I later came to know yoga more intimately; it was an evening class during my yoga teacher training after a long and exhausting day of clinical rotations as a pre-doctoral psychology intern. After I negotiated with my body, I ended up at my regular Wednesday class. The lights were off, my teacher's "fairy lights" lit the room and all I could see during my practice was my internal experience. Her voice carried me the whole time, "What expectation did you bring to the moment, let it go...Every time you want to push [your body], back out. Every time you don't want to push, try leaning in." I was aware of my mental chatter, my physical sensations, her voice that was the guide and an overwhelming experience of deepness. That night, my practice felt like I was being lifted beyond myself and grounded into the earth at the same time, like the all too common yoga phrase, "root down and lift up" to symbolize the earth element and the air element at play within one motion.

In a state of flow, I assumed my final forms, before savasana. Before final rest, I was gifted with one of my favorite class gems, a supportive adjustment by my teacher. With her adjustment to support depth in my stretch in a reclining hand-to-big toe pose (supta padangusthasana), I was able to mentally, physically, and emotionally, let go. In that next instance, my leg dropped into the deepest stretch it has ever seen and my breath carried it all the way to its limit and back. It's like she had said once before, "you can only really let go when you're supported."

Lama Rod's words communicate a truth to reclaiming our stolen and erased identities yet require a contextual environment to engage in the process of unlearning and reconnecting to our embodiment. Reclaiming the body remains a radical act of liberation, as institutional and state-sanctioned oppression are reinforced through the control of our bodies. Yoga classes became a mirror reflection, or a microcosm, of the patterns that took place both on and off of the mat, that I would later explore in community. Though, the more I became embodied in asana practice, the clearer I understood that my personal liberation would have to come from liberating the body in a cultural context and connection.

The culture needs healing that can penetrate the years of discrimination, marginalization, and systemic oppression and awaken the essence of who we are as a collective. More beautifully sung by BLC co-founder, Grant Jones, this healing should bring a sense of freedom "to live uninterrupted." Sources of cultural trauma reflect society and express themselves in the body; as above so below, as the universe so the soul, as without so within. Just as sources of pain, suffering, and trauma can be identified within the external and the internal experience, so can healing. Yoga has long been a deeply spiritual practice to engage unity with divine healing but has been repurposed in mainstream Western yogic spaces. The asana limb aims to strengthen the body for divine consciousness, but yoga practice without liberating carried grief, trauma, and collective harm is unable to be unified with spirit. Yoga for marginalized communities would benefit from enhancing asana practice with ethical principles of yoga that acknowledge the nuance of cultural trauma and healing in an environment that supports cultural visibility.

There are also implications for yoga to contribute to generative future building. Movement toward a decolonized yoga practice should include contemplative healing, where healing occurs in relationship to self and others, and its purpose is centered in healing for cultural, political, and social well-being. This would support the need for a practice that integrates cultural authenticity and self-knowledge, or more appropriately, cultural embodied knowledge – lived experiences of one's body. To that end, liberatory yoga is an ethical practice and moves toward cultural and spiritual integrity, which can offer a deeply empowering practice of self-awareness, self and community care, resilience, and accountability of dismantling systems of oppression within and without. Radical healing is reclaiming yoga as a Brown, indigenous, spiritual, and inherently liberation practice. Yoga can then re-emerge as a transformative practice in resistance and reclamation for radical presence.

Note

1 Soup joumou, a spicy Haitian squash soup that was historically only enjoyed by French slave masters and forbidden for Haitian slaves, but later reclaimed by the people after Haiti successfully revolted against slavery and proclaimed its independence in 1804.

Works cited

Adele, Deborah. *The Yamas & Niyamas: Exploring Yoga's Ethical Practice*. Duluth, MN: On-Word Bound Books, 2009.
Akbar, Maysa. *Urban Trauma: A Legacy of Racism*. Hartford, CT: Publish Your Purpose Press, 2017.
Alexander, Jeffrey C., et al. *Cultural Trauma and Collective Identity*. Berkeley, CA: University of California Press, 2004.
Barkataki, Susanna. "How to Decolonize Your Yoga Practice." *Huffington Post* (2017).
Brave Heart, Maria Yellow Horse. "Wakiksuyapi: Carrying the Historical Trauma of the Lakota." *Tulane Studies in Social Welfare* 21(22) (2000): 245–266.
Bryant, Edwin F. *The Yoga Sutras of Patanjali: A New Edition*, Translation, and Commentary. New York, NY: Farrar, Straus and Giroux, 2009.
DeGruy, Joy. *Post-traumatic Slave Syndrome: America's Legacy of Enduring Injury*. Joy DeGruy Publications Inc., 2017.
Deshpande, Rina. "What's the Difference between Cultural Appropriation and Cultural Appreciation?" *Yoga Journal* (2019).
French, Bryana H., et al. "Toward a Psychological Framework of Radical Healing in Communities of Color." *The Counseling Psychologist*, 48 (2019): 0011000019843506.
Gathers, E., Jones, G., Martin, D., Santoyo, J. F., Santoyo, J. M. *Creating Models for Social Liberation in Contemplative Spaces: The Black Lotus Collective*. Poster at Mind and Life International Symposium for Contemplative Research, 2018.
Ghandi, Shreena and Lillie Wolff. "Yoga and the Roots of Cultural Appropriation." *Kalamazoo Praxis Center* (2017).
Ginwright, Shawn A. "Radically Healing Black Lives: A Love Note to Justice." *New Directions for Student Leadership* 2015(148) (2015): 33–44.

Gray, Mel, John Coates, and Michael Yellow Bird, eds. *Indigenous Social Work around the World: Towards Culturally Relevant Education and Practice*. Farnham, UK: Ashgate Publishing, Ltd., 2008.

Owens, Lama Rod and Jasmine Syedullah. *Radical Dharma: Talking Race, Love, and Liberation*. Berkeley, CA: North Atlantic Books, 2016.

Putcha, Rumya S. "Gender, Caste, and Feminist Praxis in Transnational South India." *South Asian Popular Culture* 17(1) (2019): 61–79.

Singleton, Mark. *Yoga Body: The Origins of Modern Posture Practice*. Oxford, UK: Oxford University Press, 2010.

Yehuda, Rachel, Sarah L. Halligan, and Linda M. Bierer. "Relationship of Parental Trauma Exposure and PTSD to PTSD, Depressive and Anxiety Disorders in Offspring." *Journal of Psychiatric Research* 35(5) (2001): 261–270.

Chapter 4

Reclaiming spaces, reshaping practices

Yoga for building community and nurturing families of color

Amy Argenal and Monisha Bajaj

In this chapter, we discuss how we came together in 2016 – two mothers of color with children of South Asian heritage – to create a community-based regular family yoga practice that centers families and children of color with a South Asian teacher who pushes back against "yoga as fitness." Speaking to the experiences of organizing the yoga class, reflections from the teacher, and observations of the parents and children, we hope to share how yoga can be used to create culturally responsive spaces for families of color to develop mindful practices with their children, while at the same time, build community by nurturing and caring for those in our spaces.

In this chapter, we first situate ourselves and our positionalities. We then discuss how both the parent industrial complex and the commodification and gentrification of yoga (Das; Saapya) intersect to create skewed racial and power dynamics within spaces of family yoga. The term "parent industrial complex" has been used in popular media to discuss the multi-billion dollar industries around parenting books, child-rearing accessories, children's toys, etc. We define it in this chapter as a commodification and standardization of parenting that posits certain "must-haves" and "must-dos" for "effective" parenting, of which prenatal and family yoga classes are increasingly becoming a part. It is important to also recognize prior scholarship similar to the "parent industrial complex" that helps to frame the "yoga industrial complex". It is defined as "the web of relationships between studio systems, yoga celebrities, certifying agencies and large yoga business" (Miller 2). Miller states that it is not only about the network, but also about who is an authentic "yogi" and what that means for the continued "marginalization and exclusion of Othered yogis" (Miller 2). This is synonymous with the commodification of yoga that we discuss in this chapter.

Third, we discuss our intervention to speak back to such forces of commodification through a family yoga class centering young people of color taught by Amy's partner, a South Asian immigrant who has been teaching yoga for two decades in Nepal, Myanmar, and the U.S. We offer reflections from the instructor and parents/children on the class which, at the time of this writing, had been meeting monthly for over two years (since early 2016). Taken together, the sections of this chapter seek to interrogate – from our vantage point as mothers of color –questions posed by James Manigault-Bryant in the inaugural issue of the *Race and Yoga* journal, namely: (1) what is yoga's "relationship to racial capital," and (2) where might we seed sites that espouse "new, possible orientations to yoga that turn devoted practitioners from a world dominated by the racial fetish towards another that holds alternative realities and possibilities for social relations"? (50).

Critical postures and positionalities

Amy Argenal. I grew up in Northern California, a second-generation San Franciscan-born Latina. My father's family comes from Nicaragua and my mother's family were small scale farmers from Northern California for more than five generations. In my mid-twenties, I suffered from severe anxiety attacks and someone recommended I try yoga. I was reluctant and deeply bothered by the usually white, female instructors speaking Sanskrit in a tone that never felt quite right. At the same time a friend of mine, a South Asian woman, had just completed her yoga training and was starting her own business. It was perfect timing! I had found a yoga practice that felt authentic and helped me in my struggles in managing both physical and mental tensions.

Three years later, I moved to South East Asia (Thailand) to study in an affordable graduate program (Masters in Human Rights) and ended up in Nepal working in a school that had morning and evening yoga with the students that lived in the hostel. My future partner (at that time) was the instructor. This yoga was nothing like what I had experienced in the U.S. The children would all get together at 6 am to chant, breath, and stretch. Then for the evening yoga, there were similar breathing exercises, a few points of reflection, and a lot of singing. It was a time for the community to come together, and it was a space that I loved to start and end my day with. As we dated in Nepal, Laxman would often joke about sending our future children back to that space for them to be grounded there. Starting this class and having a space for our children to learn, breath, stretch, and chant is extremely important for our family. However, that is not the only reason, as we can do that in our home as a family. There is also power in us practicing together in community with other families.

Monisha Bajaj. I grew up in Northern California in the 1970s and 80s surrounded by a large South Asian immigrant community. My parents migrated to the U.S. from India a few years before I was born, and we visited India every one or two years. My first memories of yoga were of seeing my grandfather pull a straw mat into the front of their home and doing exercises in the morning, and my grandmother teaching me breathing or sitting postures for any ailment I had.

During my first extended stay in India as a young adult in 1998, my grandmother directed me to a yoga class at the nearby *Arya Samaj* temple, which was a room full of about 150 people seated on cushions and doing a variety of poses that could be completed while seated, following the lead of a woman at the front of the room. I was interning at a center for street-children and one of my tasks included writing fundraising appeals so the poses for relieving shoulder strain after all day at the computer were welcomed. My sense was that yoga was a part of everyday life for some South Asians, and one of the many things one could do at the temple. In my late 20s, I tried attending yoga classes at studios and at the gym in the U.S. but was repelled by White teachers butchering Hindu chants or trying to offer spiritual advice, and by a White teacher who called out her instructions in a mock Indian accent. Yoga felt more like a racial micro-aggression than an opportunity for relaxation in such settings.

However, my politics also made me wary of how yoga was being utilized in India with the rise of Hindu fundamentalism that has resulted in horrific state-sanctioned violence against Muslims, Dalits, and other groups. In 2009, while living in India for over a year conducting research for my book on human rights education programs in India, particularly for Dalit and Adivasi children, I heard about atrocities committed in the name of caste purity and the increasingly homogenized notions of what being a "Hindu" should consist of. This was the lead up to the election of the current Prime Minister of India, Narendra Modi, who did nothing to stop the violent and bloody riots in Gujarat in 2002 when he served as Chief Minister there at the time. Since his election in 2014, there have been increasing instances of violence against Dalits, Muslims (various individuals have been violently lynched in the name of religious purity for the accusation of "defiling" cows), and towards other communities.

Seeking out a way to learn yoga that did not contribute to, or endorse such larger narratives – though this is indeed a tension that we are faced with in choosing to practice something that is being hijacked both by Western consumerism *and* Hindu fundamentalist political forces – my partner and I enrolled in a month-long intensive yoga course (daily in the evenings) in New Delhi. Our class was comprised of people of all ages, fitness levels, and social identities. We were cautious about delinking our interest in yoga and its history from the political dimensions of rising Hindu chauvinism that surrounded us, and we continue to proceed with caution. I attended yoga classes on and off while in India and back in the United States, and more regularly during my pregnancy in 2013. The idea of a child-friendly space for adults and young people to practice yoga in community and taught by a South Asian instructor who didn't espouse fundamentalist attitudes, appealed to me, and, not having found any such space, Amy and I first discussed launching a family yoga class with her partner Laxman in 2015.

Engaging in yoga critically

With the Western "yoga industrial complex" on one side, and Hindu fundamentalist attempts at co-optation on the other, we have sought to engage in yoga critically by being attentive to the various dynamics at play. "Critical literacy" in this context has meant staying informed of perspectives, being clear about our intentions and alliances, and ensuring that the space doesn't get co-opted for other agendas. There are three main ideas that we have come across that are useful in considering the complex way that yoga functions both in South Asia and the West, and how it undergoes diverse forms of engagement, definition, and redefinition continually.

The first is the importance of decolonizing yoga. It is important to remember the impact colonialism had and continues to have on the way the West understands Hinduism. There are binaries that continue to exist in what "Eastern" means. There is the essentializing practice that everything yoga comes from deep-rooted tradition and is essentially wise and spiritual. As Heather writes:

> We need to decolonize our understanding of Hinduism as a singular tradition and begin to talk about Hinduisms. We need to explore non-Brahmin-centric yoga practices such as traditional Tantric, hatha yoga…We need to embrace the fact that yoga is and has been many different things to many different people and will continue to shift and change with time.

The second is the importance of interrogating caste, privilege, and marginalization in relation to the South Asian roots of yoga practices. Prachi Patankar writes:

> Caste-privileged Hindu leaders, through violent domination, have culturally appropriated a variety of diverse sects, practices, beliefs and rituals that have existed for centuries. This history, of both European influence and Brahmanic appropriation, holds true for yoga as well. It should not be assumed that all the Dalit, Bahujan, Adivasi, Muslim, Christian, Buddhist, or Sikh communities embrace Brahmanical forms of yoga as part of their culture. Representing South Asia as the birthplace of a mythical homogenous culture is a crusade of the chauvinistic upper-caste Hindus. We need to consciously learn about and highlight the rich, diverse cultures, histories, customs, and spiritual practices of the vast majority of people in South Asia, especially the Dalit and Adivasi communities who are continuing to struggle to keep their cultures alive. What we need is a constant challenge to the caste-privileged attempt to define Hindu, Indian, or South Asian culture as monolithic and *theirs*.

The third perspective that informs our approach is linked to our positionality in the United States as parents of color seeking to counter White supremacy while remaining critical of the roots of yoga and attending to social justice issues. Sheena Sood writes in her article in the *Race and Yoga* journal, and resonates with us:

> Upper-caste Hindus appropriated yogic philosophy from Indigenous cultures and molded it to construct philosophies that justify institutionalized oppression against Muslims, Christians, Dalits, Adivasis, Bahujans, Sikhs, and poor communities. Having a spiritual foundation encourages me to explore suffering and oppression on a deeper dimension. It sustains my hope and involvement in struggles for human rights. This conversation is my attempt to discuss and dismantle the oppressive, elitist, casteist values embedded in yoga to make room for a yogic theology rooted in social justice values. Practitioners

often reference the root term "yoke" in defining yoga as the union of the mind, body and spirit. For me, "yoking" has been about bridging my individual and universal soul and recognizing all of humanity as divinely connected to a universal sense of consciousness. My spiritual practice motivates me to radically imagine, inspired by Ginwright's "radical healing" concept, how we – as a human family – can experience a more honest way of healing collectively in this structurally violent society. (Ginwright 2009, 2015) (18)

Sheena Sood further writes:

Brown yogis have a unique duty to intersect our critiques and go beyond condemning Western cultural appropriation. We must follow the lead of Dalit activists and challenge Hindu nationalist attempts to claim yoga as India's ancient practice…Naming these contradictions engages Black, brown and white yogis in a deeper understanding of what healing and liberation means for all of us; it encourages us to embed new, radical meaning in our collective offering of yoga. (18)

We take up this call and hope to infuse it in our efforts however partially with the aspiration to continue to have greater coherence in our values, ideals, and practices. Attending to the fluidity and possibilities for reimagination, we have sought to create a family yoga class that can be an inclusive space, one of healing and refuge, for families of color, multiracial families, queer families, and those of various or no faiths.

Family yoga class in Oakland, California

In the latter part of 2015, Monisha suggested that we bring families of color together for a family yoga class. She asked if Amy's partner would be willing to teach it, given that he had started a class at the local library. He jumped at the idea and loved having something to start within our community in Oakland. We spread the word using Facebook groups (for example, in a group for progressive *desi* or South Asian families in the Bay Area that Monisha started) and a neighborhood blog and, in February of 2016, our first family yoga class began. We had about six families on the first day, with a varied mix of ages. Most of the families were of color, a majority with some South Asian heritage. We decided that we would run the class the last Sunday of every month, at 10:30 am, at the yoga studio that Laxman, the instructor worked at. The owner was more than happy to start and agreed to have the class be a donation-based class. It was arranged that half of the proceeds of the donations would go to the owner for use of the space, and Laxman decided to use the other half to donate to under-resourced communities in Nepal and Myanmar where he travels annually.

Over the last two years, we have had a consistent number of families joining us each month, usually between four and five families at a minimum with an

Reclaiming spaces, reshaping practices   43

increasing number of African-American, Latinx, White and multi-racial families through the neighborhood list-serves we have posted to as well as through word of mouth. Some families have come from the studio once the class was advertised on its website in mid-2017 when it became a regular offering, but the large majority came from our communities, our friends and family (including visiting grandparents that have joined the class) that we bring with us to share the space through word of mouth. Figure 4.1 below shows a sample image Amy created that we have posted to Facebook Groups for families of color and South Asian families, and that we have texted to friends to encourage participation.

The class usually starts with a brief chant, usually with the singing bowl. The instructor incorporates poses that engage the kids and also creates time for parents to do poses. He senses the energy of the families and adopts the course to meet those needs. Some classes have been designed around going through the alphabet and doing poses based off of animals with those letters, other classes have been more "traditional" adult-oriented classes with the children running around the

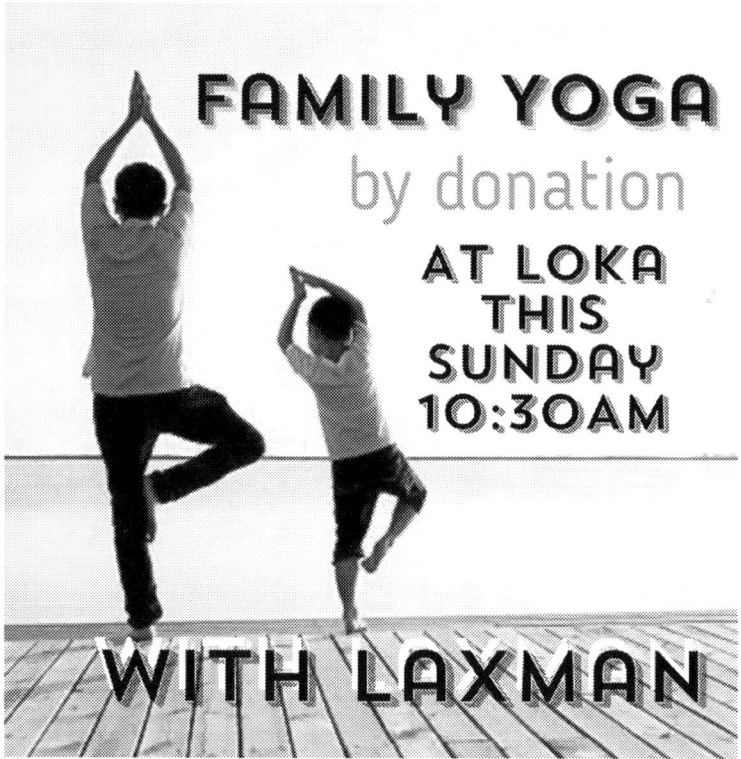

Figure 4.1 Family yoga post and image.

studio. The class always finishes with a "Namaste song" and everyone participates. The song goes like this:

> Namaste, Namaste, I am here to play
> You are special, I am special
> Namaste.

Instructor's perspectives

As mentioned above, the instructor Laxman has been teaching yoga for most of his adult life. Raised in Myanmar, Laxman served as a full-time yoga teacher in Nepal at a large English medium school in Kathmandu. He was also heavily involved in a local community group called Youth Society for Peace. Through his work with them, he has traveled all around Nepal offering yoga to marginalized and hard-to-reach communities. He has also visited a drug rehabilitation center and a senior center, teaching yoga and meditation.

Laxman centers *seva* (serving the community) in every aspect of his work. He recognizes that here in the United States he must work for remuneration, but he always tries to balance that with ways he can serve the community. The family yoga class was the ideal blend of being able to continue his *seva* while also spend time and practice with his own family.

Laxman believes that family yoga is important in this "Trump era life" where we are so busy and also so distraught. He witnesses that children do not spend enough time with their parents and family yoga can offer that time. He stated that "family yoga is a kind of play time with family. Through the imagination of poses that are about nature, the animals, and the landscapes like mountain and rivers, we play." He also shares how important it is for families to experience things together.

> It is important to understand each other through movement, in an ancient practice without any gadgets, just on the mat on the floor, closer to the ground without any distraction. Systematic movements help us to be calm and be quiet and clear in our minds. With the same movement, we are all in the same mood, it allows us to understand each other more as a family and as a community. Children see their parents' movement; parents see their children's movement. The most important thing is that the children are on the same level as their parents, on the ground, doing the same movements together, there is a real sense of sharing the feelings, the same movement done by different generations is the best way to know yourself and others. That is true understanding.

Laxman also spoke about the current trend of expensive yoga classes and why we must challenge this. He has noticed how yoga can be space for primarily "White women" but that yoga should not be owned by them. He stated that yoga

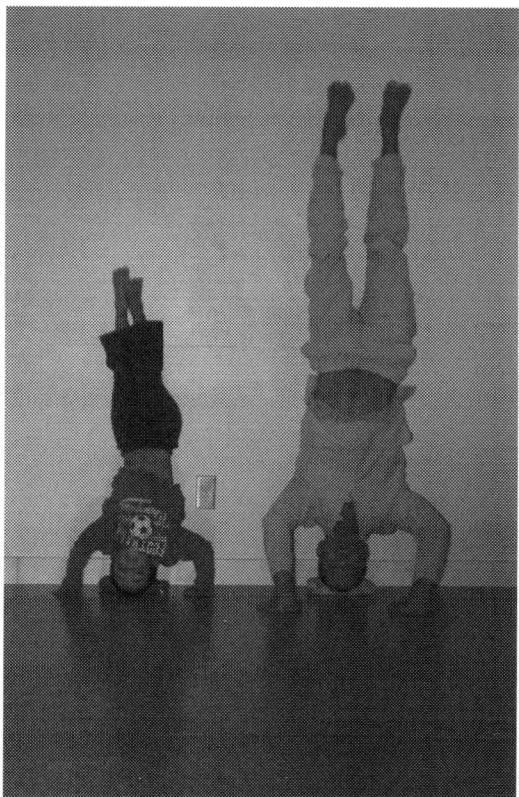

Figure 4.2 Laxman and Prashad in a pose during class.

is supposed to be a universal practice and should be free. He notices that in the United States, everything is about money. In our family yoga class, "we are practicing, and it is for us and established by us. We don't turn anyone away." The class is donation based, although the money that he makes from that goes directly to his work in Nepal and Myanmar where he runs free yoga training and camps when he goes to visit each year (Figure 4.2).

Kids/parents' perspectives

For us as mothers, finding a space that is open to families, accepting of us as women of color and affordable is so important. Amy's son, Prashad, who is five stated that he loves to do starfish pose while crawling all over his "Mama and Baba". Monisha's son, Kabir, also five years old, shared how much he enjoys when Laxman carries him like a basket and when he sings the butterfly song. Both boys love to run around the studio with all of the other kids. This is what some of the other parents shared as well. The class stresses the importance of play, and there is open time without strict rules. One parent shared that there are limited spaces where families can just be, and there is no policing of their children or their behavior. This was a theme that came up with quite a few families, the idea that they could let their children be children. They could be a family without having to fit the "perfect family mold" or without the gaze of others stereotyping children of color as rowdy or unruly. The fact that children are welcome and not only as accessories, but as integral parts of the class, is what allows the authenticity of the space. Laxman asks questions of the children throughout the class – "What is your favorite animal?" "What is your favorite color?" "What is your birthday?" and goes around to high-five their feet in the air which makes the class child-centered, interactive, and dialogic (Figure 4.3).

Some of the other reflections shared about how important it is for us to have lessons in patience. As Laxman noted above, this notion that we are always busy, is something we need to speak back to. Allowing us to engage in a practice that doesn't have a set task list is another way we can heal and be as a community. Depending on the month, Laxman may lead the kids in a train ride doing poses along the way or have everyone on their mat doing different seated poses, calling on the children to share their favorite color while they imitate a butterfly, and signing "butterfly, butterfly, what color do you like on your happy birthday?" The improvisational nature allows for everyone to be in the moment rather than having a set list of poses to be accomplished in the hour.

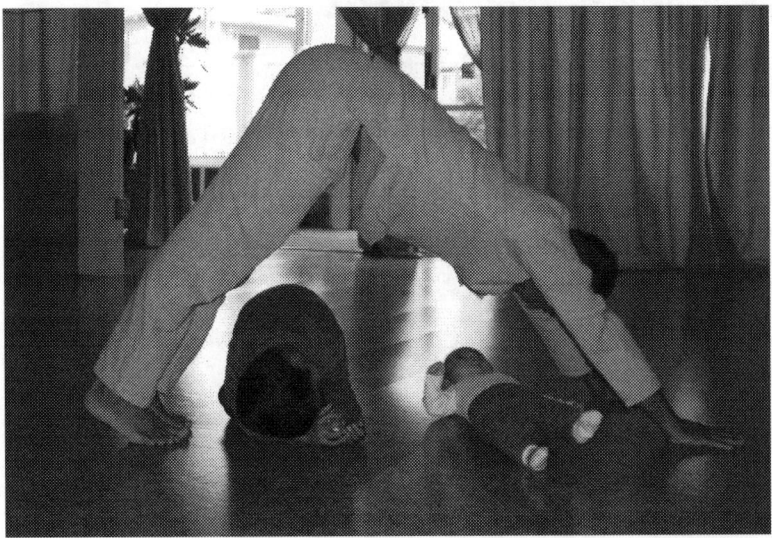

Figure 4.3 Laxman and both his children in a pose during class.

Finally, some of the participants shared about how the yoga class was a chance for us to practice something together. After class, families hang out in the studio (the next class there isn't until later that afternoon) or elsewhere, arrange play dates, go for ice cream to a nearby shop to celebrate birthdays, or strategize about issues facing them. One Sunday, a mom of South Asian boys shared how her older son was being bullied severely, and with several parents in attendance working in education, we had a long conversation about schools, strategies for engaging with teachers and schools, and brainstorming different ideas; the children ran around in the studio while we chatted.

Each Sunday, something different might transpire. On another yoga class Sunday, one of the families asked if Laxman would hold a special family yoga class for one of the children's third birthday because the daughter loved the yoga class so much. After arranging it with the studio owner, the family brought snacks and Laxman led the 15 or so children and any parents who wanted to join through yoga poses and games, followed by snacks and cake. This speaks back to what Laxman shared above about what happens when we practice something together, in community as families connected through our family yoga practice. In the words of one of the mothers who has come to the family yoga class with her daughter and her mother for three generations of collective participation:

> This was an amazing opportunity for my family to get some exercise and feel connected to a weekend activity that's from our cultural practices. It was amazing to see so many neighbors there breathing, stretching and connecting together. We need more spaces for like-minded folks to build intentional community while exploring a spiritual space!

Having a space and time for families to be together, free from scripts and oppressive norms of racial capitalism, has allowed for various connections and bonds to form. We are unsure of what the future of the space will be, but hope that it continues to be a place of nourishment, healing, and growth.

Concluding thoughts

In this chapter, we have discussed how the nexus of race, caste, gender, capitalism, and parenthood creates a space in which family yoga is commodified and appropriated for purposes other than communal well-being. We came together as colleagues, friends, and collaborators to interrupt dominant narratives of yoga through the creation of a by-donation, accessible family yoga class that centers children of color and is taught by a South Asian yoga teacher deeply rooted in traditions and practices of yoga in Nepal, Myanmar, and India. Our efforts have, in part, sought to offer experiences to our children of yoga as a collective site of practice, one that offers refuge from the larger forces of White supremacy that influence their lives as children of color.

In an era of mass consumption around childhood experiences and opportunities, family yoga has been a chance to carve out space for being together, allowing for the children to be joyful (and that has meant children running freely through the classroom or building yoga block towers to knock down if they so choose), and for families – however they are comprised – to engage in a collective practice that centers the well-being of their bodies and spirits. In a current context where children of color are under attack whether from law enforcement who target Black and Brown boys in particular; border patrol and Immigration and Customs Enforcement (ICE) tearing families apart; schooling systems that often do not center children of color's well-being; Islamophobic rhetoric and policy; and the neocolonial vestiges of beauty and worth that manipulate the minds and attitudes of our own families and communities of color, centering Brown bodies as strong, beautiful, and worthy of time and attention (at the very least once a month) has been a small form of resistance that we hope will offer our children a chance to imagine new ways of being and thinking critically in the present and future.

Works cited

Das, Kavita. "A New Initiative Seeks to Restore Yoga's South Asian Heritage." *The Aerogram* (2013).

Heather, Melissa. "Extreme Makeover: Yoga in the British Empire." *Decolonizing Yoga*, 16 April 2014. www.decolonizingyoga.com/extreme-makeover-yoga-british-empire/. Accessed 19 June 2018.

Manigault-Bryant, James. "Yoga and the Metaphysics of Racial-Capital." *Race and Yoga Journal*, vol. 1, no. 1 (2016), pp. 40–52.

Patankar, Prachi. "Ghosts of Yoga Past and Present." *BETA*, 26 February 2014. www.jadaliyya.com/Details/30281/Ghosts-of-Yogas-Past-and-Present. Accessed 20 June 2018.

Pattanaik, Devdutt. "Everybody Has an Opinion on What Yoga Is for and No One's Got It Right." *Quartz India* (2017). Web. 23 May 2018.

Sheena, Sod. "Cultivating a Yogic Theology of Collective Healing: A Yogini's Journey Disrupting White Supremacy, Hindu Fundamentalism and Casteism." *Race and Yoga Journal*, vol. 3, no. 1 (2018), pp. 12–20.

Chapter 5

The city of radical love
A Philly story of oppression, resistance, and healing

Sheena Sood and Mari Morales-Williams

Philadelphia and the Case for Radical Healing

Sitting in a dark room in the back of a community center in North Philadelphia, 65 year old Ms. Kyleah came out of *sivasana* with a calm strength and a message to share: "Yoga is not about twisting yourself, it's about connecting to yourself." In a single sentence, she was able to articulate our purpose in offering yoga as a practice of "radical healing." Shawn A. Ginwright defines "radical healing" through a lens that names the role of oppression in marginalized communities:

> Trauma conveys the idea that oppression and injustice inflict harm. Effectively responding to oppression, therefore, requires a process that restores individuals and communities to a state of well-being. *Radical healing* points to the process of building hope, optimism, and vision to create justice in the midst of oppression (Ginwright, *Black Youth Rising* 9).

Our existing social structure creates the conditions for one to either disembody from or engage in a surface level relationship to self. Conversely, Ms. Kyleah was able to name the significance of yoga as engaging one in a higher more truthful connection to the mind, body, and spirit. Her statement captures the necessity for a radical interpretation of yoga in North Philadelphia, a neighborhood impacted by high levels of state-sanctioned violence.

State-sanctioned violence is not specific to Philly, but rather part and parcel of a global regime of colonialism, racial capitalism, imperialism and militarism. Like many other post-industrial cities surviving through this matrix of domination, Philly carries generational trauma. The violence of this city's repressive regime is ingrained in the spirit of the land, in the bodies of poor people of color, and in the collective memory of Philadelphians. The regime has been the genesis of structural poverty, under-resourced schools, high unemployment, over-policing, and a lack of support for community solutions to interpersonal violence. It is in this vein that we curated the "Yoga for Spirit" series that was offered in Ms. Kyleah's neighborhood; it is in this vein that we hoped to decolonize yoga as simply a physical practice. As Black and Brown queer femme yoginis committed to sharing healing justice and liberation in our communities, we envisioned a Philly-based yoga project that was aligned with the call for "radical healing," and "healing justice"[1] more broadly. We believed offering yoga through this lens should: 1) Embody in rhetoric and practice, a decolonized and anti-racist understanding of yoga; 2) Center the most marginalized of the community/neighborhood; and 3) Deepen the capacity of local and grassroots initiatives to create cultures of hope and holistic wellness.

Roadmap of the Chapter

In the sections that follow, we begin by grounding our audience in a deeper understanding of a "healing justice" framework. We then outline watershed moments of state-sanctioned violence in Philadelphia that have accumulated in bodies and in the land. Recognizing grassroots resistance as an ever-present, balancing force, we then highlight the corresponding moments and movements of struggle against oppression that ensued. Providing this sociopolitical context supports our argument for why post-industrial cities like Philadelphia are in need of "radical healing," and how politicized yoga has been a part of that work. In chronicling different yoga offerings in the city, we pay homage to the legacy of yoga and radical healing work that inspires our own. To close, we circle back to the community center where Ms. Kyleah shared her profound wisdom. Taking a microscope to these fleeting moments of liberation and healing in "Yoga for Spirit," we hope to create a wider imagination of what radical healing can look like in Philadelphia and our broader communities.

Radical Healing and Healing Justice

> We need to be able to respond to the increased state of burnout and depression in our movements; systematic loss of our communities' healing traditions; the isolation and stigmatization of healers, and the increased privatization of our land, medicine and natural resources that has caused us to rely on state or private models we do not trust and that do not serve us (Piepzna-Samarasinha).[2]

In cultivating a cost-free yoga offering in North Philadelphia, we had hoped to build on a legacy of healing justice, a framework that was first initiated by grassroots collectives like Kindred Southern Healing Justice Collective. Their "healing justice" framework acknowledges the historical and socio-political conditions that have led to our experiences of trauma and harm. In a similar vein, Ginwright recognizes the structural oppression that low-income, people of color communities in urban areas face is made worse by the dearth of city-wide investments in community centers and the absence of coping mechanisms on a large scale (Ginwright, *Black Youth Rising*; Ginwright, *Hope and Healing in Urban Education*). In citing activist scholar Robin D.G. Kelley's *Freedom Dreams* (Kelley), Ginwright reminds us that the capacity to sustain a "radical imagination," or the "revolutionary potential of hope," is an especially challenging task in urban environments that are replete with oppressive conditions (*Black Youth Rising* 11).

Healing justice visionaries and practitioners offer radical healing as a framework to reimagine how we cultivate vibrant, healthy environments. According to Black queer healing justice veteran practitioner Cara Page and the Kindred Healing Justice Collective, "healing justice...identifies how we can holistically respond to and intervene on generational trauma and violence, and to bring collective practices that can impact and transform the consequences of oppression on our bodies, hearts and minds" (BEAM). When movements focus simultaneously on internal and external methods of change, people are able to both transform structural oppression *and* sustain our well-being. Ginwright contends:

> Healing from the trauma of oppression caused by poverty, racism, sexism, homophobia, and class exploitation is an important political act. Without a critical understanding of how the various structures of domination operate in our daily lives we cannot begin to develop meaningful forms of personal and collective resistance. Healing occurs when we reconcile painful experiences resulting from oppression through testimony and name what may seem to be personal misfortune as systemic oppression (*Black Youth Rising* 9).

These conceptualizations on "healing justice" and "radical healing" charge us all to offer healing opportunities through a social justice framework. Ginwright's analysis inspires us to prioritize individuals from structurally oppressed, urban communities in order to further develop our society's capacity to dismantle oppressive structures and envision erecting ones of liberation.

These understandings of radical healing inspire us as yogis to consider how we politicize healing for the purpose of collective liberation. In exploring various approaches to "healing justice," Ginwright discusses how *contemplative practices* build individual and collective capacity to engage and sustain social change work: "Practices like meditation, mindfulness, and yoga all prepare and strengthen individuals' capacity to stay centered in turbulent times in order to make decisions, and lead from a place of compassion and love" (*Hope and Healing in Urban Education* 28). Similar to movement facilitator and healer adrienne maree brown, we also believe in the democratic vision that "we all have the capacity to heal each other - healer is a possibility in each of us" (brown 34). Motivated by these frameworks, we curated a series of yoga offerings in the spirit of healing justice. Particular to Philadelphia, we also understood the need to recognize the unique obstacles that Black and Brown communities are forced to navigate due to state-sanctioned violence.

The Accumulation of State-Sanctioned Trauma in Philadelphia

To understand the depth of trauma within a nation, a community, and an environment, it is critical to first locate the specific historical and ongoing structural oppression a people and the land have endured. U.S. history is one of violent genocide and exploitation — state-sanctioned by the larger ideologies and systems of settler colonialism, chattel slavery, patriarchy and white supremacy. Particular to present-day Philadelphia and the greater Pennsylvania region, the displacement commences during the 1800s with the forced removal of the original inhabitants of this land, the Lenni-Lenape people, and continues into the mid-19th century with the auctioning of each enslaved Africans sold off the block between Front and Market Street.

This legacy of accumulated trauma and structural violence has continued well after the abolition of slavery, most notably in the institutions that were supposedly created to equalize Philadelphia's playing field in its post-industrial years. For instance, Carlisle, Pennsylvania was home to an Indian boarding school during the early 19th century which used violent and even fatal tactics to coerce thousands of Indigenous children to assimilate. A near century later, communities that had already been ghettoized by the real estate redlining from the 1930's to 1960s continued to experience harm through the outsourcing of factory work to underdeveloped countries, increased unemployment rates, and neglected schools (Glantz and Martinez). During the Civil Rights Era more broadly, and more specifically at the student walkout of 1967, when students and teachers in Philadelphia organized to demand the hiring of more African American teachers, better school building conditions, and African-centered curricula, the newly appointed Police Commissioner Frank Rizzo responded to this nonviolent act of resistance with brute force (Countryman). Rizzo's legacy of unabashed and "law and order" style policing endured after he served as police commissioner and mayor of Philadelphia (1972-1980).

In the 1980s, when the MOVE organization mobilized demonstrations against issues of capitalism, police brutality, and environmental degradation, those most invested in the status quo targeted the MOVE members as radical pariahs and frequently attacked and imprisoned its members. In the most brutal of these attacks, Mayor Wilson Goode and his administration[3] orchestrated a deadly assault on the MOVE organization's home. He authorized the Philadelphia Police Department to pump more than seven thousand rounds of ammunition into the MOVE home and ultimately drop a C-4 bomb on the home, killing eleven people, including five children, alongside livestock (Taylor). The bombing of the MOVE home in 1985 makes Philadelphia the only U.S. city to experience this level of militarized terror.[4]

The accumulation of state-sanctioned violence has amounted to generations of unaddressed trauma amongst Black and Brown communities. Complementing the rising cost of healthcare in the recent decades, North Philadelphia and other low-income Black and Brown neighborhoods across the city have seen their state hospitals, mental health care facilities and systems designed to treat illness and trauma in fluctuating states of financial crisis. The state's response to the full host of negligent conditions (i.e. patient abuse, crumbling edifices, etc.) has been to close these facilities rather than invest in and restructure them to better serve the communities' needs (Esack). Though the legacy and accumulation of oppression and violent harm has endured, resistance has been just as palpable.

This is not the Lost Generation: MOVE, Mumia, and Philly Youth

> This is not the lost generation. They are the children of the L.A. rebellion, the children of the MOVE bombing, the children of the Black Panthers, and the grandchildren of Malcolm; far from lost, they are probably the most aware generation since Nat Turner's; they are not so much lost as they are mislaid, discarded by this increasingly racist system that undermines their inherent worth. They are all potential revolutionaries, with the historic power to transform our dull realities. If they are lost, then *find* them (Abu-Jamal 145).
>
> - Mumia Abu-Jamal, *All Things Censored*

Given the Pennsylvania government's systemic neglect of its residents' health care needs and its willingness to inflict violence on them through the exploits of racial capitalism, Philadelphia communities have created movements that resist structural violence and that prioritize human rights and basic dignity for all people. During the late 1960's, the Black Panther Party chapters -- along with Revolutionary Action Movement cadres -- served as a catalyst for subsequent Black liberation struggles in the city and throughout the nation. Philadelphia journalist and former Black Panther Mumia Abu-Jamal[5] sought to document these movements with a prophetic regard for the revolutionary potential of young people. The MOVE Organization and Mumia fought as hard as they did to resist a police state to create a better future for all youth, with the painful understanding that childhood did not keep anybody immune from structural violence or from criminalization. In the paragraphs that follow, we integrate the narratives of the MOVE organization, Mumia, and Philadelphia youth collectives in order to showcase how they have rallied and prioritized radical healing in their struggle for Black liberation.[6]

In the spirit of love for the people and self-determination, John Africa founded the MOVE organization in 1972, which promoted the protection of all forms of life (including animals) as well as the environment. In her description of the organization, activist scholar Johanna Fernandez posits that the MOVE family's "commitment to a combination of personal, spiritual and political uplift - as well as its open denunciation of American capitalism," led them to develop "a radical vision of cooperative, healthy, and environmentally conscious living." (Abu-Jamal xxvi). In addition to calling out state violence, what made them revolutionary is how they embodied and lived out their anti-establishment politics. For example, long before it was mainstreamed as trendy, they have maintained a raw food diet, locked their hair, made their own clothes, birthed babies naturally at home, and homeschooled their children.

We lift up the MOVE family's efforts because we believe this organization serves as an early model for integrating healing and justice. Despite numerous attacks such as the 1978 siege of their family's home and the fatal 1985 bombing, MOVE is still active today. Ramona Africa, one of two survivors of the 1985 attack, has continued the struggle to free her imprisoned brothers and sisters, also known as the MOVE 9.[7] After over 40 years of sustained commitment to the freedom of her family members, by February of 2020, Ramona and other members of the MOVE organization were able to see *all* of the MOVE 9 family come home. What remains incredible to witness is that after 40 years of being trapped behind bars, their commitment to freedom, health, and resistance remains ever present. Second- and third-generation MOVE members continue the rallying call initiated by MOVE's founder: "Our organization was founded by John Africa. However, he is not our leader. John Africa has equipped each of us with the wisdom, strength, and understanding to lead ourselves" ("John Africa of MOVE – On a Move"). We see this last sentiment actualized in recent grassroots campaigns that the MOVE family has initiated and supported. For instance, current MOVE leaders like Mike Africa, Jr. has witnessed elder generations of the MOVE family, including his parents, face draconian incarceration sentences and be murdered by the state. Despite the state's attempt to separate him from his parents, throughout his youth and adulthood Mike Africa Jr. has stayed true to the values of John Africa's teachings by prioritizing the health and well-being of people (Africa, Jr.). These struggles for health and wellness have included the imprisonment of MOVE members as well as fellow political prisoner Mumia Abu-Jamal.

Sustained local, national, and international pressure from the MOVE family and various campaigns, led in part by Pam Africa, have garnered several victories in the case of Mumia, including visitation rights, and, more recently, access to adequate medical treatment for Hepatitis C. "In addition to potentially saving Abu-Jamal's life, legal advocates say the treatment mandate could help open the doors to a cure for nearly 7,000 other prisoners in Pennsylvania living with the virus over the next few years" (*Mumia Abu-Jamal Set to Begin Treatment for Hepatitis C in Prison - Hep*). In fact, based on a legal settlement that was filed for approval on November 2018, 5,000 people incarcerated in Pennsylvania prisons are eligible for access to direct-acting antiviral drugs to cure Hepatitis C (Melamed). We recognize these victories as examples of how Philadelphian activists center the human rights and health justice within abolitionist and racial justice movements.

Philadelphia youth have long been involved in their own struggles for respect and human dignity, and more recently, they have centered radical healing through campaigns for restorative justice and mental health, and political education programming. Philadelphia-based student resistance during the Black Power era, which included the 1967 Student Walkout organized by students *and* teachers, called for the Philadelphia School District to incorporate African American history in school curricula. This is an important pretext to radical healing because of the campaign's understanding of the impact that culturally-relevant curricula has on fostering positive identity development amongst the psyche of Black and Brown youth.

Building on this legacy,[8] contemporary youth organizers and their adult allies continue to organize themselves through organizations such as the Philadelphia

Student Union (PSU), Youth United for Change (YUC), Juntos, and Youth Art & Self-Empowerment Project (YASP). The city's systemic neglect and increasing criminalization of youth is observable through the 2001 state takeover of the School District of Philadelphia, the closing of 23 schools across Philadelphia in 2013, the tax abatement of Philly based corporations, and the disproportionate police-to-counselor ratio throughout the city. Following the footsteps of those who stood before them, student leaders of Philadelphia Student Union (PSU) and Youth United for Change (YUC) led another walkout of over 3,000 students in 2013 – after the city declared 24 schools were set to be closed. This helped at least one of those schools, Kensington CAPA, remain in operation. Broader coalitions for educational justice saw a partial victory in the summer of 2018 when the School Reform Commission was dismantled. Although organizations advocated for democratically electing a locally-appointed school board, Mayor Jim Kenney decided to authoritatively erect one. PSU and YUC continue to be a cornerstone in youth organizing in the city around the fight for quality education and interrupting the school to prison pipeline. More recently, their campaigns and demands have evolved to address defunding police in schools in order to invest in mental health more broadly and the need for restorative justice more specifically.

We are also reminded of an initiative taken by the students at Jubilee School in West Philadelphia that embodies this concept of healing justice. After engaging in a lesson on police brutality and visiting the tragic site of the historic 1985 MOVE bombing, fifth- and sixth-grade members felt disturbed in seeing an entire row of boarded up houses but no historic marker to commemorate the tragedy. They applied to the Pennsylvania Historical and Museum Commission to get a historical marker placed at the site of the bombing. On June 24, 2017, the results of their two-year long history lesson came to fruition when over 200 community members gathered to commemorate the unveiling of the historical marker. The children's victory is demonstrative of the capacity of urban schools to support youth organizing as a process that cultivates hope and *radical healing*. When you name trauma and oppression and you teach it, it is a basis for the Black radical imagination to help us expand our reality of oppression and gives us inspiration to consider what healing in relation to traumatic memories and multi-generational organizing can look like.

Similar to the aforementioned epigraph by Abu-Jamal that introduced this section, these campaigns teach us that our organizing efforts cannot reduce young people as victims of their trauma. Instead, we must continually embrace a multigenerational strategy for relationship-building that allows for what Roksana Mun, former Director of Strategy and Trainings at Desis Rising Up and Moving (DRUM), calls the "osmosis of experience being transferred" between youth and adult organizers (personal communication, March 3rd, 2016). This level of relationship-building reflects how our struggles toward liberation can be more holistic and inclusive of all members. When we integrate the narratives of MOVE, Mumia Abu-Jamal and Philadelphia youth through the lens of radical healing, what awakens is a broader context for how campaigns and initiatives have evolved toward liberation *and* healing.

Politicized Healing and the Revolutionary Potential of Yoga

> We have to love each other, care about each other, encourage each other and see the signs when somebody is traumatized and really having trouble. Give them a lot of attention. That is one reason why the MOVE organization has been able to maintain and sustain ourselves through all that the system has come at us with. We are not just an organization that leads to plan a rally or demonstration...we're a family.
>
> -Ramona Africa[9]

Ramona Africa's claim that love, care and intentional kinship are foundational to social movements, and our capacity to heal from systemic oppression, speaks to a premise stressed in conversations on "healing justice" -- this emphatic vision that "both organizing and healing are required for lasting community change" (Ginwright, *Hope and Healing in Urban Education* 2). We continue to lift up Ginwright's understanding of "radical healing" because it is a framework that refuses to depoliticize healing similar to how we refuse to depoliticize yoga. In addition to reminding us of the legacy of radical healing in Philly, Ramona Africa's words also encourage us, as yoga practitioners, to take radical and courageous leaps in imagining a more liberatory embodiment of yoga philosophy. As the authors of this piece, we have arrived at yoga through our own histories of trauma and healing. We experience yoga as a practice that has allowed us to heal and transform our experiences of colonial and sexual trauma. We recognize that, if decolonized and re-imagined, yoga has the capacity to be offered as a practice of radical healing. Thus, in what follows, we first call out how yoga is commodified and weaponized in the West and in South Asia. Next, we share examples of how informal networks of practitioners across the city of Philadelphia have been offering yoga through this decolonial, anti-racist lens. Included in these examples are some of our own offerings and workshops.

In its current iteration, yoga is not typically offered as a practice of radical healing. In the West especially, but also globally in South Asia, yoga has been packaged to serve a hierarchical, capitalist vision that caters to the desires of elite, heteronormative, and able-bodied communities. For example, we see this at work when the multi-million dollar yoga company Lululemon brands and charges $108 for malas - prayer beads that represent an aspect of Bhakti (devotional) yoga (Hall). The marketing of spirituality in this way is particularly damaging because it renders yoga and prayer into a material achievement and makes it exclusive to those who can afford it. As evident from this example, yoga is used to perpetuate capitalism and appropriation by white supremacist culture.

The Lululemon example also highlights the way that yoga becomes couched in a homogenized understanding of yoga as an Indian and Hindu cultural practice. While malas are not inherently tied to Hindu culture, mainstream yogic culture roots many of yoga's sacred rituals such as chanting mantras and singing bhajans (devotional prayers) in a purified understanding of Hinduism. Such interpretations are problematic because they erase the diversity of Indigenous cultures and spiritual practices, within and outside the South Asian region, that have contributed to the systematic development of yoga on a broader scale (Patankar). As Prachi Patankar - a Bahujan (lower caste) activist - reminds us, by manifesting yogic culture in this way, yoga practitioners and their cultural ambassadors perpetuate Hindu fundamentalism,[10] Brahmanical casteism, and anti-Muslim violence - mainstreaming yoga as a deeply oppressive practice. The voices that claim yoga as authentically Hindu, are "[r]ooted in the chauvinistic Hinduism among some sectors of the upper-caste minority.... [They] claim yoga as their homogenous culture—in ways that obscure the caste, class, and religious diversity and injustices among South Asians" (Patankar).

To Patankar's point, not only are South Asians of non-Hindu, lower caste communities made to distrust mainstream expressions of yoga, but this level of marginalization has a domino effect. Within a U.S. context, the most marginalized members of our communities - notably working-class people, bigger bodied and differently abled individuals, Queer and Trans folks, communities of color, and youth - are also discouraged from feeling a sense of belonging in far too many yoga studios. Aadita Chaudhury contends that the alliances that exist between white supremacists and Hindu nationalists are so dangerous that they cannot be defeated by Hindus alone; Chaudhury calls on all people, including "sub-urban yoga mums in the US[,]" to educate themselves about the secular and diverse identities in India and to "join the resistance against the oppression and abuse of the country's minorities (Chaudhury)." It is only through such willingness to interrogate yoga's deeply colonized, classist, casteist, religio-nationalist and Islamophobic tendencies that those interested in utilizing yoga for radical healing purposes will be able to achieve their goal.

Following in the legacy of movements that center healing and liberation (detailed in previous sections), we want to lift up the Black and Brown yogis in the city of Philadelphia who have made efforts to heal our communities while also resisting structural and state-sanctioned violence. This work has prioritized the significance and intersections of collective care, abolition and spiritual wellness. For example, Jazmyn Burton and jean-jacques gabriel initiated the "Get Free Fest" in 2017, a healing space driven by a three point "Get Free Manifesto": 1) We believe that yoga has the power to heal; 2) We believe that social liberation is tied to embodied individual liberation; and 3) We support Black and Brown economic mobility and freedom.[11] jean-jacques and Jazmyn have continued to recruit other yogi practitioners of color throughout the city in order to help their larger communities claim their freedom by reimagining yoga studios as a site for community building.

Sheena Sood, one of the authors of this text, got her start organizing workshops at the crux of yoga and healing justice in 2013 when she joined a few yoga teachers involved with the Campaign to Bring Mumia Home to start the Yeye Devi[12] Collective. Practitioners associated with the Yeye Devi collective began a "radical healing" project, the "Free Your Mind, Free Mumia, Free Them All" yoga series. In addition to using these community-wide yoga classes as a fundraising tool for the Campaign, the yoga offerings opened up space to have conversations that humanized political prisoners such as Mumia Abu-Jamal and members of the MOVE organization. The mission read:

> As revolutionary yoga instructor activists, we promote non-dualism, integration of that which appears to be separate. We connect the physical, mental, spiritual and emotional elements of our own health to the principles of liberation that we promote in our social environment. Given that we operate in a society that continues to systematically oppress communities of color, poor people and other marginalized groups, the Yeye Devi collective has been motivated by the apparent injustices in our society to manifest our collective duty and to unite and fight for the freedom of our people. We see our own spiritual liberation as deeply connected to Mumia's and all political prisoners' liberation, as part and parcel of our dharma [purposeful duty]. To achieve our dharma, we must heal and unite as a community.

In addition to offering a meditative and posture-based practice to attendees, the yoga series invited participants to consider how their individual liberation, a concept often discussed in yoga philosophy, is intimately connected to the emancipation of Mumia Abu-Jamal and the MOVE 9 family as well as the liberation of oppressed communities. We understood that through facilitating space for folks to develop a connection to an inner self, we were helping folks heal wounds, cultivate self-love, practice self-forgiveness and strengthen mental-emotional capacity within themselves, so they could feel holistically prepared to fight for justice.

Offering yoga in radically inclusive and healing justice frameworks has also shown up through Sheena's "Yogini Sistahs for Liberation" workshop in January 2014. "Yogini Sistahs for Liberation" sought to allow young self-identified femmes and women of color to see themselves in the practice of yoga, despite it experiencing layers of colonization. In November 2016 and March 2017 jean-jacques and Sheena curated the "Waging Wellness" yoga series, designed to help Philadelphians cope with the trauma and stress they were experiencing the ramifications of the 2016 elections. More recently, Sheena (Sood, "Cultivating a Yogic Theology of Collective Healing") has written about her personal journey with yoga and witnessing its weaponization (Sood, "Spectacles of Compassion: Modi and the Weaponization of Yoga"), and she has also developed workshops to educate others on its oppressive forces and Indigenous roots; such workshops, she hopes, can help us to critically evaluate and imagine how we can embody and offer yoga in more liberatory ways. Alongside other yoga practitioners, she currently teaches a People of Color yoga class at Studio 34 in West Philly.

Mari Morales-Williams, the other author of this text, has offered various trainings and classes with a focus on organizers, youth, and the LGBTQ community. "Sustaining Organizers through Self/Collective Care" was a training for groups like Philadelphia Student Union and their staff that provided the scientific background for the impact of various trauma (i.e. state violence, secondary trauma, organizational trauma, etc.), and framed healing as foundational work for strategic and organized resistance. The asana practice was also an opportunity for deeper community building within the staff. Vulnerable conversations about personal harm were paired with a guided meditation about the current and future well-being of the organization and its staff/members, followed by an asana practice with a restorative flow. Various iterations of this workshop were also offered to organizers from the Dream Defenders in south Florida and Palestinian organizers of Strategy and Network Development (SAND) – organizations committed to movement building for social liberation and human dignity at the local and global level. At each session, participants revealed deep gratitude for the invitation and opportunity to feel more grounded in their bodies and in truth, and more fired up in their spirit to engage in the long-haul work of movement-building.

In Mari's yoga classes for Turn Up for Freedom (T.U.F.F.) Girls, Girls Justice League, and El Centro de Estudiantes High School, each class began with interactive activities that decolonized yoga as a practice by and for skinny white women, reclaimed it as a cultural practice of Black and Brown people, and reimagined it as a process of listening, calming, and strengthening the mind, body, and spirit. In one workshop, she held practice under a tree across the street from the playground where there had been a homicide a few summers prior. The goal here was to shift away from the idea that yoga was about mental escape, but rather, a practice that can help us hold pain differently and bring a sense of breath and collective care to sites of trauma.

Within a yoga studio, Mari has also taught Queer and Trans yoga at Studio 34 in West Philadelphia with several other Queer and Trans instructors. This class serves as a safer space for people of the Queer and Trans experience to drop deeper into themselves without having to feel hyper-aware of other participants with rigid and binary perspectives of gender and the body. This class follows the trajectory of radical healing in that it was born out of the political reality that yoga studios are not immune to homophobia and transphobia. While the mission of Studio 34 is to be a center for "healing, creativity, and inclusivity," offering a class specifically for Queer and Trans individuals creates a more secure and transparent container for Queer and Trans people to bring their whole selves to the classroom, unapologetically.

In seeking to offer a yoga class at the Smith Center in Hunting Park, Philadelphia - a mostly Black working-class community, we hoped to make it accessible to a community who have been historically neglected and harmed by the state. The next section chronicles how relationship-building allowed us to cultivate our "Yoga for Spirit" series at the Smith Center, and revealed critical lessons for continuing this work in other cities like Philadelphia.

Yoga For Spirit: Lessons Learned for the Future of Radical Healing

The Smith Center is located in the Hunting Park community in North Philadelphia. Like many industrial neighborhoods of the 1980's, Hunting Park lost much of its economic base as manufacturing companies left town to become multinational corporations, while local government divested from the community. Underground economies emerged as a means of survival for remaining residents. A 2010 *Philadelphia Weekly* feature on Hunting Park captures some of the public perception of the neighborhood: "….the area gained notoriety as one of the most dangerous open air drug markets in the city. To the west, a menacing pageant of prostitutes, pimps and assorted street hustlers lined up and down Old York Road" (Murtha).

It is within this social and economic context that a recreation center was initially welcomed by local residents - in part. Some residents were hesitant about a large center establishing itself without community input or leadership (personal communication, 2016).[13] This was reflected in how the center has struggled to attract a larger constituency. The Police Athletic League (PAL) operated the center from 2007 to 2011, but it was eventually turned over due to lack of community participation. In 2011, the individual proprietor who built the center and contracted it out to the PAL, revamped its mission and restructured its staff overhead. Mari joined this staff as an education director from 2013-2014, and saw first-hand how little communication there had been between the Smith Center and local residents. Despite leaving her position, she maintained a relationship with the Center due to a sense of commitment to the community surrounding the center. Over the years, she saw programming gradually grow in what it offered youth from K-12, but there was relatively little to no programming for adults.

After conversations with several community members to gauge an interest in yoga, Mari and Sheena developed a proposal for a class to help fill in the gap in programming. We agreed to offer yoga twice a week for thirteen weeks, and to provide water and fruit to engage in community building post-class. Within two weeks, our proposal was approved by the Smith Center. Our target audience were female-identified adults, although no one would be turned away on the basis of gender. In total we had about 12 participants, where a typical class had 3-4 students between the ages of 18 and 70. Mari and Sheena co-taught the first class, and then alternated Tuesdays and Thursdays. At each session, the music was much less about interrupting the silence of the room; but about providing sonic healing through the voices and rhythms of our ancestors and singing bowls. On certain days, this sounded like Anoushka Shankar or Sweet Honey In The Rock. Other days, it might be Tracy Chapman or Jamila Woods, Black folklore singers whose lyrics call out structural oppression, lift up Black girl magic, and affirm that "[we're] talkin' about a revolution/It sounds like a whisper" (Chapman).

From the first day that our Yoga for Spirit series began, in October 2016, our intention was to create a culture of collective care and radical healing. In arriving at the series with previous history with community members, open hearts, naturally-scented incense/candles, carefully curated playlists, and nourishing snacks, we hoped to not simply share a healing practice with participants but also to build transformative relationships centered around healing collectively in the same space. Although we knew attendance was low and often remarked on the need to do better with outreach, the sacred and intimate connections we were building in that dark room, at the end of the hallway, were medicinal and restorative. At least 2-3 women from the neighborhood, many of whom were busy providing for their families during the work days and weekends, were consistent with their attendance. Many of them felt the class to be a space of refuge from the ongoing struggles of the outside world, *and a* place to collectively strategize responses to said struggles. One of the regular attendees, Imani, remarked on the effect that practicing consistently had on her sense of purpose at work and relationship to her family, friends and co-workers. Working in a hospital, a typically a high-stress environment, Imani said she noticed a difference in how she responded to conflict at work when she was practicing yoga on a regular basis, that she was able to keep calm and respond to it by offering solutions rather than internalizing the stress that co-workers were experiencing. She also noted staying away from drama and gossip for the sake of personal peace. She was grateful to her yoga practice for equipping her with tools of resilience and readiness for social spontaneity.

Beyond cultivating a healing environment in the space, we prioritized making ourselves available for participants to debrief the way they connected to various asanas (yoga poses) and the insight they gained by connecting to a deeper, more interior space within their being. It is in this context that Ms. Kyleah reflected to us her understanding of yoga as a practice that is more about connecting to yourself than it is about twisting yourself. One evening as we were debriefing class and Ms. Kyleah's consecutive attendance, she remarked how meaningful Yoga For Spirit was to her: "This is the only hour in the week that I get for myself."

We believe our intention setting with the series made for a different kind of environment from the majority of mainstream yoga spaces. By prioritizing an approach that allowed conversations and exchanges between teachers and students before and after class and connecting the practice to the political and personal nature of our work and relationships, the intention in the space and the structure of the classes served as a precondition for yoga to embody the tenets of radical healing.

Most of our takeaways stem from what it means to give access (both in terms of location and cost) to some of the most impacted people in Philadelphia. As people who have the least access to social services, offering yoga and community building as an act of radical healing make our time spent politically urgent. However, over time we learned that location and cost were not the only issues of access. When we debriefed with Imani about why she felt we did not have a higher attendance, she attributed this to the intimidation that people in the neighborhood might have about yoga. Although we are not white, we are young, petite, able-bodied femmes who have the physical appearance of what a "yoga body" is supposed to look like. Given our tight work schedules, we were forced to rely on word of mouth and on the outreach coordinator (a young white male). From this, we learned the importance of using outreach to educate about body positivity/possibilities, and to be more intentional and creative in checking our privileges. For instance, what if we had offered Ms. Kyleah a small honorarium to help us recruit more seniors? She is an older and well-respected leader in the neighborhood who shattered the "yoga body" myth that only served the tastes and desires of white supremacy. Most significantly, she understood our goal for radical healing in a fundamental way.

Conclusion

Healing is an embodied process that allows us to move from trauma to wellness, from fear to courage, from hopelessness to confidence and optimism. In thinking about the possibility of what radical healing can look like in Philadelphia, we root our intentions in recalling the legacy of resistance in Philadelphia and how it has, for so long, nurtured a space for healing from the layers of collective trauma. Philadelphian educators, artists, healers and spiritual leaders have fueled resistance by prioritizing the wholeness, the self- and cultural awareness, health and well-being of their greater communities. Despite the layers of trauma and harm woven into the city's most marginalized neighborhoods, this legacy of organizing through a framework of spiritual healing and cultural justice has persisted through the cultivation of faith-based, artistic and healing spaces across time and space.

While Yoga for Spirit represents a fraction of this work, it can also be seen as a microcosm of the limits and possibilities of it. The limits highlight the nuanced nature of access, the need for politicized yoga taught by practitioners that represent body, ability, and gender diversity, and continued grassroots education that yoga is for everybody. It is our hope, that the possibilities of this work affirm these values, and encourage other wellness practitioners to study the geo-political context of land and the people in which they serve, in order to more holistically cultivate community-building as a part of the practice. In conclusion, radical healing through yoga gives life and credence to a vision gifted to us by the radical humanist, Grace Lee Boggs: Instead of only seeing ourselves only as victims, we begin to see ourselves as part of the continuing struggle of human beings, not only to survive but to evolve into more *human* human beings (Boggs 255). Breath by breath, moment to moment, we believe this evolution is necessary for humanity, from Philly to Palestine, and beyond.

Notes

1 We recognize overlaps in how both the "radical healing" and "healing justice" frameworks conceptualize trauma through a political lens and treat it as a wound that is caused by structural violence, often inherited through historical, generational harm. We, therefore, use these concepts interchangeably.

2 The quote above is referenced by Leah Lakshmi Piepzna-Samarasinha and credited to the Kindred: Southern Healing Justice Collective, and Cara Page, one of the guiding forces behind its founding in 2007. As a response to the crisis of trauma, violence and social oppression - which was especially apparent in the aftermath of Hurricane Katrina -

healers and organizers of color based in the Southern United States came together to establish Kindred. The collective worked to center body work, counseling and healing through a social justice framework.

3 In addition to Goode's administration, the Philadelphia branch of the FBI authorized this attack (Coard 30).

4 Rather than addressing the impact of the trauma that was inflicted on Black Philadelphians and the MOVE family by the bombing, the city of Philadelphia has invested its energy in normalizing the celebration of murderers like Frank Rizzo and Wilson Goode, Sr., as is indicated by the statues and streets that memorialize their legacies.

5 Mumia Abu-Jamal is a Philly native and former member of the Black Panther Party chapter in North Philadelphia. He is a journalist, radio host and award-winning prison scholar. In 1981, Mumia Abu-Jamal was arrested and convicted for the murder of Officer Daniel Faulkner. After over thirty years of death row threats from the state, the campaign succeeded in removing Abu-Jamal from death row. Abu-Jamal was placed into general population at the State Correctional Institution (SCI) - Mahanoy in 2012 to carry out a lifelong sentence. Activists on the ground still consider this a bittersweet victory since this is essentially death by incarceration.

6 In naming Black liberation, we do so from the radical perspective that Black liberation is deeply entwined with all oppressed peoples' liberation. It calls for the global reordering of power structures through revolutionary change.

7 The MOVE 9 refers to the 9 family members who were imprisoned for one police officer's death after the August 1978 confrontation in Powelton Village. They include Delbert Orr Africa, Janet Hollaway Africa, Janine Phillips Africa, Charles Simms Africa, and Edward Goodwin Africa. According to the official website of the MOVE 9, Merle Africa and Phil Africa were "murdered by the system in the toxic death jails of Pennsylvania." Due to sustained pressure from the organization and its allies, Debbie Africa was released in June of 2018, Michael Davis Africa, Sr., in October of 2018, Janet and Janine Africa in May 2019, Eddie Africa in June 2019, Delbert Africa, in January 2020, and the last surviving member, Chuck Sims Africa, in February 2020.

8 In 1967, in response to poor school conditions, racist school practices, and a lack of curriculum on African American history and culture, a coalition of active students that included the organized a massive student walk-out that included students from all corners of the city.

9 "Stay Woke, Stay Whole Healing Manual" is an internal document for Black Youth Project (BYP) 100 created for its national chapter-based membership.

10 Although India is legally a secular state, non-Hindu citizens experience religious and cultural nationalism at the institutional level. For instance, schools in the state of Uttar Pradesh have mandated yoga as part of their daily curricula. Though the state officials suggest this mandate is not about imposing organized religion on students, the chanting of "aum/om" during these sessions contradicts this claim. This is indicative of the attempt to conflate yoga with Hinduism.

11 The "Get Free Manifesto" was originally available at the following website: https://www.getfreefest.com/. This website has since expired.

12 The Yeye Deve collective was founded by 4 yoga instructors: Jazmyn Burton, Maiga Milbourne, Sheena Sood and Jamila Wilson. In Yoruba, Yeye refers to "mother." In Sanskrit, Devi is the term for Goddess. We chose to lift up language from African and Asian spiritual traditions in initiating this work because we wanted to center our enlightened ancestors in this work.

13 Mari Morales-Williams gathered this sentiment from an informal conversation with a community elder who resides in the Hunting Park neighborhood.

Works Cited

Abu-Jamal, Mumia. *All Things Censored*. Seven Stories Press, 2001.

---. *Writing on the Wall: Selected Prison Writings of Mumia Abu-Jamal*. Edited by Johanna Fernandez. City Lights Publishers, 2015.

Africa, Jr., Michael. "'They Can Only Stretch the Bond. They Can't Break It.'" *Colorlines*, 21 November 2018. https://www.colorlines.com/articles/they-can-only-stretch-bond-they-cant-break-it.

BEAM. "What Is Healing Justice?" *Black Emotional And Mental Health Collective*, 2017. http://www.beam.community/healing-justice.

Boggs, Grace Lee. *Living for Change: An Autobiography*. 2nd ed. edition. University of Minnesota Press, 2016.

Brown, Adrienne Maree. *Emergent Strategy: Shaping Change, Changing Worlds*. AK Press, 2017.

Chapman, Tracy. *Talkin 'bout a Revolution*. Elektra, 1988.

Chaudhury, Aadita. "Why White Supremacists and Hindu Nationalists Are so Alike." *Al Jazeera*, 13 December 2018. https://www.aljazeera.com/indepth/opinion/white-supremacists-hindu-nationalists-alike-181212144618283.html.

Coard, Michael. "MOVE 30: Inside the May 1985 Assault on Osage Avenue." *Philadelphia*, May 2015. https://www.phillymag.com/news/2015/05/12/move-30-year-anniversary/.

Countryman, Matthew J. *Up South: Civil Rights and Black Power in Philadelphia*. 9th edition. University of Pennsylvania Press, 2007.

Esack, Steve. "Gov. Tom Wolf Closing Residential Mental Health Facilities, 734 Workers to Be Impacted, in Budget Crunch." *Themorningcall.Com*, 12 January 2017. https://www.mcall.com/news/pennsylvania/mc-pa-wolf-closing-state-hospitals-20170112-story.html.

Ginwright, Shawn. *Black Youth Rising: Activism and Radical Healing in Urban America*. Teachers College Press, 2009.

---. *Hope and Healing in Urban Education: How Urban Activists and Teachers Are Reclaiming Matters of the Heart*. Routledge, 2015.

Glantz, Aaron and Emmanuel Martinez. "For People of Color, Banks Are Shutting the Door to Homeownership." *Reveal from The Center for Investigative Reporting*, February 2018. https://www.revealnews.org/article/for-people-of-color-banks-are-shutting-the-door-to-homeownership/.

Hall, Alena. "Here's Why Lululemon Is Charging $108 for Meditation Beads." *Huffington Post*, 7 December 2017. https://www.huffpost.com/entry/heres-why-lululemon-is-charging-108-for-meditation-beads_n_6464434.

"John Africa of MOVE – On a Move." The MOVE Organization, 2019. http://onamove.com/john-africa/.

Kelley, Robin D. G. *Freedom Dreams: The Black Radical Imagination*. Beacon Press, 2003. https://www.amazon.com/Freedom-Dreams-Black-Radical-Imagination/dp/0807009776/ref=sr_1_1?keywords=freedom+dreams&qid=1553292099&s=gateway&sr=8-1.

Melamed, Samantha. "5,000 Inmates with Hepatitis C Sued Pa. Prisons. Now, They're on Their Way to Getting Treatment." *The Philadelphia Inquirer*, 20 November 2018. https://tinyurl.com/y2krzklt.

Mumia Abu-Jamal Set to Begin Treatment for Hepatitis C in Prison - Hep. 7 April 2017. https://www.hepmag.com/article/mumia-abujamal-set-begin-treatment-hepatitis-c-prison.

Murtha, Tara. "Hunting Park Bounces Back." *PhiladelphiaWeekly.Com*, 5 January 2010. http://www.philadelphiaweekly.com/news/hunting-park-bounces-back/article_ece6a3bc-6dad-5ac1-9574-5a143ae8418c.html.

Patankar, Prachi. "Ghosts of Yogas Past and Present." *Jadaliyya*, 26 February 2014. http://www.jadaliyya.com/pages/index/16632/ghosts-of-yogas-past-and-present.

Piepzna-Samarasinha, Leah Lakshmi. "A Not-So-Brief Personal History of the Healing Justice Movement, 2010–2016." *MICE Magazine*, 20 October 2016. http://micemagazine.ca/issue-two/not-so-brief-personal-history-healing-justice-movement-2010%E2%80%932016.

Sood, Sheena. "Cultivating a Yogic Theology of Collective Healing: A Yogini's Journey Disrupting White Supremacy, Hindu Fundamentalism, and Casteism." *Race and Yoga*, vol. 3, no. 1 (2018). escholarship.org, https://escholarship.org/uc/item/0wn4p090.

---. "Spectacles of Compassion: Modi and the Weaponization of Yoga." *Jadaliyya*, May 2020. https://www.jadaliyya.com/Details/41048.

Taylor, Keeanga-Yamahtta. *From #BlackLivesMatter to Black Liberation.* Haymarket Books, 2016. https://www.haymarketbooks.org/books/778-from-blacklivesmatter-to-black-liberation.

Chapter 6

Body science of survivorship

Mapping the neurological impacts of interlocking systems of oppression and co-designing equitable solutions through movement and breath

Morgan Vanderpool

As you read, please breathe at a rhythm and volume that supports you in staying as connected as possible to your capacity for choice-making: choosing to move, breathe, stretch, and connect in a way that serves and supports your survivorship – the badass you that has persisted, resisted, and brilliantly adapted to be here, alive, in this moment.

This piece is written in honor of the badassery of your survivorship, and in reverence of the complexities of neuroplasticity.

Introduction

I welcome you, the brilliant kaleidoscope of both badass survivor of, *and* complicit participant in systems of violence. We are complex beings, that is for sure. I wholeheartedly trust that if you are choosing to read this, you have the absolute best intentions to be of service to the cultivation of healing, freedom, and justice. I also acknowledge that we are all inherently human, we will all cause harm along the way, and there is space to restore that too.

It is my hope through this piece to share from both the wisdom and the limitations of my unique identity as a White, queer, non-binary, multi-lingual, nerd, clinical social worker, and dancer, who is a survivor of queerphobia, sexual and gender-based violence, and who is in active recovery from White Body Supremacy and White saviorism (Menakem, 2017). I also hope to share from the profound wisdom I've been gifted through the trust and connection that has been extended to me in health-centric, justice-centric, and trauma-sensitive relationships over the years, in many states and countries. I've learned from folx whose complex and brilliant survivorship has exponentially expanded my understanding of the awe-inspiring strength, adaptability, and deep-seated resilience of our nervous systems' capacity to survive and thrive.

In this piece, it is my intention to focus on how embodied movement and breath practices are the foundation to how we can pragmatically and healthfully engage in resistance and system change (starting with your own nervous system). I will offer a neuroscientifically-based, integrative approach to attending to the impacts of survivorship of systems of oppression, through engaging in trauma-sensitive

~Written in honor of the badassery of our survivorship,
and in reverence of the complexities of neuroplasticity.~

movement and breath practices that build nervous systems robust enough to do the work together, while designing relationships that unwire oppressive paradigms, and inclusively co-construct new ones ("Body-Based Intersectional Countertransference").

Problems and solutions

Wiring ourselves for freedom and connection starts from an understanding of the innermost formation of our genetic code and our nervous systems' brilliant survival adaptations.

This further implores us to understand the impact of oppressive systems on our neurological conduction and accompanying body sensations, to better guide how we interact and wire with ourselves, others, and the systems around us.

Through this process, we can explore cultivating patterns of breath and movement that have the capacity to foster anti-oppressive relationships. This comes with the complications of recognizing that all the while, we are interacting within, and doing our best to disrupt, hijack, and defrag systems of oppression. We have the opportunity to recode and rewire our relationships for equity, connection, mutual understanding, and sharing of power. We have some massive work to do, and, thankfully at this point in history, we have the backing of neuroplasticity and epigenetics on our side to understand the complexity of the challenges and the solutions.

The systems we've survived

Below is a condensed list of the multiple systems we've all survived. We've survived each system proportionate to, and in accordance with, the positionality of our mixed/multiple identities. When we take into account how they all come together, we can more comprehensively understand the moment-to-moment survival adaptations that our bodies have instinctively calculated to continue to persist. This multi-systems lens increases our capacity to perceive, process, and include the vast multiplicity and miraculous adaptations in how each of us has wired for survival.

These systems individually, and in combination with one another (in the non-exhaustive list below) holistically cause a lack of access to a felt sense of the following: safety, ease, connection, being seen, heard, and validated, and the agency/ability to make change. The systems include: *Colonialism, racism, queerphobia, ageism, capitalism, cisnormativity, sexism, religious and political oppression, immigration systems, patriarchy, lack of inclusion due to neurodiversity, body size politics, colorism, xenophobia, educational elitism, lack of access to communication/language, commodification of humans, living beings, and nature.*

All of these systems are perpetuated by the violence built off of transgenerational othering, that is supported by the neurological capacity to disconnect and unfeel the reality of another. Due to the inherent interconnected nature of

*~Written in honor of the badassery of our survivorship,
and in reverence of the complexities of neuroplasticity.~*

humanity, I propose that every single one of us is uniquely surviving the violence that the systems above, individually and intersectionally, create. We can greatly benefit from learning the nuances of our neurological survival patterns and how they can unconsciously keep systems of violence in motion within ourselves and in relationships.

Survival, em-bodied and em-brained

Below I describe piece by piece our genes, nervous systems, key areas of our brains, breath, muscles/rhythms, and how our felt senses of self are set up to co-communicate, and how they have been impacted by systems of violence that create experiences of trauma. These pieces of the map are vital to know so that when we are investing in relationships centered on anti-oppression, we can operate from a realistic map of our neurological functioning. Such realism supports cultivating compassion for both our limitations and capacities. Additionally, the map supports us in being able to name which part of ourselves is neurologically being activated, or turned off, so we can be real about what neurological tools we bring to build anti-oppressive solutions, and what neurological infrastructures can get in our way, despite our best intentions.

Epigenetics

The genetic expression for every protein in our body is impacted by our life experience and is then passed down to our progeny. The way my system operates is inherited from my ancestral line, and so is yours. Our ancestors, within us via our DNA, are aiming to support us by offering us the code and gene expression (manifesting in the structure of our whole body/brain and our thoughts, perceptions, and behaviors) that preserved their existence. We may never have directly experienced the trauma of our ancestors (that which they caused, and that they survived), yet our bodies have been built on their architecture.

When we spend time in relationship with one another in the present, it's a convening of our ancestry. My epigenetic makeup (the combination of my racial, gendered, socioeconomic, political, religious, etc., ancestry) may have co-protected yours, and it may have put your ancestral code at extreme risk. It's necessary to consider that if my ancestors have participated in perpetuating a type of violence that you survive daily such as racism, capitalism/poverty, sexism, or queerphobia, then I will be felt by you as a threat inherently, and appropriately, due to your epigenetic survivorship. In choosing to be in relationship with one another, we are inherently navigating the survival responses of our ancestors within our bodies, and in relationship with each other. This is all playing out moment to moment, breath to breath, and we are being asked to give space for our ancestors to breathe with us, be with us in real time, and to compassionately recognize the survival responses within our epigenetic lineage of survivorship and complicit perpetratorship (Caldwell & Leighton, 2018; Menakem, 2017).

~Written in honor of the badassery of our survivorship,
and in reverence of the complexities of neuroplasticity.~

Gratefully, we can lean on the freedom that is offered through our epigenetic flexibility. We can practice trusting that our choices, behaviors, actions, and relationships will also shape the genetic expression of our bodies and the next generations. Thanks to epigenetics, we know we are influential in coding the future genetic architecture we wish to create.

Survival systems

Our bodies are brilliantly equipped with automatic survival systems that react on our behalf without our conscious consent in habitual patterns informed by our epigenetics. They will engage when our sensory systems perceive a felt sense of threat to our body's or identity's integrity. A felt sense of threat originates from our body picking up on signals (neurocepted internally or perceived externally) that we will be unseen, unheard, or invalidated by manifestations of the systems of violence outlined above (Porges, 2017). These survival responses are brilliantly adaptive, and can also be incredibly frustrating and disruptive to equitable, systemic change.

These responses are in large part (85%) fed by afferrently (body-to-brain) conducted signals along the vagus nerve. They are activated in concordance with the perceived amount of agency and necessity to self-protect that each body may have in any given situation. It's my long-term observation that the vagus nerve is one of the most beautiful systems in our body. Its primary purpose is to neurocept internal signals within our body and send them to our brain for interpretation of how safe or unsafe, well or unwell, we feel, moment to moment based principally on breath rate, heart rate, gut signals, tone of voice, facial expression, and physical sensation. In the big picture, our brain filters how our body is feeling, and our body's felt state is foundational to how our brain synthesizes our present-moment status of well-being. In summary, our body signals inform our felt sense of well being five times more potently than our mind's conduction to our body (Dana, 2018; Menakem, 2017; Porges, 2017).

Below are five principal survival responses described briefly: Fight, Flight, Freeze, Submit, Fawn (FFFSF). They each manifest via a spectrum of body sensations, movement, breath rate, words, perception, and mindset.

> *Please pause.*
> Before reading further, please take the space and time to honor your body's and your ancestors' bodies' wisdom, for the moments in which these responses have assured our survival.

- Fight (resist/defend)
    - You may feel muscles prepped for action, short quick breath, heat/flushing, rage/anger/frustration, penetrating gaze, posturing to get bigger/take up space, clenched fists.

*~Written in honor of the badassery of our survivorship,
and in reverence of the complexities of neuroplasticity.~*

- Flight (avoid/deny)
  - An almost instantaneous lack of capacity to stay present with thoughts, feelings, ideas. Anxiety. Lack of eye contact. Leaving a place or disengaging from others.
- Freeze (lack of action/movement)
  - Possibly feeling stuck, immobile, muscles unable to move, sedentary, inactive, heaviness, depression of the nervous system.
- Submit (going along to get along, body going soft to decrease harm)
  - Includes a possible sinking feeling, swirling sensations/thoughts, floating, following someone else's desire/direction due to your body feeling as if they have access to more agency/power than you. You may be able to subconsciously predict the needs of a person in power and comply to meet them without active consent. Particularly complicated response in the context of sexual assault, as the survivor's body will comply non-consensually to get through the assault.
- Fawn (copy or mentally/physically emulate the behaviors of the powers that be)
  - Typically talked about the least and may be twinned with submit, creates the most confusion and shame because within a fawn response, we adopt the mentality and behaviors of those who are in power around us, even if their behavior is violent and/or against our own morals. You may feel dissociative, disconnected, or disembodied.

The above FFFSF responses predictably manifest in a series of physical sensations, muscle contractions or movements, breath rates and volumes, physical posturing, eye movements, facial expressions, and tones of voice. When activated, they will streamline our neurology for survival, turning on certain systems and turning off others. The FFFSF survival responses activate and communicate on our behalf every moment of every day, as we are co-wiring and firing in relationships with every breath we breathe (Dana, 2018; Levine, 2010; Porges, 2017; van der Kolk, 2014).

In my observations, the majority of us have not spent the time to explore the nuances of these sensations in a way that has felt supported. Nor have we practiced prioritizing naming them as dynamics that are pervasively playing out in our relationships. Our FFFSF responses typically bring up an intensity of body sensations that we've been socially conditioned to hide from ourselves and others. Yet there are innumerable benefits when we start to get to know our own FFFSF responses and practice engaging with them from a pragmatic place of efficacy.

Survival responses and breath

One of the principal ways we can practically and efficaciously gain connection with our FFFSF responses is through increasing our attentiveness to, interoceptive

*~Written in honor of the badassery of our survivorship,
and in reverence of the complexities of neuroplasticity.~*

awareness of, and engagement with, our breath (interoception being the practice of sensing the internal sensations of our body) (Porges, 2017).

Our survival responses are primarily navigated by our autonomic nervous system, which has two branches: the sympathetic branch, which is principally responsible for our fight and flight responses; and the parasympathetic branch, which activates with a felt sense of ease or safety. The parasympathetic branch facilitates resting, digesting, connecting, and restoring our cells and ensuring our immune systems can stay active (Levine, 2010). Anatomically, there are certain muscles that are innervated, i.e., neurologically connected to, our sympathetic and our parasympathetic branches. Our pectorals and our trapezius muscles are sympathetically innervated and our diaphragm, intercostals, and abdominals are parasympathetically innervated (Dana, 2018; Farhi, 1996).

In the context of survivorship of systems of violence/complex trauma, our breath patterns are one of the key components that initiate and sustain our FFFSF responses. Breath in the context of FFFSF tends to have patterns of holding, erratic rhythms, atrophy of muscles through lack of use, and tension from overuse. And if habitually engaged in FFFSF responses, the muscles aren't utlized in a way that creates a sense of autonomously chosen breath patterns, but rather patterns that are neurologically engaged without our active/conscious consent (Rothschild, 2000).

Thus, on a practical level, I propose that when we are initiating opportunities for restoration of our bodies to engage in trauma-sensitive and equity-oriented work, one of the most direct tools that we can apply is to practice engaging a breath rhythm that we are actively choosing moment-to-moment. Breathing a rhythm that is predictably felt, and sustainably adaptable to the precise work that we are doing in the moment, is key to keeping our nervous systems engaged in the present. Generative breath is only possible when we are not forcing or assigning ourselves to breathe in a certain way, but rather creating choice-based breath rhythms. Everyone's body has survived through its own muscular pattern of disconnection and tension, overuse and underuse. Thus, forcing atrophied, neurologically disconnected, or tight muscles to move in a prescribed way will be felt as a threat internally, and instigate an FFFSF response. Thus it is imperative that we choose to breathe in a way that is both understanding of the patterns that we have learned through our own survivorship, and meets the need of our present moment context.

In relationship, this type of chosen breath pattern is an exponentially potent practice to assure that we are attuning physically, and neurologically communicating, with those who are in close proximity to us. When we assure our own felt sense of ease and connection, we can create space for others to do the same, even amidst challenges and discomfort. And although we may have been taught certain ways to breathe from embodiment practices like yoga, due to our neurodiversity of survivorship, each survivor requires access to breathe in a way that is most adaptable for them moment-to-moment, to cultivate the greatest potential for relational resonance.

~Written in honor of the badassery of our survivorship,
and in reverence of the complexities of neuroplasticity.~

Additionally, as we choose a breath rhythm that is adaptive to the present moment, and less likely to be repeating an FFFSF response, our body posture, eye contact, tone of voice, and many other physical elements shift. As they shift, we decrease the likelihood that we will co-trigger FFFSF responses in relationship to one another and more parts of our brains that are necessary to stay fully engaged, stay on ("Body-Based Intersectional Countertransference").

Next, I will highlight some of the key areas of our brains, and principal functions of our nervous systems, that are the key players in our survival of interlocking systems of oppression.

Survival "em-brained" – the structural nitty gritty...

- Amygdala: Our internal alarm system
    - As with all parts of our brain, it is wired based on our lived experience and via epigenetics' imprint. It's a small almond-sized area of our brain located in our base brain. It adapts in its sensitivities in response to moments in which our survival systems have engaged. It automatically takes charge for our survival and receives most of its signals from body sensations. When actively sounding the alarm (when our FFFSF response is active), fewer resources get allocated to the subsequent areas of our brain.
- Insula: I am, I exist
    - A midbrain structure, located in both the right and left hemispheres. Its job is to perceive body sensations and translate them into a felt and understood sense of self. It is the seat of our own self-sensing, and our felt sense of worth.
- Broca's area: Speech production
    - Located on the lower portion of the left frontal lobe of the brain, it is in charge of motoric language production. When the amygdala is activated, the Broca's area is one of the spaces that does not have full conductivity. So in those instances of a felt sense of threat, we tend to end up saying things we wish we didn't or can't say the things we wish we could, and in a large way our language patterns follow our survival patterns.
- Prefrontal cortex: Our "highly evolved" mind
    - The most frontal region of our brain, last to have evolved, and responsible for executive function – new learning, reason, logic, planning, perspective-taking, and mental resonance. It receives much less activity when our amygdala is activated. This doesn't mean that we aren't thinking or perceiving or trying to plan, but rather that its function is informed by FFFSF responses, rather than being open/available for its full function (Levine, 2010; Sapolsky, 2017; van der Kolk, 2014).

~Written in honor of the badassery of our survivorship,
and in reverence of the complexities of neuroplasticity.~

Survival em-bodied: Body-based neurological functions

- Interoception
  - The neurological function of body sensations/processes arriving along afferent (body-to-brain) pathways, to the mind for interpretation and understanding. Interoception is occuring whether we are aware of it or not. Our body's sensations are consistently informing our mind's perception of our felt sense of safety, well-being, and emotional state.
- Proprioception
  - The neurological function of sensing our body in space. How much space we occupy, and the relationship of our body within, and to, our own bodies, the space, and the people around us. The capacity to accurately feel our height, width, reach, strength, steadiness, and physical support.
- Neuroception
  - Neuroception describes the way our autonomic nervous system subconsciously responds to situations as safe or dangerous. Also described as the process through which the nervous system evaluates risk outside of your conscious awareness, primarily through body sensation

(Dana, 2018 & Porges, 2017).

Practical application of em-brainment and em-bodiment

So how do all these functions and structures communicate in the context of wiring our nervous systems for equitable relationships and intersectional trauma sensitivity?

From understanding that our bodies' internal sensations are informed by our epigenetic survival wisdom, we can create relational space where any sensation, movement, word, tone of voice, breath, or environmental stimuli can trip our amygdala to sound the alarm for our FFFSF response, and the FFFSF response in another. Honoring that neurodiversity is foundational for us to understand that at any moment we could have a lessened sense of connection to our sense of self (insula losing connectivity), and that we may be verbally communicating in a way that has helped us survive or self-preserve via FFFSF (Broca's area informed by amygdala function). It's vital for us to be clear that the above patterns could neurologically reinforce a system of violence in relationship to self and in relationship to others.

Each distinct breath, vocal tone, and word we utter carries a different weight or impact, depending on our transgenerational and intersectional survivorship. Here lies an opportunity for growth in our relationships, to be able to hear and validate the FFFSF responses active in our language expression, while doing the attentive

~Written in honor of the badassery of our survivorship,
and in reverence of the complexities of neuroplasticity.~

work of talking in a way that makes it accessible for everyone to be heard and understood. Spending the time to use words and tones that don't preserve positionalities and ways of thinking that have been protected by systems of power is vital to this work. And a reminder, our words and tones are generated from our breath patterns and interoceptive felt sense of self.

A note on silence…if your body has assured its survival through a freeze or submit response, it's likely that your adaptive survival response has been silence. It's natural; we shut up because of how often we've been unheard by systems of power. Doing this work with integrity stems from doing the kind of embodiment work that neurologically, via breath and movement, equips us to battle the multiple layers of neurological wiring developed to enforce the codes of silence.

Additionally, our insula receives reduced activity when we experience a felt sense of threat to being unseen or unheard by relational systems of power. In those moments we have a harder time accessing a felt sense of self that permits us to know we exist, and thus have a solid felt connection to who we are, outside of our survival responses. This work is tricky sometimes because we can get to know our sense of self as congruent with our survival responses, yet if our survival responses lead, then we will be working without a solidly firing insula, effectively engaged Broca's area, or a fully online prefrontal cortex.

Another tricky element at play at this level of analysis, is that our awareness of interoceptive processes (our capacity to feel our moment-to-moment felt sensations) is diminished during times of threat of being unseen, unheard, or invalidated. Feeling all the sensations involved with surviving trauma is not always to the benefit of our survival, due to system overwhelm (Porges, 2017). So, purposefully strengthening our interoceptive capacities, grounded in adaptable movement and breath, is a big component of developing the neurological agility necessary to stay present and keep our sophisticated neurological structures online.

Interoceptive capacities are strengthened through moving and breathing in ways that we intentionally initiate for ourselves. This centers the opportunity to consistently create, and consent to, present-moment felt sensations. We can practice this through increasing awareness of how we are breathing, focusing on how our muscles and joints feel, or sensing the surfaces we are connected to. When engaging in practices like this, you may notice sensations of your FFFSF responses simultaneously with the present-moment felt sensations that you are initiating. The potency of your interoceptive practices will be strengthened by creating sensations that are in addition to, or unique from, the bodily sensations associated with your FFFSF response (Emerson, 2011).

Interoception is additionally enhanced or emboldened through moving and breathing in ways that you choose, that have not been assigned by someone else, but those chosen in concordance with the present-moment physiological state of your body. For example, stretching or strengthening as little or as much as it feels accessible to you moment-to-moment, and moving at a rhythm or pace that is authentically yours (Emerson, 2011).

*~Written in honor of the badassery of our survivorship,
and in reverence of the complexities of neuroplasticity.~*

Via cultivating present-moment felt sensation, through choice-based movement and breath, we create an attuned relationship with the afferent (body-to-brain) conduction of our nervous system. Through consistent interoceptive and proprioceptive practices, we neurologically layer a more predictable and trustworthy relationship with our felt sense of self, and a sense of agency and connection, all the while increasing the likelihood that our insula and prefrontal cortex stay online (Emerson, 2011; van der Kolk, 2014).

Another supportive element of practicing choice-based movement and breath has to do with increasing our proprioceptive capacity. In the context of survivorship of complex trauma and systems of oppression, our body learns all too well that our physical and relational boundaries get crossed during times of having power executed over us, violations of our body's integrity, and when our felt sense of self is compromised. As a result, it can be challenging to have an accurate or predictable sense of how little or how much space we occupy or take up. Simultaneously, it can feel very unpredictable to move in space with others in a way that feels resonant or consensual. We can attend to this proprioceptive impact through practicing movement and breath that support us in sensing the felt structural extents of our body, the soundness or efficacy of our muscles, and practicing noticing where our body starts and stops physically, and the space we physically occupy. Physical practices that support us in feeling our edges, our reach, and our strength can give us a keener awareness of a body-based understanding of our boundaries, limitations, and capacities.

Increasing our proprioceptive and interoceptive capacities creates a cleaner and stronger connection for accessing our body as a guide to how to engage in relationships that honor our individual and shared survivorship.

Survival responses and positionality: A focus on intersectional balancing

- *A description to combine how the relationships of the 16 (non-exhaustive) intersecting systems of oppression are experienced and communicated in relationships, via our five survival responses.*

For each aspect of our identity, we engage a distinct combination of FFFSF in response to each system of oppression. We each may have had a myriad of responses to each system, e.g., fought sexism, fawned to racism, avoided colonialism, submitted to capitalism, etc. This multiplicity in survival responses could be calculated, or interpreted as 16 (the number of systems listed above) multiplied by five (the number of survival responses), equaling up to 80 neurological responses that could be co-occurring within us, at any moment. It can be especially confusing and complicated when we have distinct survival responses to the same system. For example, if I have a history of having survived via subconsciously submitting and fawning to racist practices as a white-skinned person, and having fought and frozen to queerphobia as a queer person, which could be unique from

*~Written in honor of the badassery of our survivorship,
and in reverence of the complexities of neuroplasticity.~*

a straight person or a person of color, for example. Within this perspective, we are challenged to create space for the immense diversity of neurological responses inherently present. Because when it is not fully accounted for, it creates a hotbed for conflict and misunderstandings in relationships ("Body-Based Intersectional Countertransference").

One of the complexities, or a double-edged sword, of neuroplasticity of survival is when it complicitly supports systems of violence staying in place. An interesting lens through which to explore survival behavior is through that of the folx who are typically protected via the systems of violence due to their privileged statuses. Folx with protected positionalities can tend towards a flight, freeze, submit, or fawn response to the presence of systems of oppression. That allows for the system to continue to play out, and can be classified as complicit perpetration of, and participation in, those systems. For example, a White person with a conditioned freeze response to the presence of racism, in a community within which they hold a position of power, leads to inaction and silence. This is foundational to the important understanding behind how White silence equals violence (Diangelo, 2018).

Any social movement that is intentionally built and designed for anti-oppressive practice requires a nuanced approach to be able to suss out how our survival responses are communicating with one another. Folx with protected or privileged positionalities within collective work must work to increase our capacity to validate our felt sense of a co-activated FFFSF response, while staying relationally connected to sharing power. We must be prepared to encounter and anti-oppressively attend to, responses such as someone fawning to us in a position of power, or the discomfort of someone rightfully fighting us to validate their survivorship. All the while, we must equitably and proportionally honor our own survivorship's FFFSF responses. Particularly for folx with protected identities, we are challenged to be self-reflective about how our bodies show up embedded in systems of violence, because we are conditioned to not feel their impact. We are also asked to explore how we might fawn to the systems of power that folx with less protected identities fight to survive each day. If someone with a protected identity is perceived as fawning or submitting to systems of violence, instead of resisting them or working for them to change, then that person will be felt as a threat by folx surviving those systems of oppression, and be a complicit corroborator with the system of violence.

I have observed that we can get distracted from resolving our collective relationship with the systems of violence, and can get hyperfocused on our individualized survival responses, and how they play out interpersonally, rather than intersectionally. Neurological intersectionality invites us to reassess or adjust the common polarized, binary view of victim and perpetrator of systems of oppression. It offers us a shift to consider each one of us as a unique balance of survivor and non-consensual participant in systems of oppression. We can work to foster accountability for self or others who are FFFSF'ing from a position that reinforces a system of oppression, consciously or subconsciously. Especially when in relationships with bodies and identities that have been put at risk by bodies that look, sound, and move like our own. Coconspiratorship, in deconstructing systems of

~Written in honor of the badassery of our survivorship,
and in reverence of the complexities of neuroplasticity.~

power, is built off of a commitment to validate survival responses to systems of oppression, and practicing moving and breathing in ways that wire for options that balance out our FFFSF responses.

A foundational piece that I feel we are being called to create within the networks of folx focused on our individual and collective liberation, is to apply equitable deference to the survival responses that carry an exponentially more complex amalgamation, and valid intensity of survival responses. One of the layers of accountability for collective liberation is to do the internal work to assess how direct or indirect your survivorship of systems of violence has been. For example, if your body has experienced a lesser frequency of the 80 biological responses due to direct threat from systems of power, then it is your responsibility to invest in cultivating your interoceptive window of tolerance for validating the pain of oppression you've bypassed through the protected aspects of your identity. The equilibrium of sharing power stems from the capacity to sense how much the folx who you are in relationship with are navigating highly-impactful FFFSF responses, and how much extra energy you could inherently have due to the elements of your identity that are protected.

> A note to the reader...This may be a prime time to explore taking a pause. To breathe, to notice the body sensations you're experiencing, and maybe create some movement that supports the present moment felt sensations you are experiencing.

Unifying neuroscience, embodiment, and equitable nervous system restoration

As adrienne maree brown purports, in systems change work, we have to "move at the speed of trust" (p. 42). If I trust and understand my survivorship, then I have a greater capacity to learn to trust yours and intrinsically honor all the intersecting components of it. In other words, I've gotta practice keeping my insula and my prefrontal cortex engaged. I must feel myself so I can accurately feel another, or move and collaborate with another.

We have a rich opportunity to become familiarized with the movement and breath patterns of our intersectional survival responses, and practice creating enough felt sense of agency within our own body, through choice-based movement and adaptable breath rhythms, so that we may adapt our pace of movement to increase the likelihood of connection and collaboration with our fellow survivors.

I would like to propose that a strong foundation for systems change will be built by investing energy in practicing moving and breathing individually, and with one another, in a way in which our survivorship is honored. Our level of trust and connection in relationships arises when we take the time to breathe and move together, while necessitating attention to the amount of systemic risk faced by the bodies that we are in relationship with. We are co-creating a neurological felt sense of connection, when we are being seen, heard, and validated proportionately

~Written in honor of the badassery of our survivorship,
and in reverence of the complexities of neuroplasticity.~

and equitably for our body's epigenetic survivorship. That is when our whole selves are seen, heard, and included.

I want to be a part of communities which are advocating for practices that increase moment-to-moment interoceptive awareness, building a capacity to move at a pace where we can attune to the epigenetic origin of a sensation, while practicing adapting our movement and breath rate so that it creates space for connection with self and connection with others, without forcing it to be a certain way. We can build this reality through creating robust enough interoceptive capacities that allow us to be present with the neurological challenge that comes along with creating anti-oppressive and equitable conversations, relationships, and systems.

A reflection on the term "healing" as it fits in with surviving systems of oppression: Grievously, the western health system pathologizes the natural survival responses of individuals and communities most impacted by systems of oppression. Our natural responses to systems of violence have long been diagnosed as disorders, when in reality they are, more often than not, miraculous adaptations of nervous systems wiring for survival. The lens of this paper invites us to consider how much space we can give to recognize the adaptable genius of our nervous system, and honor its brilliance and its limitations.

In conclusion, we can build our path forward on a mutual understanding that each of us neurologically calculates and epigenetically codes, how we effectively and ineffectively survive the kyriarchy of power structures within which we coexist, on a moment to moment basis. We can simultaneously honor that our FFFSF responses are based on our bodies doing the best they know how to make sure we take our next breath, while being able to hold each other accountable for our FFFSF responses through equitably giving relational deference to the folx who carry the higher complexity of survivorship, and working to center their access to neurological connection in relationship.

We can simultaneously trust that neuroplasticity is at our disposal to create anti-oppressive relationships, and that it requires an incredibly powerful, concerted focus to employ it effectively for long-term engagement in equity work founded on dismantling and defragging our nervous system's relationship with White Body Supremacy. The complexity of the work requires that we are moving and breathing in ways that cultivate robust nervous systems and restore the interoceptive capacity that make it possible for us to stay neurologically connected amidst the immense challenges involved in multi-systems, embodied equity work.

> I would like to express a huge thank you for every breath, movement, and action that you dedicate to nervous system restoration and the cultivation of anti-oppressive relationships.

The following questions are available to help ground what you have just read, so that you can digest, apply, and incorporate the content into your practices and relationships.

~Written in honor of the badassery of our survivorship,
and in reverence of the complexities of neuroplasticity.~

FFFSF

You could explore the felt sensations of the following:

- Fight: met with softening/releasing muscular tension, exploring effective action, or leaning on our interconnectedness and co-labor-ation.
- Flight: met with engagement with sensation and staying present within discomfort.
- Freeze: met with choosing stillness and movement when useful.
- Submit: met with exploring balanced physical boundaries, acts of interdependent and autonomous choices.
- Fawn: met with choosing to move for my body, and exploring authentic self-expression.

Breath

- What could it feel like to effectively choose to breathe with my diaphragm, intercostals (all of them), and abdominals in a way that meets my present moment experience? Via exploring rhythm, location of muscular movement, volume, etc., of my breath?
- How often do I practice healthfully oscillating between breathing with my pectorals and my trapezius muscles, and my diaphragm, intercostals, and my abdominal muscles?
- What could it be like to take the time to create space to assure that I am choosing an autonomous and resonant breath rhythm, while the folx who you are in relationship with are able to do the same?

Movement

- How do I move on a day-to-day and moment to moment basis? Which systems am I reinforcing with that movement?
- What kinds of movement and breath practices can I incorporate into my life that support releasing my dependence on survival responses and engage sustainably in trauma restoration and equity cultivating work?

Epigenetics

- What material do I need to read and engage with to understand the survivorship of my ancestors and the ancestors of those with whom you are in relationship? And with whom you desire to be in equitable relationship?
    - Resources available in works cited: DeGruy, Million, Hernandez-Wolfe, Caldwell and Leighton, and Menakem.
- What are my FFFSF responses to my epigenetic history? And to that of my ancestors who have engaged with systems of violence?

~Written in honor of the badassery of our survivorship,
and in reverence of the complexities of neuroplasticity.~

- How do I engage in a trauma sensitive relationship with that history? And how does that history engage with the history of those with whom I am in a present-day relationship?

Intrapersonal and interpersonal relationships

- How do/can my daily choices release the behaviors and movements that perpetuate my participation in systems of oppression?
- How do I breathe, move, think, and act to survive the systems of violence? And what options could I explore to opt out of those behaviors and thought patterns that perpetuate the violence of being unseen, unheard, and invalidated, for myself and others?
- How can I better explore finding my own windows of relational challenge to experiment with resonant relational rhythms? Slowing down or speeding up to sync up with the present-moment need for connection and co-labor-ation?
- How have I adapted to survive each system of oppression? And are those adaptations aligned with my most authentic self and how I desire to show up in the world?
- How do I breathe, move, think, and act to perpetuate the systems of violence that oppress others?
- How often do I ensure that I am moving in synchrony with my own body? Moving in synchrony with others? And adapting my rhythm to effectively link up with them? (Menakem, 2017.)

Systems

- What systems am I Fighting? Fawning? Freezing? Avoiding? Submitting to? How am I doing it?
- What kind of work do I need to commit to in order to better understand how folx with identities unique to mine have survived systems of oppression/violence and how those survival patterns are related to my own survival history?
- For the protected identities that embody, how can I address my fawn, freeze, flee, and submit to the systems I'm protected by to practice staying present enough to engage in disrupting the system in my interpersonal relationships and sphere of influence?

Works cited

"Body-Based Intersectional Countertransference". Uploaded from Morgan Vanderpool's YouTube channel. https://www.youtube.com/watch?v=hLj7WwIZhT8, 15 May 2020.

brown, adrienne maree. *Emergent Strategy*. Chico: AK Press, 2017.

Caldwell, Christine and Leighton, Lucia Bennet. *Oppression and the Body- Roots Resistance & Resolutions*. Berkeley: North Atlantic Books, 2018.

~Written in honor of the badassery of our survivorship,
and in reverence of the complexities of neuroplasticity.~

Dana, Deb. *The Polyvagal Theory in Therapy- Engaging the Rhythm of Regulation*. New York: W.W. Norton & Company, Inc., 2018.

DeGruy, Joy. *Posttraumatic Slave Syndrome- America's Legacy of Enduring Injury and Healing*. Portland: Joy DeGruy Publications, Inc., 2005.

Diangelo, Robin. *White Fragility- Why It's so Hard for White People to Talk about Racism*. Boston: Beacon Press Books, 2018.

Emerson, David. *Overcoming Trauma through Yoga-Reclaiming Your Body*. Boston: North Atlantic Books, 2011.

Engler, Mark and Engler, Paul. *This is an Uprising- How Nonviolent Revolt is Shaping the Twenty-First Century*. New York: Nation Books, 2016.

Farhi, Donna. *The Breathing Book- Good Health through Essential Breath Work*. New York: St. Martin's Press, 1996.

Hernandez-Wolfe, Pilar. *A Borderlands View on Latinos, Latin Americans and Decolonization- Rethinking Mental Health*. Lanham: Jason Aronson, 2013.

Levine, Peter. *In an Unspoken Voice- How the Body Releases Trauma and Restores Goodness*. Berkeley: North Atlantic Books, 2010.

Menakem, Resmaa. *My Grandmother's Hands*. Las Vegas: Central Recovery Press, 2017.

Million, Dian. *Therapeutic Nations- Healing in an Age of Indigenous Human Rights*. Tucson: University of Arizona Press, 2013.

Porges, Stephen. *The Pocket Guide to the PolyVagal Theory- The Transformative Power of Feeling Safe*. New York: W.W. Norton & Company, Inc., 2017.

Rothschild, Babette. *The Body Remembers- The Psychophysiology of Trauma and Trauma Treatment*. New York: W.W. Norton & Company, Inc., 2000.

Sapolsky, Robert. *BEHAVE- The Biology of Humans at Our Best and Worst*. New York: Penguin Books, 2017.

van der Kolk, Bessel. *The Body Keeps the Score- Brain, Mind and Body in the Healing of Trauma*. New York: Viking, 2014.

~Written in honor of the badassery of our survivorship,
and in reverence of the complexities of neuroplasticity.~

Chapter 7

Pedagogy of movement
Yoga in migrant projects from a race and class perspective

Firdose Moonda

Introduction

Yoga, as a cultural phenomenon, has never been more globally popular especially as evidence-based research into its benefits has increased. Apart from its use as a physical exercise, yoga is also used as a complementary treatment for a variety of mental health conditions such as stress and anxiety[1].

This is important because the world is sadder, angrier, more fearful, and stressed than ever before (Gallup 2019), and those feelings are expected to increase in the aftermath of the Coronavirus pandemic. Although the issues of undocumented migrants have taken a backseat, as global unemployment rises, and conflicts in Syria, Libya, and Yemen, amongst others, continue, the number of refugees from developing countries is expected to grow. So, too, is xenophobic rhetoric and far-right populism on the rise (Hunyadi & Molnàr, 2016).

In 2017, the United Nations (UN) put the total number of international migrants at 258 million, which included a record high of 70.8 million forcibly displaced people. Of those, 180 million migrants come from the Global South and 165 million are hosted in high-income countries. Europe is home to 78 million migrants.

The definition of the word migrant is technical, but post-2015, when more than a million people entered Europe by irregular means (IOM, 2015), the term is linked to class. A migrant, unlike an expatriate, is seen as someone who has fallen foul of border control regulations in rich countries (Trilling, 2019). As a result, migrants are considered among the "most vulnerable members of society," (UN, 2017, p.1) who are at greater risk of human rights' violations, abuse, and discrimination (Edwards et al, 2018). The rate at which migrants have access to psychological help is lower than that of host populations because of language barriers, cultural differences, and cost (Selkirk et al., 2014). In the United Kingdom (UK), restrictions on access to the National Health Service (NHS) results in many migrants not seeking treatment and being at risk of their conditions worsening (Rafighi et al., 2016). A study of the relationship between trauma, post-migration problems, and the psychological well-being of migrants (Carswell et al., 2011) showed that health initiatives aimed at this population should address overall well-being, including issues of alienation.

There are several overlaps between the needs of migrant populations and the uses for yoga in health and social care. Increasingly, yoga is being recommended as a suitable, low-cost, high-impact intervention for at-risk communities even though the demographic profile of most yoga practitioners has been found to be middle-class, White women (Biswas, 2012:96). The intersection of these phenomena forms the basis of inquiry for this study. It aims to understand how yoga is taught to mostly non-White migrants in a Western setting, considering the race and class differences between teachers and students, to assess who benefits from those initiatives and to analyze whether the effectiveness of these programs can be accurately measured.

This chapter begins by explaining the theoretical approaches that underpin this study with a particular focus on pedagogy to examine the relationship between teachers and students and how yoga has been taught over time. The case study, which contrasts the approaches of two organizations who offer yoga interventions to migrant communities, will examine the methods and effectiveness of these programs using critical pedagogy, critical race theory (CRT), and the White-saviour industrial complex (WSIC).

Participant observation was conducted between October 2018 and July 2019, at Ourmala, an organization that offers weekly classes to refugees and asylum-seekers concurrent with the academic calendar in London, and the OMPowerment Project, which runs 35-hour yoga leadership training courses for migrants. An emic approach studied yoga as an experience with a range of perceptions and emotions that are difficult to quantify (Sharf, 2000:268). This research aims to describe actions and effects from the perspective of yoga teachers and participants and to humanize the subjects. In so doing, it runs the risk of bias as the researcher becomes part of the calibration process (Sklar 1991:8) which makes self-reflexivity important. As a yoga teacher, a migrant from South Africa, a country with a history of legalized racial segregation, a person of color and a woman, my own background and race and the relationship I had with the organizations may have colored the experiences I had with the organizations and affected my critique.

At both programs, I was involved in trade exchanges in order to gain access to classes and participant interviews. This involved compiling both organizations' Monitoring and Evaluation (M&E) reports for 2019. At Ourmala, I worked with Jordan Royster, an MSc Inequalities and Social Sciences Student at the London School of Economics. The OMPowerment Project allowed me free access to their Facilitation Training, valued at £250, in exchange for my work on the M&E. I also assisted in the planning for their London training session which included securing a venue and recruiting participants.

Ourmala provided a sample size of 53 participants and ten months of class observations, while the OMPowerment Project contained five participants and six days of training. The differences in numbers and time period make an exact comparison between the two organizations difficult, but there is sufficient overlap in their aims and methods to compare their approaches.

Research context and theoretical approaches

In academia, yoga studies are interdisciplinary, with scholars from history, philosophy, anthropology, and biomedical science and other disciplines, as demonstrated by this collection, all contributing to research. This section zones in on recent work which considers the way yoga has been commercialized and sold as a tool of self-governance as well as how it has been taught over time.

The West's interest in the orient and yoga coincided with religion being driven out of the public sphere through the separation of church and state and secular ideals of the Enlightenment. This paved the way for the privatization of faith (Carrette & King, 2005:37). In the 1980s, with global markets deregulated, the term "spirituality," which referred to a non-religious way of being, became aligned with economic demands and corporate consumerism (Carrette & King, 2005:44–45) and yoga was mythologized and mass-marketed (Jain, 2014). The act of self-care was given an elevated status which turned yoga into a technology of the self (Foucault, 1988), a form of governmentality that shifts the responsibility of wellbeing from state and institutional structures onto individuals, who are expected to self-manage and seek constant self-improvement (Godrej, 2017:781). It can be argued that in going through these shifts, yoga has been appropriated, symbolically displaced (Antony, 2018), and commodified.

The race and class barriers to accessing yoga are most widely studied in the United States where the discourse has intensified from White domination to White supremacy. The interlocking forces of orientalism and settler colonialism, a term used to describe the takeover of American land by White settlers who sought to enhance their own wealth and power through the removal of indigenous peoples and their traditions (Blu Wakpa, 2018:2), have resulted in the eclipsing of ethnic minority groups and established Whiteness as the norm. Together, settler colonialism and orientalism uphold White privilege (Blu Wakpa, 2018:4) and create an entitlement that can lead some White people to see their role as to educate and save those they see as less fortunate (Bandyopadhy and Patil, 2017:651–653).

The relationship between teacher (*guru*) and student (*śiṣya*) is key in yoga, as historical evidence shows. In the Classical Indian period transmission of knowledge was oral and the *guru–śiṣya* relationship involved the cohabiting of a teacher with his students. The *guru* instructed his *śiṣya* in moral codes and was also the conduit to the student's exposure to higher consciousness (Raina, 2002:173). In literature, the significance of a teacher for a successful yoga practice can be found in the 17th century *Śivasaṃhitā*, which warns that without a *guru*, a yoga practice can be fruitless and even dangerous (Mallinson and Singleton, 2017:71). The advent of tantric lineages required students to undergo initiation and the *guru's* role was to pass down secret *mantras* to his students. Members of other lineages were not privy to the same *mantras* and this led to competition and hierarchy among *gurus* (Raina, 2002:176). Modern yoga put *gurus* and their followers in a different geographic relationship and eliminated the necessity of personal contact (Singleton and Goldberg, 2013:1). Instead, *gurus* could institutionalize their teachings (Newcombe, 2007) and influence students through certified training programs. Scholarship on the growth of the *guru* industry has looked at those teachers who have created empires, such as Iyengar, who linked his training to adult-education systems in Birmingham, Bikram Choudhry, who attempted to copyright the intellectual property rights for his 26-posture hot yoga sequence (Fish, 2006), and Pattabhi Jois, who continues to have altars dedicated to him in *Aṣṭāṅga* studios despite a sexual abuse scandal (Griswold, 2019). However, these high-profile teachers make up a small minority of the teaching population. Most modern yoga teachers are relatively unknown and their pedagogical practices are largely understudied. It is this type of teacher and their role that this paper will consider.

The literature on yoga pedagogy looks at teaching methods when dealing with specific types of students, such as those over 65 years old (Krucoff et al, 2010) or those in prison (Auty et al, 2015). This work establishes the roles of teachers, for example as "guardians of safety" (Krucoff et al., 2010:899) to older students but does not examine the social relationship between teachers and students. Bourne (2010) studied intercultural teaching in Vedic chanting classes in South India and found that teachers' approaches changed when dealing with Western students, who viewed the class as a commodity, rather than a part of everyday life. In response, the teachers told personal narratives to explain things to Western students in greater detail and provided written copies of the chants, while local students received impersonal teaching and oral transmissions. This study has not been done in yoga. Antony (2016) looked at Western teachers instructing Western students and found that teachers either replaced Sanskrit words with English terms or colloquialisms for ease of understanding or used Sanskrit to try and inspire a deeper understanding of the practice, discussed the physiological benefits of poses, rather than any spiritual aspects of yoga, and varied sequences to avoid boredom and satisfy customer demand. This study demonstrates examples of orientalizing and commodification by both teacher and student. A culturally-adapted Cognitive Behavioural Therapy was trialled with Farsi-speaking refugees from Afghanistan and Iran and proved effective in treating stress and anxiety (Kananian et al, 2017). All of these studies have small sample sizes and limited scope and do not directly address race and culture in yoga.

An exception is Biswas (2012:102), who examined yoga in Prospect Heights in the early 2000s, after the 9/11 attacks and at a time of social disunity as a consequence of gentrification. White privilege was juxtaposed against Black, working-class disadvantage and teachers believed they could facilitate social harmony and healing. This marks a starting point for my work, which seeks to explore the race and class dynamics in more detail.

The way in which yoga is taught to migrants will be examined through the lens of critical pedagogy and CRT, as outlined by Paolo Freire (1970) and Delgado and Stefancic (2001:9–11). Freire's theory of pedagogy divides society into two sectors: the oppressors, who benefit from structural and social inequalities, and the oppressed, who are victims of such constructs. Although Freire initially rejected using race as the basis of this distinction and preferred to use class, he later revised his thoughts and asserted that racism could not be understood without class as a framework (Freire, 1970:14). He considered how the oppressor exerts their ideas onto the oppressed, believing themselves to have the unique power and knowledge to facilitate transformation and regarding the capacity of the oppressed with suspicion (Straubhaar, 2014:382). This leads to the "banking" system of education in which students are seen as empty vessels, into whom information can be deposited. Freire proposes challenging the oppressors' notion of superiority through a critical pedagogy, which involves students' own knowledge and experience.

CRT also hinges on power and traces current inequalities to historical practices of racial exclusion, argues that racism is an ordinary part of life, and looks at how multiculturalism is reduced to a sideshow which avoids addressing issues of social justice. CRT challenges the assertion that Whiteness is the normative standard and seeks to contextualize the lived experiences of people of color, by contesting stereotyping (Taylor, 1998:123). Kimberly Crenshaw's work on intersectionality (1991), which identifies intragroup differences to problematize generalized identity politics, provides a multi-dimensional approach which aims to understand the particular kinds of exclusion faced by individuals.

Finally, Teju Cole, who took CRT further when he coined the phrase White-saviour industrial complex (WSIC) in an article in The Atlantic,[2] provides another layer to unpack race relations. Cole critiqued the ambitions of privileged, White Americans to "make a difference," without doing due diligence by consulting with the people they wanted to assist. He explained the WSIC as overlooking macro-issues such as government policy and structural inequality and simplifying activism to satisfy fantasies of heroism (Cole, 2012).

> The White saviour supports brutal policies in the morning, founds charities in the afternoon and receives awards in the evening. The White Saviour Industrial Complex is not just about justice. It is about having a big emotional experience that validates privilege (Cole, 2012).

By presenting this case study, this chapter aims to understand whether race and class differences between yoga teachers and students influences the way the practice is taught and whether its benefits are fully explored and experienced.

Case study

This case study uses participant observation to examine the work of Ourmala and the OMPowerment Project, both registered charities based in the UK, which offer yoga to migrants. The organizations were selected because of their contrasting pedagogic approaches. Ourmala teaches regular weekly classes during school term-time as an ongoing service for migrants while the OMPowerment Project offers once-off training aimed at equipping migrants with the tools to teach in their own communities. Ourmala was founded in 2011, offers 11 weekly classes in London, and has an established presence in the London refugee community. Participants are referred to Ourmala via their General Practitioner or a third-party organization such as the Red Cross and receive a travel refund on attendance. The OMPowerment Project began in 2017 and has held training sessions in refugee camps in Greece, Palestine, Norway, Myanmar, and Kenya. This was its first project in London. The differences in the organizations were helpful in sourcing more than one method of yoga teaching and understanding the relationship between teachers and students over varying periods of time. This study will look at the content of the organizations' trauma-informed teacher-training modules and their on-the-ground teaching methods. It will also consider participants' experiences through the M&E program of each organization.

Data collection

Data collection took place in six phases between October 2018 and July 2019, as illustrated in Figure 7.1 below. An observation notebook was kept in each phase. All hard copies, including questionnaires and transcripts, are in secure storage and all data has been anonymized.

I performed various, unpaid roles at Ourmala, including administrative assistance at their classes, assistant teaching, and lead teaching. In February 2019, I completed Ourmala's online course, Healing Yoga for Refugees, Asylum-Seekers, and Displaced People and was certified to teach in the Ourmala style. Between April and May 2019, I undertook the M&E process with Ms. Royster

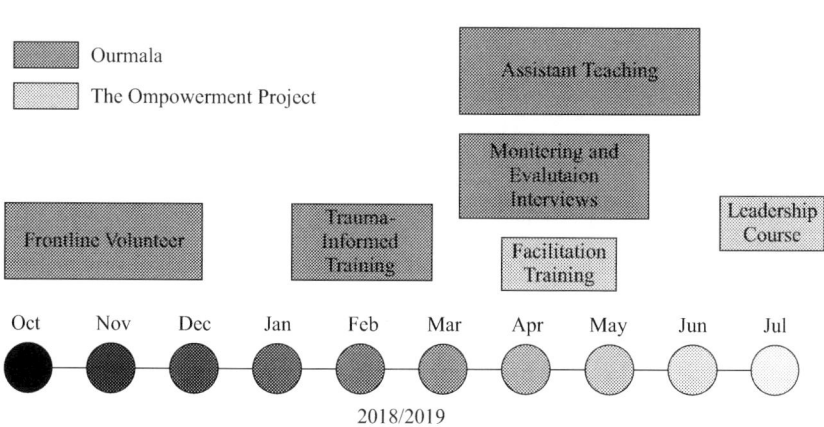

Figure 7.1 Timeline of data collection

which allowed us to gather data for the organization's annual report. To do this, we attended nine of the 11 classes at least twice over a five-week period, conducted questionnaires, observed and participated in classes, and held a focus group. We sent out an online survey for teachers and teaching assistants, in which I did not participate.

The M&E process was underpinned by confidentiality and informed consent. Ourmala's yoga program evaluation questionnaire was designed by CEO Emily Brett and asked participants their level of agreement, from strongly agree to strongly disagree, with 20 statements relating to their physical and mental state and their feelings of social integration before and after a yoga class. These included asking participants whether they felt happy, sad, stressed, relaxed, or lonely. An additional six questions were used to obtain demographic details. I designed a further five-question survey with additional questions about participants' experience of yoga including their self-practice and similarities between yoga and their own culture. All participants were invited to a focus group which was held on May 28, 2019.

I completed the OMPowerment's Facilitation for Trauma and Transformation training online between April and May 2019 and submitted the assignment questions. I worked with CEO Julia Midland to organize the London training session for six days between July 17 and July 29, 2019. Observations took place throughout that period. Participants were asked to fill in a questionnaire based on the Freiberg Mindfulness Inventory (FMI) and Harvard Trauma (HT) Questionnaire before and after the course. On three of the six days, they completed daily mood scales before and after the yoga practice. A focus group was held on the final afternoon.

During the teacher trainings, I made notes on three areas:

- The type of yoga taught
- Language
- Awareness of the role of the teacher and their relationship with students

While attending classes, I recorded observations across four categories:

- Class structure
- Language
- Interactions between teachers and students and among students
- Participant feedback

Sampling

Fifty-three Ourmala participants were involved in the observation period and M&E. Of those, 33 (79.6%) identified as female and 12 (20.4%) as male. Ages ranged from 20 to 69. Eighteen nationalities and seven religious denominations were represented with the biggest group from Eritrea (15 people) and followers of the Greek Orthodox faith and the second largest (12 people) from Bangladesh, and Muslim. The majority of participants, 29, identified as Black (54.7%). There was also Asian, White, Indian, and mixed-race representation across 13 other participants (24.5%).

The OMPowerment Project had five participants, three who identified as female and two as male. Ages ranged from 29 to 60. There were five nationalities represented and two religions with the majority of the participants not following any faith. Four of the five participants identified as Black, and one as White.

Two participants took part in both the Ourmala and the OMPowerment Project studies which brought the total sample size to 56. Of this group, more than half the participants, 31, identified as Black (55.4%) and a further 13 as a race group other than White. The total number of non-White participants was 44 (78.6%). Five participants did not disclose their race and nine others identified as White (16.1%).

The Ourmala teacher survey received responses from nine teachers, three assistant teachers and five people who are both teachers and assistants, totalling 17. I excluded myself from the Ourmala survey because I did not want my own qualitative answers to impact the findings. Of those responders, 16 identified as White. The OMPowerment Project's leadership course is run by a lead teacher, who is White, and one assistant, which was me. In total, 19 teachers and/or assistants were part of this research and of those, 17, or 89.5%, identified as White. I included myself in the overall quantitative demographic statistics because my role as assistant at the OMPowerment Project was significant enough for me to be counted as a member of the teaching group (Figures 7.2–7.8).

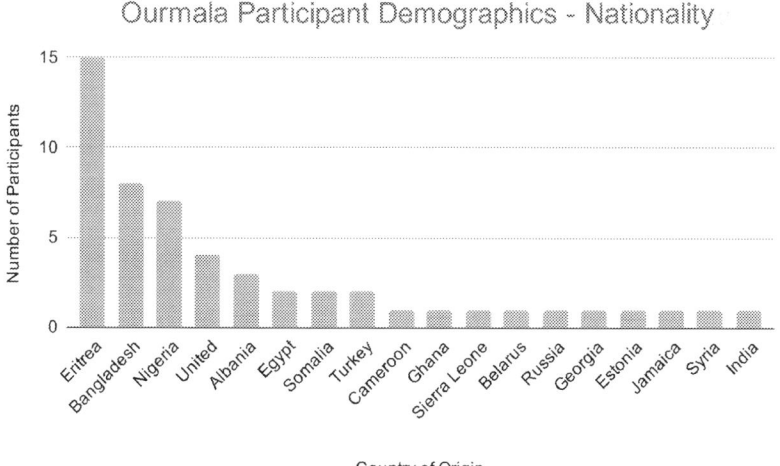

Figure 7.2 Ourmala participant demographics – nationality

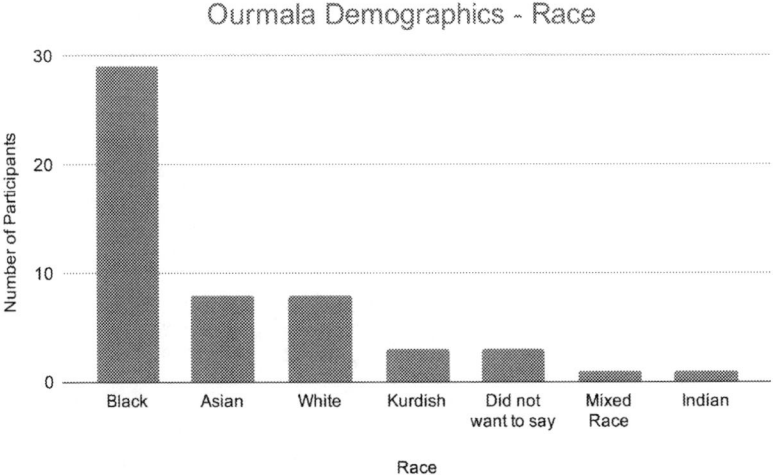

Figure 7.3 Ourmala participant demographics – race

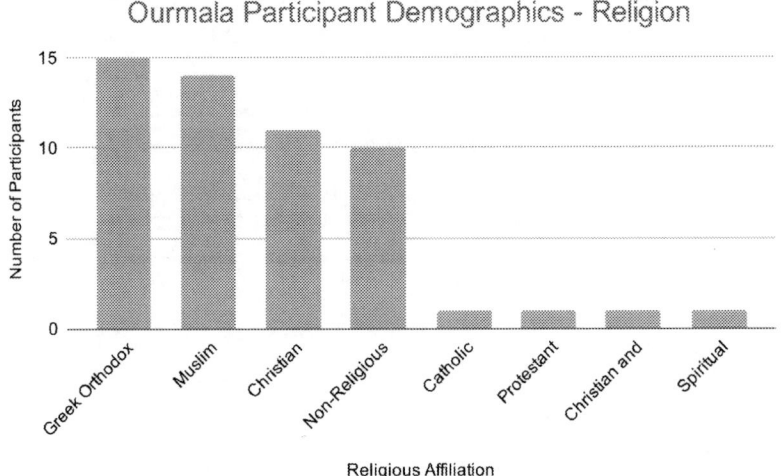

Figure 7.4 Ourmala participant demographics – religion

Pedagogy of movement 91

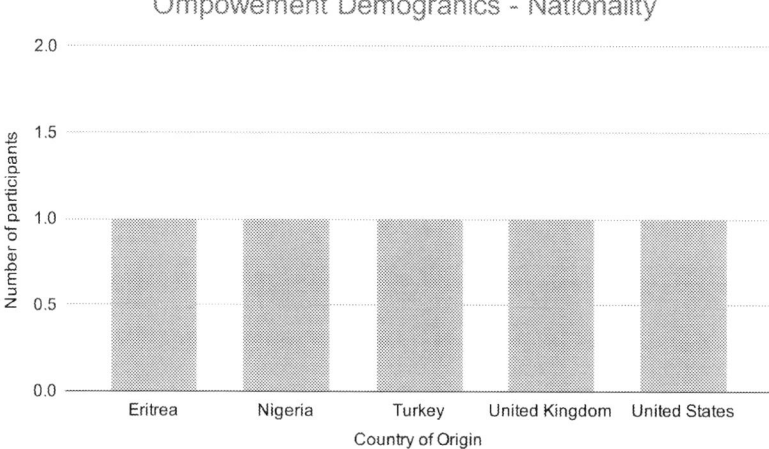

Figure 7.5 OMPowerment participant demographics – nationality

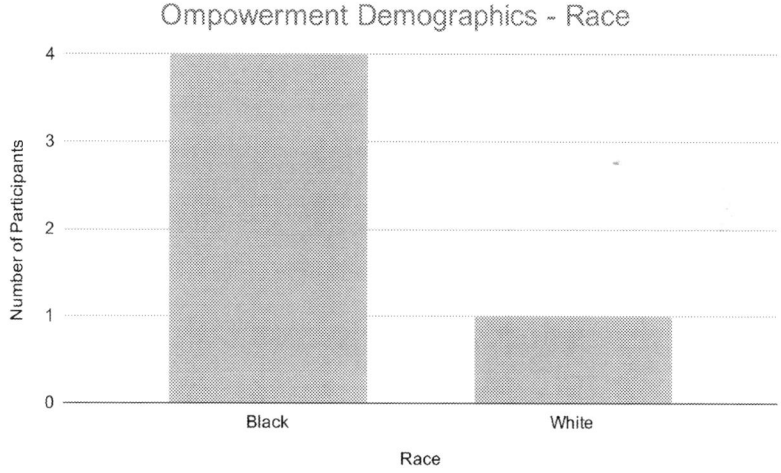

Figure 7.6 OMPowerment participant demographics – race

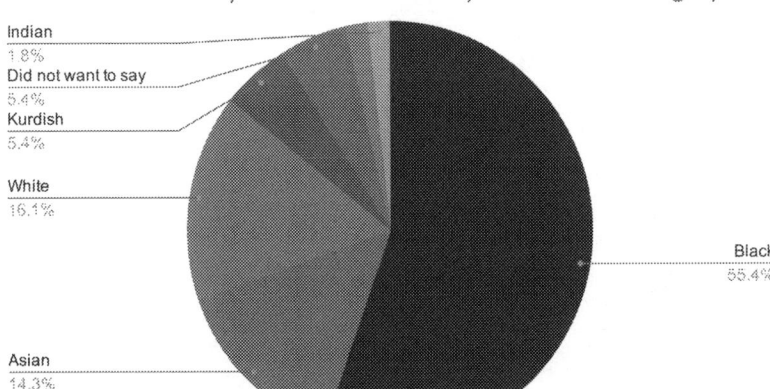

Figure 7.7 Ourmala and OMPowerment – participant race demographics

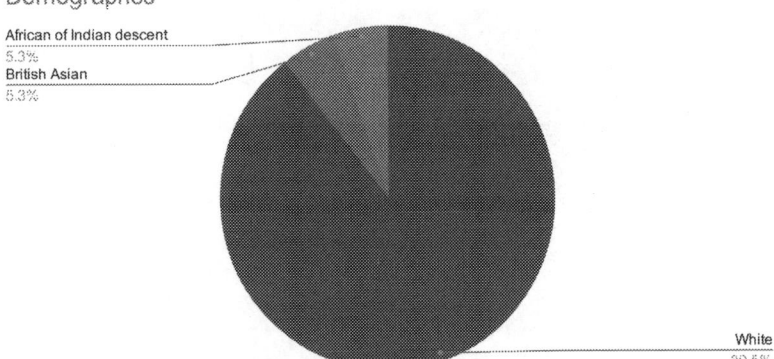

Figure 7.8 Ourmala and OMPowerment – teacher and assistant teacher race demographics

Teacher-training module observations

Ourmala's training consisted of six, 90-minute videos. The bulk of the content dealt with Ourmala's approach to trauma-informed training, based on the work of Dr. Stephen Porges, who conceptualized polyvagal theory to explain the science of trauma.[3] The second session was presented as a yoga class taught in Ourmala-style by Brett. Trainees were required to confirm they had watched each session and complete a short survey in order to be certified.

The OMPowerment Project's training was made up of two streams, each divided into four modules with written material and video content. Four modules focused on self-awareness, two dealt with refugee awareness and the final two with trauma. There were self-enquiry assignment questions for each module, which needed to be submitted before certification.

Admission into either course was open to anyone interested in working with refugees or other at-risk groups.

Ourmala's yoga program combines movement with regulated breathing. They seek consistency of teaching across all their class, based on the *Aṣṭāṅga* primary series and require participants to hold poses for five breaths. Modifications are offered for each pose, including for participants who practice while seated on a chair. Ourmala also claims to offer soft-skills linked to yoga such as discipline through punctuality and has strict rules for latecomers, who are not allowed to enter the class or obtain a travel refund if they are more than 15 minutes late. "This is how our society works. If there is a cultural difference where this is not the case, then it can be really helpful to practice this," Brett said.

The OMPowerment Project teaches self-regulation through tools of grounding, centering, and orienting. This encourages participants to feel connected to the present moment, by feeling the earth beneath their feet, connecting to their core with their hands on their belly, and orienting by looking around the room and picking objects in a particular color or repeating the date and time to create awareness of where they are. Yoga poses are taught through a series of "gateways," which serve as an introduction to a larger repertoire. Participants can move in and out of poses at their own pace and create their own forms of movement. Participants are provided with templates for classes to practice on their own. All classes must end with a final resting pose (*śavāsana)*.

Ourmala's classes should be taught in simple, clear language which steers away from scientific terms to avoid "overwhelming" participants with words. Ourmala also tries to assist participants in learning conversational English. There is an emphasis on pronouns, body parts, and pose names. During the Ourmala-style class, Brett pointed to her toes, wiggled them, and said, "These are my toes." She then pointed to an imaginary participant's toes and said, "Those are your toes," emphasizing the difference between "my," and "your." Ourmala classes should start with the opening chant of the *Aṣṭāṅga* sequence: "*Vande Gurunam Charanaravinde, Sandarshita Svatma Sukava Bodhe."* The direct translation of this is, "I bow to the lotus feet of the supreme *guru*, which awakens insight into the happiness of pure being." However, Ourmala translates it as, "We are here together and we are here as individuals." Brett said the accurate translation was "too abstract" to explain to participants.

The OMPowerment Project facilitation aims to limit command language and offer invitations instead. For example, instead of saying, "Stand at the top of your mat," say, "I invite you to come to the top of your mat." It cautions against alignment cues such as "keep your hips level," which seek to bring the participant into a textbook form of a pose. "Notice how you feel," is an oft-repeated phrase. Metaphorical language is discouraged to ensure cultural sensitivity, because teachers may not be aware of taboo subjects among a particular group of people.

Ourmala asks teachers to reflect on their reasons for teaching in the project and to familiarize themselves with situations which require signposting to other institutions, such as if a participant discloses suicidal thoughts. During a class, Ourmala hands out color-coded consent discs which participants use to indicate if they want to be physically adjusted or not. Participants place the discs next to their mats with their choice, either green for yes or red for no, facing upwards. They are allowed to change their choice at any time during the class

The OMPowerment Project's modules on privilege cover implicit bias and trainees are made to interrogate their own position in terms of race and class. The OMPowerment Project advises teachers not to offer physical adjustments unless expressly asked by a student and to ensure that consent is obtained each time a physical adjustment is provided.

Both programs emphasize the need for teachers working in a trauma-informed environment to prioritize self-care and seek continued mentorship.

Class observations

Nine of Ourmala's 11 weekly classes were observed at least twice each during the M&E process. I also made notes during the classes taught between October and June. The OMPowerment Project was observed in full on the six days it ran between July 17 and 29, 2019. Observations are categorized into class structure, language, interactions, and student feedback.

One of the nine Ourmala classes followed the *Aṣṭāṅga* primary series exactly. The others contained elements of the series and included a warm-up, standing postures, balances, backbends, supine poses, and *śavāsana*. Participants were encouraged to become familiar with a set sequence and repeat that weekly. This proved problematic when the majority of participants at a particular class were observing the *Ramadan* fast, which meant they abstained from food and drink for a period of at least 17 hours but the practice was not modified to accommodate for this. When asked why the teacher said, "We do the same thing every week and that's how it is". Several participants complained of thirst and exhaustion during that month.

The OMPowerment training course was set up across six days which all started with a yoga practice, followed by discussion, pose breakdown, and practice-teaching in which participants taught each other. During the led classes, the facilitator offered several versions of each pose, including the choice not to practice the pose at all and pick another. At first, participants were reluctant to choose anything other than what the facilitator was demonstrating but by the third day, participants made small self-adjustments in the poses. During the practice-teaching sessions, participants initially used the same words they heard in the morning practice but in later sessions, found their own ways of expressing instructions. The words grounding, centering, and orienting were always used.

No Ourmala classes began with the *Aṣṭāṅga* primary series opening chant and at four classes there was no chanting at all. One class included the chant *Om*, which was explained as the "sound of God". A Christian participant at this class had earlier expressed reservation about attending and asked if "God will be angry with me for doing yoga." She was told that yoga was not religious.

In Ourmala classes, teachers spoke louder and slower than they did in regular conversations, especially when using pronouns. Participants were often asked if they remembered pose names and were praised when they did. At one class, the teacher taught participants the names of some muscles and bones, such as biceps or shoulder blade, playfully tested them each week, and complimented those who offered correct answers.

At the OMPowerment Project participants were provided with explanations for words they did not understand such as "resources," which was explained as tools. Invitation language was used to encourage choice.

Ourmala teachers rarely remembered participants' names and often mistook Eritrean participants as being from Ethiopia. All venues except one had an area for participants to socialize if they arrived early. When they did, they sat together. Teachers and assistants greeted participants but seldom sat with them. At one venue, participants were not allowed to enter the studio until a set time, while teachers were let in at any time. On one occasion, participants were made to stand outside in the rain before their allocated entry time. Participants occasionally brought teachers samples of food from their culture, which included *injera* (a flatbread made from Teff flour) from the Eritrean participants and samosas and sweetmeats during *Ramadan* from the Muslim participants.

The OMPowerment Project had a lunch break each day, with food provided for participants. Teachers and participants who chose to stay at the venue during this time always sat together. In casual conversation, participants often complimented the lead teacher's clothing or physical appearance. One participant asked the lead teacher whether her hair was "naturally so beautiful."

A further significant event took place at the end of the 2018 calendar year when Ourmala could no longer offer participants travel refunds based on their postcode. Instead, participants were required to disclose their residential status to determine if they were entitled to a refund. Those with indefinite leave to remain (and therefore access to universal credit) would not be given travel refunds at all while those still seeking asylum could claim refunds to cover the cost of their transport. This resulted in a decrease in class numbers. By April, funding had been secured but refunds were still conditional on residential status. Participants with refugee status were entitled to a £5 refund while asylum-seekers could continue to claim their full travel refund. Class numbers picked up thereafter.

Participant feedback: Ourmala

The Ourmala questionnaire sought to measure whether participants experienced a difference in their physical and mental states and their feelings of social integration after a yoga class. Indicators of mental health were expressed in the statements: depressed, stressed, happy, hopeful, relaxed, anxious/nervous, and confident. Indicators of physical health were indicated as: pain in the body, headache, comfortable in my body, better posture, tired, and strong. Social integration markers were: English is good, have a support network, able to make friends, and isolation/loneliness. Ms. Royster and I recorded participants' responses before and after classes and calculated all reported changes. We found that 90% of participants experienced at least one improvement in an indicator of mental health, 87% in at least one indicator of physical health, and 53% in at least one indicator of social integration. A small percentage, 4%, experienced a decrease in one indicator of mental health, 3% in one indicator of physical health, and none in social integration.

Sixteen participants attended the focus group which was recorded and transcribed. Participants' responses were anonymized. The main topics discussed included reasons for doing yoga, physical and mental health benefits derived from yoga, challenges of coming to class, relationships with teachers, and how yoga relates to participants' cultures.

Participants described several improvements in their health since beginning yoga, including relief from body pain and better sleep, with two participants reporting decreased use of sleeping tablets. Most used the word "calmer," to describe their mental state and thanked the program for allowing them to experience "less stress." A widely agreed benefit was the social aspect, especially because participants spend large amounts of time alone at home.

> "We get to see people. Most of the time, none of us get out of the house."
>
> B.

Travel time and travel costs were cited as the biggest challenges to attending yoga classes. Commutes ranged between 45 minutes and two hours. Some participants asked for an increase in travel refunds, especially for those who only receive £5. This led to a discussion about the disclosure of residential status, which participants found triggering.

> It's embarrassing. As soon as I show my ID card, I can see judgment. I'm scared of going to an office where they ask for my ID. I feel like don't exist. I feel like I don't matter.
>
> A.

A, who identifies as White and is from Albania, is an asylum-seeker and began to cry when this topic came up. She was comforted by several Black, Eritrean participants who said their status as refugees should be an example to A that her situation could change.

All participants asked for more classes and said that the schedule should not be run alongside the school calendar because it broke the rhythm of their practices, especially over the summer holidays which extend for several weeks. K said he found it "takes too long to learn things again."

More than half the participants, 54%, in the survey had a self-practice, but those at the focus group said their efforts to practice at home were irregular and difficult because of lack of space and comfort. H said she tried to go to a public class but, "saw so many young women, fit and beautiful that I got shy and left." D suggested participants practice together in a park but none of the others were willing to because they felt "embarrassed," to do yoga outside. The biggest reason for not being able to practice alone was the absence of a teacher.

> When I don't have a teacher, I can't do it. I come here and I do it here. When I go home, I want to try but there's nobody who says, "do it like this." I try myself but I forget.
>
> L.

Participants' used adjectives such as "kind," "helpful," "supportive," and "amazing," to describe their teachers and acknowledged teachers' expertise.

> "She will teach me how to support my body."
>
> B.

All participants experienced formal yoga for the first time in the UK but said certain poses reminded them of their childhoods. The Eritrean participants demonstrated an activity that they did at ceremonies at home but when asked if they would like to incorporate it into their yoga classes said it was "too silly."

Participant feedback: The OMPowerment Project

The OMPowerment Project's Before and After Questionnaires measured changes in participants' states of mind. The FMI contains 13 statements about current experiences and participants indicated whether they experience those states rarely, occasionally, fairly often, or almost always. The categories in which participants reported the most positive change after the training were "I am able to pause before reacting," and "I feel connected to my experience in the here and now." The HT contains 32 questions which asked participants how often they experience particular emotions or states. Three of the five participants went from experiencing poor sleep "extremely often" before the training to "only a little" after the training and from feeling they had "only a little" capacity to help others before to feeling they could help others "quite a lot" after. The mood scales showed that all five participants felt more awake, energized, and calm after a yoga practice than before.

The focus group was held with all five participants. The main topics discussed were how participants' experiences of yoga had changed over time, what changes they noticed in themselves, comparisons between the OMPowerment Project and other yoga programs, and their plans on completion of the training.

N used the word "strict," to describe her previous experience of yoga while D encountered a "cultural wall with the understanding of what yoga is." M found the yoga she practiced before to be "White and middle-class and genderized as well, just women." Through the OMPowerment Project training, the participants discovered ways to personalize yoga. D said he could "do it in my own way," J felt he was allowed the "freedom to express myself," and M encountered, "different types of people within yoga which has made the practice more open."

The participants reported being more aware of their emotions and reactions and being able to self-regulate by using techniques they had learnt in yoga. M said she had grown "stronger and more resilient," and D said he paid more attention to his responses in situations which made him angry or uncomfortable because it is sometimes "not necessary to vent emotions." H experienced a change in her level of confidence, through learning to teach.

> In the beginning, I was very nervous, but in the middle, I started to teach and I felt confident. This is a big change for me. I have been learning yoga for four years, and I've never done any teaching. Before I just used to copy the teacher, but now I understand the technique.
>
> H.

All participants agreed that the element of teaching was the biggest difference between the OMPowerment Project and other yoga programs they had attended. The combination of participant-led yoga and teacher facilitation impacted J's self-esteem.

> In this environment, you bounce off each other and give each other inner strength. The teachers give you inner strength and make you believe in yourself and your abilities and what you can and can't do.
>
> J.

All participants expressed an interest in teaching in their own communities and in practicing together and assisting each other to improve their teaching skills.

Teacher survey

The link to an online survey was distributed to all Ourmala teachers and teaching assistants. The questions were open-ended, which allowed teachers to write out responses. Seventeen responses were received and the similarity among answers allowed for the results to be categorized into three central themes: reasons for joining Ourmala, challenges of teaching an Ourmala class, and recommendations for improvement.

Eight respondents said they joined Ourmala because it "felt good," to teach yoga to refugees and seven others said they were interested in making yoga accessible to disadvantaged communities. Seven respondents said the language barrier was the most challenging aspect of the role, six that timekeeping and disruptions were problematic, and a further five that they struggled to manage different abilities in a class.

All the teachers and assistants expressed satisfaction and accomplishment after teaching an Ourmala class, using words such as fulfilled, inspired, uplifted, affirmed, invigorated, and grateful to describe how they felt after teaching. When asked if participants had taught them anything, the bulk of teachers' answers included the words resilience, patience, generosity of spirit, and the universality of good values.

Analysis and discussion

The data will be analyzed using Freire's theory of critical pedagogy, CRT, and Cole's extrapolation of WSIC to examine whether there is a power dynamic in teaching yoga to migrants, if this dynamic is racially constructed, and if teachers subscribe to the notion of White-saviorism. Finally, the ability to accurately assess the impact of the yoga programs on participants' overall wellbeing will be considered, taking into account race and class differences.

Applying Freire's division of society, the teachers can be seen as the oppressors and the participants as the oppressed. In pedagogic terms, the oppressors are privileged and believe they have the power to positively impact the oppressed (Straubhaar, 2014:382). By completing a trauma-informed teacher training, albeit with no eligibility criteria or examination requirement to pass, yoga teachers believe they have the knowledge to help migrants. At Ourmala, this knowledge comes from the scientific validation of polyvagal theory, which also leads to the assumption that migrants are, on the whole, trauma-sufferers. While there is some literature to substantiate this (Edwards et al, 2018), it remains generalist and ignores the complex matrices of challenges facing migrants and the barriers they face in accessing yoga. For some participants, religion was a significant barrier to entry, for others, like H, who left a public class because she felt different to other participants, image was a problem, and for several more, who opted not to attend classes when the travel refund policy was changed, there were financial concerns. An intersectional approach (Crenshaw, 1991) would more accurately identify participants' individual needs and could result in a more accessible and flexible yoga program. The OMPowerment Project made attempts to individualize the practice and gave participants' agency through teaching each other but still contained some must-dos. For example, final resting pose must be taken, no matter how long or intensely a participant had practiced. Therefore, yoga in these programs is taught to migrants in a way that follows Freire's banking approach.

This means oppressors establish a paternalistic form of control and do not trust the capacity of the oppressed or believe that they have the resources or knowledge to educate themselves (Straubhaar 2014: 382). The oppressed respond by constantly seeking the approval of the oppressor and downplaying their own skills.

The overall result is the creation of dependency. There is evidence of all this at Ourmala, beginning with the teacher-training's incorrectly translated chant that has been deliberately simplified because of an assumption that the concepts are too complicated for migrants. In practice, this was not done but teachers used other chants. This represents the orientalizing and settler-colonizing of yoga as a way to further reinforce the teachers' advanced knowledge (Blu-Wakpa, 2018). The Ourmala teachers infantilized participants through loud, slow speech and an emphasis on pronouns when teaching the names of body parts, tested participants' knowledge, and showed surprise when participants answered correctly, which both delighted and validated participants. Participants were grateful to teachers and sought their approval through gestures like bringing the teacher food, and dismissed their own practices, such as the Eritrean women who called their jumping, "silly." The participants believed that the teachers knew better, even when it came to participants' own bodies, such as B. Participants expressed dependency on teachers, were "embarrassed" about their own ability, and in L's case, believed they could not practice yoga without a teacher. At the OMPowerment Project, the teacher's role of facilitating healing by providing participants with the tools of self-regulation inferred that the teacher has the key to unlock participants' potential. The participants relied on teachers to instil them with a sense of self-belief, as J said, and even when they began teaching, used particular words they had learnt in the sessions. This also matches Freire's banking-approach to education.

To move to a problem-posing approach, Freire argued that the oppressors must undergo personal transformation (Straubhaar, 2014: 381). This is lacking in Ourmala's teacher-training, which only posed one question about the reasons for wanting to teach in their program and did not seek or critique the answer. The OMPowerment Project's modules on self-enquiry required introspection on a teacher's race, class, and social position but did not offer solutions beyond awareness for how to deal with this when teaching. Therefore, teaching yoga in migrant communities perpetuates a pedagogy of the oppressed with a clear division of power between teachers and students. I will now consider if that divide is racially constructed.

The sample size in the two projects showed that the majority of migrant yoga practitioners were non-White (78.6%) and a greater proportion of yoga teachers were White (89.5%). Even those migrants who identified as White could be considered closer in social status to other migrants than to White teachers, as could be seen in Ourmala's focus group when participants of different races showed solidarity over their residency status. For the most part, there was a racial divide between teachers and students. That would not be a concern if it did not also subscribe to CRT, as will be shown below.

Some aspects of the programs showed an ordinariness of racism in which Whiteness was established as the norm (Taylor, 1998: 123). Ourmala's assumption that participants would not understand the importance of timekeeping because their culture may be different, the lack of effort by teachers to remember names, their frustration with participants' poor English or abilities, and the conflation of people from Eritrea being from Ethiopia, are examples of this. Teachers could be said to view participants as noble savages of sorts, with wholesome values. The words they used to describe what participants taught them such as "generosity of spirit," illustrates this and while it may not appear outwardly negative, it fails to recognize the complexity of participants as multidimensional people. There were also instances of segregation, most glaringly at the venue, where teachers were allowed to enter the room at any time but participants were made to wait outside, but also during social time at other venues when participants and teachers did not mingle. At the OMPowerment Project, a smaller group meant there was less segregation and participants' feelings of inclusion were more widely expressed, but participants were still in awe of teachers, as shown in the comment about a teacher's appearance.

The teacher-student relationships also demonstrated elements of Cole's WSIC. When teachers were asked why they chose to join Ourmala, the majority expressed self interest which resembles Cole's explanation of how "a nobody from America or Europe can go to Africa and become a godlike saviour or, at the very least, have his or her emotional needs satisfied" (Cole, 2012). The answer to the question of who benefits from the program therefore also includes the teachers.

Ultimately, the benefits expressed by participants cannot be discounted. Participant feedback across both projects was overwhelmingly positive. Improved sleep and the socialization were cited as the biggest benefits, but participants experienced several other mental and physical health improvements. What cannot be known without a more scientific approach is how much those benefits can be attributed to yoga and how much is based on the participants' perceptions that yoga works in their best interests. Both programs gave participants the message that they have the power to control their emotions and reactions, and the feedback reflects the participants' desire to prove their success in yoga to their teachers. A more cynical suggestion would be that the feedback was a consequence of participants receiving travel refunds, especially when taking into account the drop in class numbers when the refund policy was changed.

This reality, which reduces participants to an economic underclass, served as the motivation for some teachers to become involved with the program. The teachers viewed the participants as disadvantaged and unable to access yoga, which may be true, but the programs lacked the element of consultation which Cole believes should take place before aid is offered. At best, these programs are a form of WSIC, which creates a program that suits teachers more than students such as Ourmala's term-time only scheduling or both programs' emphasis on teacher self-care; at worst, they could result in an inappropriate and potentially harmful practice such as the classes that took place during *Ramadan*. The OMPowerment Project aimed for more engagement with participants but the duration of its training sessions means this was short-lived. The timing of the training meant it was beyond the timeframe of this study to follow up with The Ompowerment Project participants but future work could examine their methods of teaching and whether they apply oppressive or critical pedagogies. Both programs promote self-responsibility (Godrej, 2017) but do not question the structural inequalities which put participants and other migrants in situations where they cannot rely on institutional support. There was no evidence of teachers protesting against restrictions on immigration, for example, which could, as Cole says, make a real difference.

Conclusion

The surge in the popularity of yoga and its use as a treatment for a range of physical and mental health conditions and the growing number of migrants moving from developing countries to developed ones may not immediately appear to have much in common. However, yoga interventions are increasingly being proposed as inexpensive and holistic ways of treating physical and mental conditions, which migrants are at a greater risk of encountering, and as a means of promoting social integration. This approach does not take into account the culture of modern yoga, a practice which has become dominated by the White middle class. This paper set out to investigate whether that dominance affects the way yoga is taught in two migrant yoga programs in London. It asked who the beneficiaries of such programs are and assessed if race and class differences affect how accurately the success of such yoga programs could be measured.

Critical pedagogy, critical race theory, and the WSIC were used as the framework for this analysis. Data was collected through participant observation of the trauma-informed teacher-training programs at Ourmala and The OMPowerment Project, in regular weekly classes at Ourmala, and in the six-day OMPowerment Project training session. Ourmala's program reinforced teacher superiority and created dependency through an assumption of unique knowledge and the use of language, while The OMPowerment Project promoted agency but transferred responsibility of well-being onto participants. A teacher survey revealed that most Ourmala teachers joined the program for an improved sense of self. Combined with examples of the ordinariness of racism, this showed a perpetuation of the WSIC. The OMPowerment Project aimed to create teachers out of participants but more research needs to be done to know whether this was successful.

Participants' perceptions of their own benefits cannot be ignored and the majority reported improvements in physical and mental health and in their sense of integration but it is difficult to know how much these benefits can be attributed directly to yoga. The relationships between teachers and participants, based on the participants seeking praise and wanting to prove themselves, also makes it difficult to assess the true effectiveness of the yoga program. This does not mean the program lacks efficacy but points to the challenges of measuring human experience. Directions for future research would include follow-ups with The Ompowerment Project participants and studies of yoga interventions among other population groups which could increase our knowledge on cultural relationships and power dynamics in yoga.

Notes

1 The scientifically proven benefits of yoga include gaining flexibility and strength in upper and lower limbs (Sivaramakrishnan et al., 2019), easing neck pain (Allende et al., 2018), back pain (Highland et al., 2018), joint pain associated with arthritis (Middleton et al., 2018), and lowering hypertension (Wolff et al., 2013). Yoga is also effective in reducing stress (Chaoul & Cohen, 2010) and depression, improving poor sleep (Balasubramaniam et al, 2013), treating anxiety (Sharma & Haider, 2013), trauma (van der Kolk, 2014), substance abuse (Khalsa et al., 2008), and increasing psychological wellbeing and behavioural functioning in prison populations (Auty et al, 2015).
2 Cole was responding to a documentary made by Invisible Children Inc about Ugandan rebel leader Joseph Kony, who led the Lord's Resistance Army. The film was part of a campaign to have Kony arrested.
3 Polyvagal theory refers to the branches of the vegas nerve which connects organs including the brain, heart, lungs, and intestines, and shows the connection between reactions in the body to social experiences. It provides an understanding of the "biology of safety and danger" (van der Kolk, 2014:78) and suggests ways of self-regulating.

Bibliography

Alexander, G., Innes, K.E., Bourguignon, C., Bovbjerg, V.E., Kulbok, P. and Taylor, A.G. (2012). Patterns of yoga practice and physical activity following a yoga intervention for adults with or at risk for type 2 diabetes. *Journal of Physical Activity and Health*, 9, pp.53–61.
Allende, S., Anandan, A., Lauche, R. and Cramer, H. (2018). Effect of yoga on chronic non-specific neck pain: An unconditional growth model. *Complementary Therapies in Medicine*, 40, pp.237–242.
Alter, J. (2004). *Yoga in Modern India: The Body Between Philosophy and Science*. Princeton: Princeton University Press.
Antony, M. (2016). Tailoring nirvana: Appropriating yoga, resignification and instructional challenges. *International Journal of Media & Cultural Politics*, 12(3), pp.283–303.
Antony, M. (2018). That's a stretch: Reconstructing, rearticulating, and commodifying yoga. *Frontiers in Communication*, 3, pp.1–12.
Askegaard, S. and Eckhardt, G. (2012). Glocal yoga: Re-appropriation in the Indian consumptionscape. *Marketing Theory*, 12(1), pp.45–60.
Auty, K., Cope, A. and Liebling, A. (2015). A systematic review and meta-analysis of yoga and mindfulness meditation in prison. *International Journal of Offender Therapy and Comparative Criminology*, 61(6), pp.689–710.
Balasubramaniam, M., Telles, S. and Doraiswamy, P.M. (2013). Yoga on our minds: A systematic review of yoga for neuropsychiatric disorders. *Frontiers in Psychiatry*, 3, pp.1–16. doi:10.3389/fpsyt.2012.00117
Bandyopadhyay, R. and Patil, V. (2017). 'The white woman's burden' – the racialized, gendered politics of volunteer tourism. *Tourism Geographies*, 19(4), pp.644–657.
Barrett, C. (2016). Mindfulness and rehabilitation: Teaching yoga and meditation to young men in an alternative to incarceration program. *International Journal of Offender Therapy and Comparative Criminology*, 61(15), pp.1719–1738.

Bilderbeck, A.C., Farias, M., Brazil, I.A., Jakobowitz, S. and Wikholm, C. (2013). Participation in a 10-week course of yoga improves behavioural control and decreases psychological distress in a prison population. *Journal of Psychiatric Research*, 47, pp.1438–1445. doi:10.1016/j.jpsychires.2013.06.014

Birch, J. (2011). Meaning of haṭha in early haṭhayoga. *Journal of the American Oriental Society*. 131(4). pp.527–554.

Biswas, P. (2012). Social sutra: Yoga, identity, and health in New York's changing neighborhoods. *Health, Culture and Society*, 3(1), pp.95–111.

Blu Wakpa, T. (2018). Decolonizing yoga? and (Un)settling social justice. *Race and Yoga*, 3(1), pp.1–19.

Bogic, M.M, et al. (2012). Factors associated with mental disorders in long-settled war refugees: Refugees from the former Yugoslavia in Germany, Italy and the UK. *British Journal of Psychiatry*, 200(3), pp.216–223.

Bourne, J. (2010). Pedagogic practice, culture and the globalization of yoga teaching. *Journal of Applied Linguistics and Professional Practice*, 7(1), pp.11–26.

Bowers, H. and Cheer, J. (2017). Yoga tourism: Commodification and western embracement of eastern spiritual practice. *Tourism Management Perspectives*, 24, pp.208–216.

Burnett-Zeigler, I., Schuette, S., Victorson, D. and Wisner, K. (2016). Mind–body approaches to treating mental health symptoms among disadvantaged populations: A comprehensive review. *Journal of Alternative and Complementary Medicine*, 22(2), pp.115–124.

Carrette, J. and King, R. (2005). *Selling Spirituality: The Silent Takeover of Religion*. London: Routledge.

Carswell, K., et al. (2011). The relationship between Trauma, post-migration problems and the psychological well-being of refugees and Asylum seekers. *International Journal of Social Psychiatry*, 57(2) pp.107–119.

Chaoul, M. and Cohen, L. (2010). Rethinking yoga and the application of yoga in modern medicine. *CrossCurrents*, 60(2), pp.144–167.

Cole, T. (2012). The white-savior industrial complex. *Atlantic*. Available at: https://www.theatlantic.com/international/archive/2012/03/the-white-savior-industrial-complex/254843/ [Accessed 6 Sep. 2019].

Cramer, H., Ward, L., Steel, A., Lauche, R., Dobos, G. and Zhang, Y. (2016). Prevalence, patterns, and predictors of yoga use. *American Journal of Preventive Medicine*, 50(2), pp.230–235.

Crenshaw, K. (1991). Mapping the margins: Intersectionality, identity politics, and violence against women of color. *Stanford Law Review*, 43(6), p.1241.

Danylchuk, L. (2019). *Yoga for Trauma Recovery*. New York: Routledge.

De Michelis, E. (2004). *History of Modern Yoga*. London: Continuum.

Delgado, R., and Stefancic, J. (2001). *Critical Race Theory: An Introduction*. New York: New York University Press.

Duffield, M. (2005). Getting savages to fight barbarians: Development, security and the colonial present. *Conflict, Security & Development*, 5(2), 141–159.

Edwards, J., Anderson, K. and Stranges, S. (2018). Migrant mental health, Hickam's dictum, and the dangers of oversimplification. *International Journal of Public Health*, 64(4), pp.477–478.

Eliade, M. (1969). *Yoga: Immortality and Freedom*. Princeton: Princeton University Press.

Factor-Litvak, P., Cushman, L., Kronenberg, F., Wade, C. and Kalmuss, D. (2001). Use of complementary and alternative medicine among women in New York City: A pilot study. *Journal of Alternative and Complementary Medicine*, 7(6), pp.659–666.

Field, T. (2011). Yoga clinical research review. *Complementary Therapies in Clinical Practice*, 17, pp 1–8. doi:10.1016/j.ctcp.2010.09.007

Fish, A. (2006). The commodification and exchange of knowledge in the case of transnational commercial yoga. *International Journal of Cultural Property*, 13(2), pp.189–206.

Foo, S., Tam, W., Ho, C., Tran, B., Nguyen, L., McIntyre, R. and Ho, R. (2018). Prevalence of depression among migrants: A systematic review and meta-analysis. *International Journal of Environmental Research and Public Health*, 15(9), p.1986.

Foucault, M. (1988). Technologies of the self. In L.H. Martin, H. Gutman and P.H. Hutton, eds., *Technologies of the Self: A Seminar with Michel Foucault*. Amherst: University of Massachusetts Press: 16–49.

Freire, P. (1970). *Pedagogy of the Oppressed*. London: Continuum.

Gallup Inc. (2019). Gallup 2019 global emotions report. *Gallup.com*. Available at: https://www.gallup.com/analytics/248906/gallup-global-emotions-report-2019.aspx [Accessed 6 Sep. 2019].

Gandhi, S. (2017). Yoga in popular culture. *Religion and Popular Culture in America*, Third Edition, 3(1), pp. 337–350.

Ganpat, T. and Nagendra, H. (2012). Integrated yoga therapy for improving mental health in managers. *Industrial Psychiatry Journal*, 20(1), p.45.

Godrej, F. (2017). The neoliberal yogi and the politics of yoga. *Political Theory*, 45(6), pp.772–800.

Griswold, E. (2019). Yoga reconsiders the role of the guru in the age of #metoo. *New Yorker*. Available at: https://www.newyorker.com/news/news-desk/yoga-reconsiders-the-role-of-the-guru-in-the-age-of-metoo?fbclid=IwAR3olkE--d6sH3deAUxsSDyFxq390w1EMnLgmLaMJpalyQ77Tju3aTWjRz0 [Accessed 25 Jul. 2019].

Highland, K., Schoomaker, A., Rojas, W., Suen, J., Ahmed, A., Zhang, Z., Carlin, S., Calilung, C., Kent, M., McDonough, C. and Buckenmaier, C. (2018). Benefits of the restorative exercise and strength training for operational resilience and excellence yoga program for chronic low back pain in service members: A pilot randomized controlled trial. *Archives of Physical Medicine and Rehabilitation*, 99(1), pp.91–98.

Hinton, D.E., Rivera, E.I., Hofmann, S.G., Barlow, D.H. and Otto, M.W. (2012). Adapting CBT for traumatized refugees and ethnic minority patients: Examples from culturally adapted CBT (CA-CBT). *Transcultural Psychiatry*, 49(2), pp.340–365. doi:10.1177/1363461512441595

Hunyadi, B. and Molnár, C. (2016). Central Europe's faceless strangers: The rise of xenophobia in the region. *Freedomhouse.org*. Available at: https://freedomhouse.org/report/special-reports/central-europe-s-faceless-strangers-rise-xenophobia-region#.XXIHFZNKhZ0 [Accessed 6 Sep. 2019].

IOM (2015). Irregular migrant, refugee arrivals in Europe top one million in 2015: IOM. *International Organization for Migration*. Available at: https://www.iom.int/news/irregular-migrant-refugee-arrivals-europe-top-one-million-2015-iom [Accessed 7 Sep. 2019].

Jain, A. (2014). *Selling Yoga: From Counter-Culture to Pop Culture*. New York: Oxford University Press.

Kananian, S., Ayoughi, S., Farugie, A., Hinton, D. and Stangier, U. (2017). Transdiagnostic culturally adapted CBT with Farsi-speaking refugees: A pilot study. *European Journal of Psychotraumatology*, 8(1390362), pp.1–10.

Karmalkar, S. and Vaidya, A. (2017). Effects of classical yoga intervention on resilience of rural-to-urban migrant college students. *Indian Journal of Positive Psychology*, 8(3), pp.429–434.

Khalsa, S., Khalsa, G., Khalsa, H. and Khalsa, M. (2008). Evaluation of a residential kundalini yoga lifestyle pilot program for addiction in India. *Journal of Ethnicity in Substance Abuse*, 7(1), pp.67–79.

Koch, A. (2014). Competitive charity: A neoliberal culture of 'giving back' in global yoga. *Journal of Contemporary Religion*, 30(1), pp.73–88.

Kothari, U. (2006). Critiquing "race" and racism in development discourse and practice. *Progress in Development Studies*, 6(1), pp.1–9.

Krucoff, C., Carson, K., Peterson, M., Shipp, K. and Krucoff, M. (2010). Teaching yoga to seniors: Essential considerations to enhance safety and reduce risk in a uniquely vulnerable age group. *Journal of Alternative and Complementary Medicine*, 16(8), pp.899–905.

Mallinson, J. (2014). Haṭha Yoga. *Brill Encyclopedia of Hinduism*, 3, pp.770–781.

Mallinson, J. and Singleton, M. (2017). *Roots of Yoga*. London: Penguin.

Markula, P. (2004). "Tuning into One's Self:" Foucault's technologies of the self and mindful fitness. *Sociology of Sport Journal*, 21(3), pp.302–321.

McCall, M. (2014). In search of yoga: Research trends in a western medical database. *International Journal of Yoga*, 7(1), p.4.

McCartney, P. (2019). Spiritual bypass and entanglement in Yogaland (योग तान): How neolberalism, soft hindutva and banal nationalism facilitate yoga fundamentalism. *Politics and Religion*, XIII(1), pp.137–175.

Middleton, K., Ward, M., Haaz Moonaz, S., Magaña López, M., Tataw-Ayuketah, G., Yang, L., Acevedo, A., Brandon, Z. and Wallen, G. (2018). Feasibility and assessment of outcome measures for yoga as self-care for minorities with arthritis: A pilot study. *Pilot and Feasibility Studies*, 4(1).

Morgan, G., Melluish, S. and Welham, A. (2017). Exploring the relationship between postmigratory stressors and mental health for Asylum seekers and refused Asylum seekers in the UK. *Transcultural Psychiatry*, 54(5–6), pp.653–674.

Newcombe, S. (2007). Stretching for health and well-being: Yoga and women in Britain, 1960–1980. *Asian Medicine*, 3(1), pp.37–63.

Newcombe, S. (2009). The development of modern yoga: A survey of the field. *Religion Compass* 3(6): 986–1002.

Newcombe, S. (2017). The revival of yoga in contemporary India. In: J. Barton ed. *Oxford Research Encyclopedias: Religion*. Oxford: Oxford University Press, pp. 1–55.

Palbag, S. (2018). Integration of yoga in modern healthcare system: A dream to reality. *BLDE University Journal of Health Sciences*, 3, (1). pp.9–11.

Pandya, S. (2016). Millenarianism and yoga: A spiritual approach to mental health. *Journal of Spirituality in Mental Health*, 19(2), pp.151–168.

Pratap Singh, A. (2017). Yoga for mental health: Opportunities and challenges. *MOJ Yoga & Physical Therapy*, 2(1), pp. 1–6.

Pumariega, A., Rothe, E. and Pumareiga, J.B. (2005). Mental health of immigrants and refugees. *Community Mental Health Journal*, 41(5), pp.581–597.

Rafighi, E., Poduval, S., Legido-Quigley, H. and Howard, N. (2016). National health service principles as experienced by vulnerable London migrants in 'Austerity Britain': A qualitative study of rights, entitlements, and civil-society advocacy. *International Journal of Health Policy Management*, 5(10), pp.589–597.

Raina, M. (2002). Guru-Shishya relationship in Indian culture: The possibility of a creative resilient framework. *Psychology and Developing Societies*, 14(1), pp.167–198.

Rogers, R.A. (2006). From cultural exchange to transculturation: A review and reconceptualization of cultural appropriation. *Communication Theory*, 16(4), pp.474–503.

Ross, A., Friedmann, E., Bevans, M. and Thomas, S. (2013). National survey of yoga practitioners: Mental and physical health benefits. *Complementary Therapies in Medicine*, 21(4), pp.313–323.

Samuel, G. (2008). *The Origins of Yoga and Tantra: Indic Religion to the Thirteenth Century*. Cambridge: Cambridge University Press.

Selkirk, M., Quayle, E. and Rothwell, N. (2014). A systematic review of factors affecting migrant attitudes towards seeking psychological help. *Journal of Health Care for the Poor and Underserved*, 5(1), pp.94–127.

Sharf, R. (2000). The rhetoric of experience and the study of religion. *Journal of Consciousness Studies*, 7(11–12), pp.267–287.

Sharma, M. and Haider, T. (2013). Yoga as an alternative and complementary therapy for patients suffering from anxiety: A systematic review. *Journal of Evidence-Based Complementary & Alternative Medicine*, 18, pp.15–22. doi:10.1177/2156587212460046

Shetty, A. (2016). Yoga as physical therapy intervention and future direction for yoga research. *Journal of Yoga & Physical Therapy*, 6(2).

Singleton, M. (2007). Suggestive therapeutics: New thought's relationship to modern yoga. *Asian Medicine*, 3(1), pp.64–84.

Singleton, M. (2010). *Yoga Body The Origins of Modern Posture Practice*. Oxford: Oxford University Press.

Singleton, M. and Goldberg, E. (2013). *Gurus of Modern Yoga*. Oxford: Oxford University Press.

Sivaramakrishnan, D., Fitzsimons, C., Kelly, P., Ludwig, K., Mutrie, N., Saunders, D. and Baker, G. (2019). The effects of yoga compared to active and inactive controls on physical function and health related quality of life in older adults- systematic review and meta-analysis of randomised controlled trials. *International Journal of Behavioral Nutrition and Physical Activity*, 16(1).

Sklar, D. (1991). On dance ethnography. *Dance Research Journal*, 23(1), pp.6–10.

Straubhaar, R. (2014). The stark reality of the 'White Saviour' complex and the need for critical consciousness: A document analysis of the early journals of a Freirean educator. *Compare: A Journal of Comparative and International Education*, 45(3), pp.381–400.

Strauss, S. (2005). *Positioning Yoga Balancing Acts Across Cultures*. Oxford: Berg.

Taylor, E. (1998). A primer on critical race theory. *The Journal of Blacks in Higher Education*, 19, pp.122–124.

The Good Body. (2018). Yoga statistics: Staggering growth shows ever-increasing popularity. *The Good Body*. Available at: https://www.thegoodbody.com/yoga-statistics/ [Accessed 6 Sep. 2019].

Trilling, D. (2019). How the media contributed to the migrant crisis. *Guardian*. Available at: https://www.theguardian.com/news/2019/aug/01/media-framed-migrant-crisis-disaster-reporting [Accessed 6 Sep. 2019].

United Nations, Department of Economic and Social Affairs, Population Division (2017). International Migration Report 2017: Highlights(ST/ESA/SER.A/404).

Van der Kolk, B. (2014). *The Body Keeps the Score: Brain, Mind, and Body in the Healing of Trauma*. New York: Penguin Group.

White, D.G. ed. (2012). *Yoga in Practice. Princeton Readings in Religions*. Princeton: Princeton University Press.

Wolff, M., Sundquist, K., Larsson Lönn, S. and Midlöv, P. (2013). Impact of yoga on blood pressure and quality of life in patients with hypertension – a controlled trial in primary care, matched for systolic blood pressure. *BMC Cardiovascular Disorders*, 13(1).

Chapter 8

White hygiene, White womanhood, and wellness in the United States

Rumya S. Putcha

In December 2018, actress and lifestyle influencer Gwyneth Paltrow made headlines after she seemed to suggest that she was responsible for popularizing yoga as a wellness activity in the United States. "Forgive me if this comes out wrong," Paltrow demurred, "but I went to do a yoga class in L.A. recently and the 22-year-old girl behind the counter was like, 'Have you ever done yoga before?' And literally I turned to my friend, and I was like, 'You have this job because I've done yoga before.'"

Paltrow's self-aggrandizing response isn't completely wrong; for more than a decade, she has built a personal brand by urging other White women to eat, exercise, and live exactly as she does. She's among a group of White well-to-do women who have made self-help and "wellness" into a highly individualistic and often unethical billion-dollar industry of aspiration. A minute or two spent browsing Goop.com offers a window into Paltrow's vision of health: One can purchase a wide variety of luxury lifestyle products including a $15,000 gold dildo (now marked down to $11,500) and an $80 crystal-infused water bottle. One of the most popular items on the site is a dietary supplement dubbed "High School Genes"; priced at $90 for a 30-day supply, it's billed as a "comprehensive nutritional regimen designed to provide intense support for normal glucose and energy metabolism, as well as cellular health."

Goop also offers advice columns on sexual health, in many cases suggesting diets or enhancements that are not only prohibitively expensive, but also run directly counter to medical advice.[1] Goop's questionable and often irresponsible recommendations, which are now available through a Netflix series, The Goop Lab, have earned Paltrow consistent criticism for years, but she has stood firm, insisting that her exorbitantly priced products are simply an opportunity for consumers to exercise "autonomy over their health." Paltrow's ongoing success typifies the North American and neoliberal capitalist belief in health as a personal, individualistic enterprise – a consumer experience that can be bought, sold, and of course promoted on social media platforms, like Instagram. It's a symptom of the same phenomenon that in recent decades has fueled everything from anti-vaccine propaganda to essential-oil proselytizers to yoga and mindfulness devotees. This attitude toward health is deeply narcissistic, of course, and it is also dangerous.

White hygiene and White womanhood

In this article, I focus on the rise of yoga and mindfulness industries, also known euphemistically as "self-care" or "wellness" cultures within the context of the United States. Drawing on over a decade of ethnographic work in commercial yoga studios in Chicago, Boston, and Houston, I interrogate the imperatives of health alongside the racialized and gendered definitions of beauty (see Prasad 2015, Aizura 2009). Within this frame, I examine how and why yoga bodies have become synonymous with White women and their wellness. Rather than seeing the successes of yoga industries as coterminous with liberatory work, I argue that such assemblages reveal the most recent adaptation of White hygiene, a mechanism by which White hegemony and its reliance on White woman's purity remains intact in 21st century Euro-American settings. Below, I will first lay out a brief history of White hygiene in relation to the beauty and fitness industries and then connect this legacy to the larger gendered dynamics of health and wellness cultures in the United States.

One could easily argue that Paltrow is far from the first celebrity to introduce the United States to the individualistic, cost-prohibitive, and beauty-centered idea of health that yoga industries typify. As soon as product endorsements and cheap print media existed, so did a steady stream of wealthy White women – celebrities – whose bodies and therefore whose health or fitness routines inspired the masses, or at least those who could afford it. One of the earliest celebrities to endorse yoga-for-health, for example, was Norma Jean Mortenson, better known as Marilyn Monroe, who is said to have credited yoga-inspired exercise routines for her much-admired physique (see Figure 8.1).

The earliest examples of aspirationally fit women's bodies emerged well before Monroe, though, in the early 20th century, where the influence of film culture and modern dance elevated dancing female bodies from the entertainment realms of vaudeville and burlesque (see Srinivasan 2007). No longer base and bawdy, dance in colonial-cosmopolitan spaces like New York, London, and Paris was now art performed by well-bred White women like Ruth St. Denis and Louise Brooks – and in many cases it was an art built upon racist and Orientalist themes, often involving dancers who appeared in black- or brownface (see Figure 8.2).

These dancers were also among the first to introduce consumer forms of exercise and fitness to the US, notably in Los Angeles. This is the circuit that brought us Jane Fonda in the 1970s to 1980s, Suzanne Somers in the 1990s, and today, Gwyneth Paltrow. In other words, there is a long, complicated history behind the sexualized construction of healthy womanhood through White bodies – the primary mechanism by which White hygiene is made material. This history stretches from early dancer-actress-icons like Joan Crawford through the housewives looking to "relax" in the postwar era (see Figure 8.3), to the insta-yogis we see today. And as many historians have noted, this assemblage constructs clear connections between hygiene and sanitation within the home and White women's bodies (see Simmons 1993).

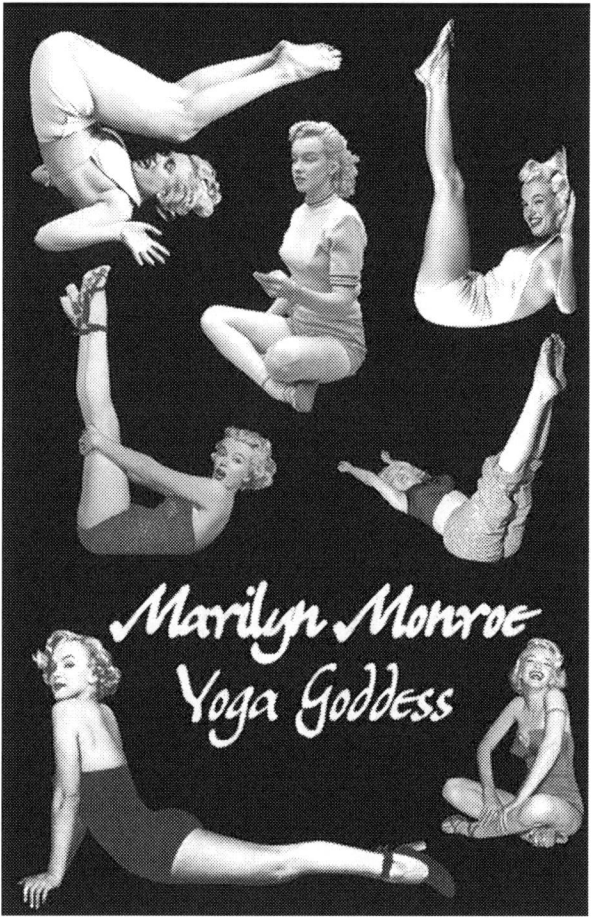

Figure 8.1 Promotional photographs of Marilyn Monroe, 1948.

After *Eat, Pray, Love*

Recent wellness fads, however, aren't necessarily the result of celebrity exercise regimens or the media-fed desire for a "hot" body. In many ways, the 2006 bestselling self-help novel/travel diary by Elizabeth Gilbert, *Eat, Pray, Love*, popularized a way of living that has since come to shape notions of beauty, health, and practices of womanhood in the US context. Joining a larger body of work set in the global South in the post-9/11 era, the memoir particularly valorized yoga, but also alternative forms of medicine and "self-care" as a means by which White women could "find themselves" as well as claim their sexuality outside of the confines of marriage. Feminist scholars like Shefali Chandra

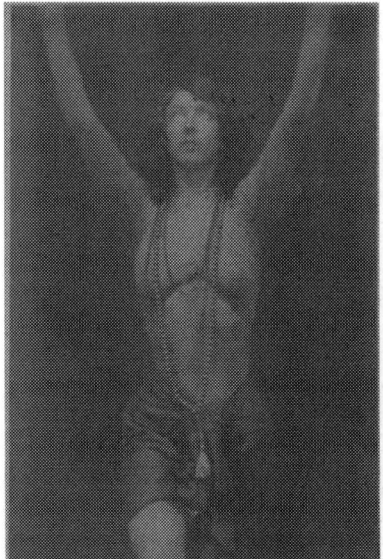 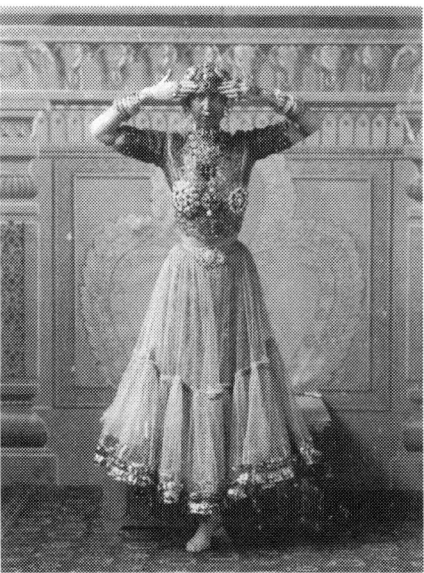

Figure 8.2 Ruth St. Denis performing in brownface in Yogi (1911) and Nautch (1908) debuted in Vienna. Courtesy New York Public Library.

have noted the capitalist and imperialist logics at the heart of such engagements; "Skillfully navigating between twentieth-century imperial history, the rise of the War on Terror, and a barely contained obsession with Hindu female sexuality, each of these texts is driven by the conviction that India, and Indian women, will heal the mind and body of the white woman. India enables the American woman to cure herself" (Chandra 2014, 488). *EPL* was the book that launched the yoga-as-exercise craze – aided and abetted by North American athleisure brands like Lululemon – repackaging an old Orientalist tale of White folks traveling to formerly colonized places, consistently framed as "dirty," to rejuvenate, feel sexy, and learn tolerance, but always on their terms, of course (see also Craik 2020).

Since the advent of Instagram celebrity/influencer culture, this is the logic of leisure-wellness that underscores the steady onslaught of Instagram posts under the tags #selfcare, and which for all intents and purposes has demonstrated that black- or brownface no longer requires face paint, just the vapid excuse of "good intentions" backed by all the monetary advantages of whiteness. In many ways, this is how health and wellness for White women operates as an extension of White hygiene, today often occluded by the reductive logics of "cultural appropriation." These are the social mechanisms which brought us preternaturally fit, "yogini" Madonna during her Ray of Light phase and today positions women like Paltrow as heir apparent to the racial power dynamics that encourage White women to embrace self-indulgent consumer-driven ignorance and call it "enlightenment."

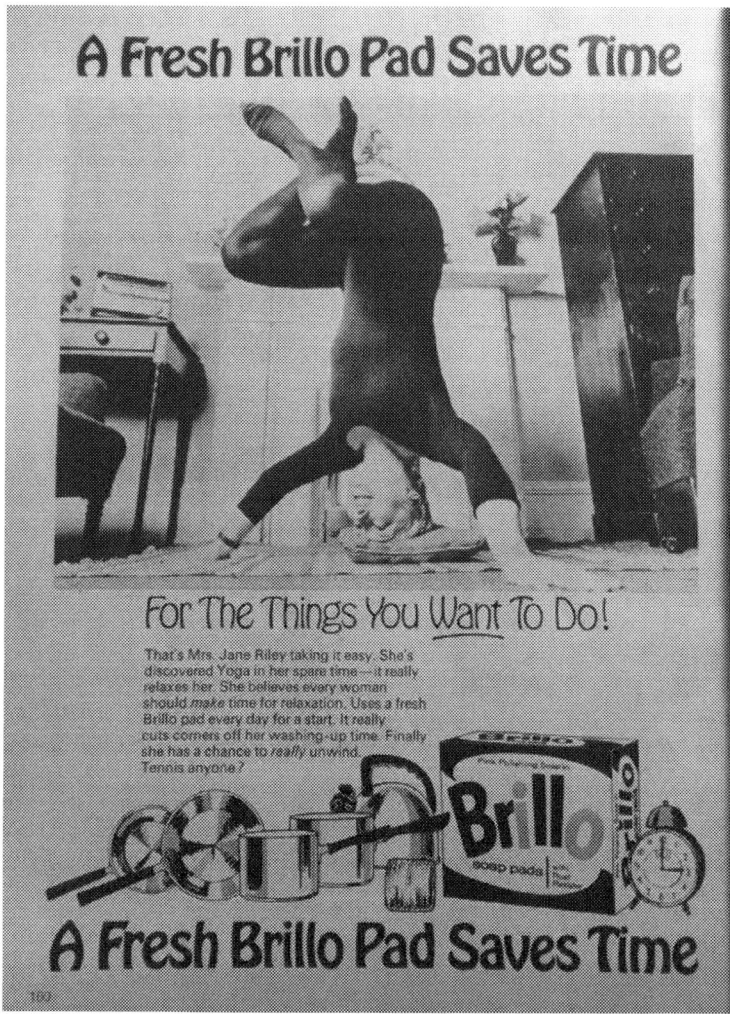

Figure 8.3 Brillo advertisement, 1968.

Whiteness and wellness in the United States

Claims to wellness or self-care as something that can be bought or sold, taken on or off at will exposes the nefarious logics of American imperialism and its narcissistic impulses. Furthermore, when aligned with so-called women's issues, like access to healthcare, claims to feminism tend to excuse impact and instead center intentions. This mechanism, by which White women are taught to see themselves as perfect victims in turn feeds the self-centered and neoliberal rhetoric of "my best interest at any cost." This is what some feminists have theorized as imperial feminism – a recognition that "white, Eurocentric [women] have sought to establish [themselves] as the only legitimate [form of] feminism" (Amos and Parmar 2005, 44). Put another way, the mechanisms by which "White women wellness" operates in the 21st century is just the latest iteration of imperialist thought by which White women capitalize on their racial privilege to get their own needs met, and in the process, uphold the very White hegemonic patriarchy that plagues our society at large.

If you have been following the conversation on wellness trends and its target demographics, the data is unequivocal: economically privileged women in the U.S., White women, turn to performative wellness trends, like yoga, to participate in the production of an elitist womanhood through Orientalist escapism and virtue-signaling, most notably in contemporary settings like social media (see Birdee et al. 2008 and Park et al. 2015). However, there's a darker, less apparent outcome for this trend: Keeping in mind underreporting rates among populations that lack access to adequate healthcare and especially mental healthcare, recent studies (see Smith et al. 2015) have suggested a link between affluence and personality disorders. In other words, yoga and its related practices have arguably become a wellness activity wealthy White women turn to in order to cope with mental health. This new finding is puzzling – indeed, it is hard to separate cause from result at the moment, that is, are more wealthy White women experiencing mental health issues because of the pressure to conform to unattainable body image standards? Or are we simply hearing more about mental health epidemics in this demographic because our society is more attuned to wealthy White woman wellness needs? The answer is likely "both."

Instagram and its influencers clearly capitalize on the aspirational aspects of the fad by selling the idea that participation in yoga not only improves mental health, but also, paradoxically, offer followers and consumers a sense of individuality. For example, a common phrase among White women who participate in commercial yoga industries is that it has helped them "find themselves" and "accept" their bodies. However, this is the same fitness culture that has borne witness to unprecedented rates of eating disorders, including a new diagnosis known as "orthorexia nervosa" – an obsession with eating healthy or "clean." Despite the supposed logic of self-love and acceptance, yoga cultures appear to be engendering new and dangerous forms of conceit and controlling tendencies.

To this point, studies on yoga often note the incongruous logic that seems to underpin White women's attachment to fitness trends like yoga – a logic that reveals that the "love and acceptance" attitudes are quite superficial and even destructive. Indeed, in yoga studios, one can observe that White women's claims are not about acceptance, but rather a desire for a "safe space" – a euphemism for homosociality – a recognition that women feel less safe when men are present and that White folks feel safer around other Whites. Many White women describe feeling safer around other White women, but can't quite reconcile how their sense of safety relies on exclusionary and often structural forms of inequity.

A case study from my ethnographic research in Texas offers a useful example: In response to learning that her suburban, $100/month yoga studio had come under fire for harassing and then banning non-White members, one upper-middle-class woman, a human-resources director named Alyssa, defended the studio by asserting that she is "just a White woman trying to fight mental illness through yoga. [The studio] helped me a lot. It's a good place, even if it has done things some people find bad [discriminatory]." Alyssa knew that she was supporting a business which was openly and perhaps actionably biased, but she did not care as long as *her* personal wellness needs were being met. Attitudes like this among the majority White cis-female demographic who participate in health and wellness industries are not rare, despite their troubling insistence on ignoring their own complicity in systems of injustice and marginalization. Indeed, White women's well-being, including social and economic mobility, can and will be achieved at all costs, and in many cases they will willingly endorse differential treatment.

We know that discrimination produces cascading effects across communities, and Alyssa's example clearly demonstrates how White hygiene today underwrites structural or institutional racism. Though she might be only one person, her willingness to excuse illegal forms of bias so easily offers unsettling insight into her work in human resources. HR departments oversee civil rights and workplace equity matters; how effectively can she address these matters in light of her comments?

In this regard, the research on institutional racism tells a larger story about how White women's social and economic mobility is predicated on the disenfranchisement and continued oppression of historically marginalized populations. This research demonstrates how the so-called "velvet ghetto" or majority women industries, like human resources, education, nursing, and more recently fitness industries like yoga, but also Cross-Fit, which are all also majority White, actually underscore broader economic trends in the US. Across these industries, there is a constant – White or aspirationally White women performing their bodily capital, in both racist and ableist forms in order to preserve their own position and power. In many ways, this is not a new story, even as the research on White women's involvement in enslavement and egregiously White supremacist organizations like the Ku Klux Klan and today, its modern-day auxiliaries such as the Daughters of the Confederacy or the Junior League, garner renewed attention (see Jones-Rogers 2019).

Conclusion

Differential access to healthcare, including wellness care in the United States, and the logics of White hygiene it lays bare, thus exposes what Kimberlé Crenshaw once aptly diagnosed as "the false tension between feminist and antiracist movements" – a mechanism media studies scholars like Chenjerai Kumanyika characterize as a willful ignorance; a kind of blindspot not born of a lack of knowledge, but outright denial in the face of evidence and truth. Indeed, attitudes like "my health at any cost" must be understood within a longer history of how White hygiene shapes public health and in contemporary settings, for example, leaves communities of color, like Flint, Michigan, without clean drinking water and bears witness to higher rates childhood diabetes in minority/low-income areas – areas which lack access to both safe recreational spaces and parks and/or grocery stores. It is not a coincidence that yoga studios tend to exist in upper-middle-class and majority White areas, next to some sort of "clean eating" juice/coffee bar. What today might appear to an untrained eye as an ambient form of exclusion otherwise marketed by Paltrow as a wellness must-have, is intimately tethered to a larger story of public health and racial injustice, up to and including the kinds of medical experiments conducted on people of color in the early 20th century, as well as the ableist logics of abortion access that values cis-white women's bodies above all. As historians like Harriet Washington and Thomas Leonard have both demonstrated in their work, access to health, even in its progressive forms, remains inextricably intertwined with 19th-century racial science, the rhetoric of eugenics, and social Darwinism, which in the US context remains obsessed with maintaining White women's innocence at all costs.

So, at the very least, Alyssa's comments capture the limits of one person's understanding of how systemic racism might affect access to health and wellness for historically marginalized populations. But at the very most, attitudes like "my health at any cost" are logical extensions of a capitalist order which equates wealth with access and access with health. It is not only individual access to health and wellness that is essential, no matter how often we are sold the neoliberal idea that "it's your workout." Individual health outcomes are inseparable from community health support, and so we must begin to see what is good for everyone and available to everyone as a must for a healthy society.

In the end, the cult of White hygiene and its gendered imperatives must be understood as both a cause and a result of a White supremacist social order. Though its genesis makes sense in a place like the US, which has so often and willingly ignored women's rights to bodily autonomy, such trends still place queer, trans, non-white, and disabled folks at far greater risk. Once we move beyond facile interpretations of yoga as a self-care or uncomplicated wellness activity, it is but a truism that access to healthcare remains shaped by forms of bias that privilege the health of those who look, walk, and talk like those offering care.

Note

1 See for example the recommendations on Goop's website related to yoni eggs and vaginal health.

Bibliography

Aizura, A. 2009. "Where Health and Beauty Meet: Femininity and Racialisation in Thai Cosmetic Surgery Clinics". *Asian Studies Review* 33(3): 303–317.

Amos, Valerie, and Pratibha Parmar. 2005. "Challenging Imperial Feminism". *Feminist Review* 80: 44–63.

Birdee, G.S., Legedza, A.T., Saper, R.B., Bertisch, S.M., Eisenberg, D.M. and Phillips, R.S. "Characteristics of Yoga Users: Results of a National Survey". *Journal of General Internal Medicine* 23(10): 1653–1658.

Chandra, S. 2014. "'India Will Change You Forever': Hinduism, Islam, and Whiteness in the American Empire". *Signs* 40(2): 487–512.

Craik, Jennifer. "'Feeling Premium': Athleisure and the Material Transformation of Sportswear". *Fashion and Materiality*, London: Bloomsbury Visual Arts, 214–232.

Jones-Rogers, Stephanie E. 2020. *They Were Her Property: White Women as Slave Owners in the American South*. New Haven: Yale University Press.

Leonard, Thomas C. 2017. *Illiberal Reformers: Race, Eugenics, and American Economics in the Progressive Era*. Princeton: Princeton University Press.

Prasad, Srirupa. 2015. *Cultural Politics of Hygiene in India, 1890–1940: Contagions of Feeling*. Basingstoke: Palgrave Macmillan.

Ross, A., Friedmann, E., Bevans, M. and Thomas, S. National Survey of Yoga Practitioners: Mental and Physical Health Benefits. *Complement Therapy Medicine* 21(4): 313–323.

Simmons, Christina. 1993. "African Americans and Sexual Victorianism in the Social Hygiene Movement, 1910–40". *Journal of the History of Sexuality* 4(1): 51–75.

Srinivasan, Priya. 2007. "The Bodies Beneath the Smoke or What's Behind the Cigarette Poster: Unearthing Kinesthetic Connections in American Dance History". *Discourses in Dance* 4(1): 7–47.

Tang-Smith, E., Johnson, S.L. and Chen, S. 2015. "The Dominance Behavioural System: A Multidimensional Transdiagnostic Approach". *Psychology and Psychotherapy* 88(4): 394–411.

Washington, Harriet A. 2008. *Medical Apartheid: The Dark History of Medical Experimentation on Black Americans from Colonial Times to the Present*. New York: Harlem Moon.

Weigman, Robyn. 1995. *American Anatomies: Theorizing Race and Gender*. Durham, NC: Duke University Press.

Chapter 9

Incomplete
Impeding the settler colonial project through Yoga for Black Lives

Stephanie D. Hicks

I was not thinking about yoga's relationship to settler colonialism when I started Yoga for Black Lives (YBL)...at least, not explicitly. I was heartbroken and confused, walking a downtown Chicago sidewalk, fumbling with my cell phone to send a text message.

It was a hot day in July when Philando Castile was shot and killed by police officer Jeronimo Yanez in Minnesota[1]. The day before, police officers shot and killed Alton Sterling in Baton Rouge, Louisiana[2]. Black people had just begun grieving Sterling when the Facebook video of Castile's shooting and death, filmed by his partner, Diamond Reynolds, went viral. I got the news like everyone else – through the internet – as I was on my way to assist my yoga teacher and friend at an outdoor rooftop yoga class. My mind turned to the event, and the students we would be teaching. Mostly White, affluent, tight-bodied yogis who wanted – and were able to pay – to practice asana[3] on a downtown Chicago rooftop as the sun set. The event featured a DJ pumping music into headphones that each student would wear, making this a "silent" rooftop yoga class. It seemed pointless to teach the class, offensive even. And at the same time, the practice seemed like *some* response to the umpteenth death of a Black person at the hands of police. I stopped mid-sidewalk, and completed a text message to my closest friends: "If I taught a yoga class for Black people mourning Black folks killed by the police, do you think people would come?" Immediately, they responded in the affirmative. I kept walking.

By the time I reached my teacher at the rooftop venue, I was holding my heartbreak, anger, confusion, and part of a plan. Her face held the same questions I was struggling with, "What is happening in the world?" "Why teach this class?" I told her I wanted to teach a donation-based class that centered Black people who had lost their lives at the hands of police. She thought it was a great idea, but it did not change the fact that we were scheduled to teach a rooftop full of privileged yogis. We chatted, and decided to go on with the class. My teacher alluded to what was happening in the world in her class theming. I went straight home after, and I continued to plan.

What began as an intention to hold one donation-based yoga class to support organizations in Chicago that were resisting state violence against Black people turned into a series of yoga classes held in theaters, community arts organizations, and schools. The first YBL class was held in a downtown Chicago yoga studio. The studio's owner donated the studio space, and I was able to lead a practice for my loved ones that, I think, provided some channel for our rage and grief while affirming community. It also raised some much-needed funds for a local protest against the Chicago Police Department's violence towards Black communities[4]. After that, I started a YBL website, began fielding requests to teach YBL classes in various community spaces and, most importantly, continued to give money to Chicago organizations and defense funds that were resisting.

Throughout 2016, and into 2017, I taught several YBL classes, some as a part of ongoing "residencies" with organizations, some as one-off endeavors. I was working on my dissertation at the time and although it was hectic, looking back on it now, that period was one of the most satisfying and joyful in my practice of yoga thus far. But as YBL expanded beyond my loved ones – close friends and family, many of whom are activists of color – I began to notice sharp racial differences in the makeup of YBL classes. Maybe this should not have surprised me; Chicago is a diverse but segregated and gentrified city and I was teaching in many different neighborhoods, each with their own communities. As YBL gained some traction, though, I found myself teaching classes in majority-White spaces. White teachers even offered to host and teach the classes. While YBL classes were never closed to non-Black people, I began to think more about why I started YBL and its purpose, and what role White people have in it.

Thoughtful scholars have critiqued western yoga as a continuation of the process of colonization, upholding White supremacy and capitalism through a host of violent practices (Page). Yoga in the West has become synonymous with the predominantly White, cis-gendered, upper-middle-class, able-bodied women who teach and practice asana in corporate studios in urban areas (Kaushik-Brown). In urban communities of color that are experiencing intense gentrification, yoga studios have become symbols of the process, signaling the removal/push-out of Black and Brown people while ushering in young White professionals eager to develop the space for their benefit.

So what does it mean to continue Yoga for Black Lives classes with White yogis as sponsors, teachers, and attendees? Do these White people act as takers-of-space, both in urban communities, and within the practice? Does allowing them to take part in YBL de-center Black people and the harm they have experienced? Does it further that harm? Is it incumbent on practitioners of color in a space like YBL classes to care about White people's contributions, or should they be creating their own spaces of resistance? Are all of these questions a sign that I, a Black woman yoga teacher, care a bit too much about White people and their feelings? I am writing to think through these questions, in hopes that they will help me vision a path forward for Yoga for Black Lives.

In order to respond to any of these questions, I felt it necessary to think about the relationships that support my yoga practice, and thus support YBL. I also talked to people who have taken YBL classes, both people of color and White people.

My primary yoga teacher is a White woman. She is dedicated to self-study, to the study of yoga philosophy, and to continually deepening her practice and unpacking Whiteness as it affects her life and the lives of others. I trusted her exasperation and anger on the day of our rooftop yoga class, just as I have trusted her support of YBL. She has championed it, promoted it, volunteered to assist in classes, and volunteered to teach without pay to make sure all proceeds went to YBL (though to date, only I and one other teacher have led YBL classes, and we were both Black women). She has made space for me to take YBL into places I would not have been able to without the backing of a White person.

Similarly, the first yoga teacher and studio owner to offer their space for a YBL class was a White woman. It is not lost on me that, because of structural and institutional racism, a White yogi is more likely to have space and resources to offer than a practitioner of a different race in most US cities. Immediately after I expressed my intention to hold the first class, she reached out to me offering her studio and all its resources, asking for nothing in return. When I held that first class, the room was filled mostly with Black people and people of color. There were only a few White people. I knew them all personally, and knew they trusted me as a yoga teacher and friend. I also knew that they were committed to racial justice.

Months later, when I found myself teaching a series of YBL classes at a community arts center, I noticed that as the series progressed, the numbers of students in classes grew, but the number of White people attending also grew. One evening, I began class as I usually do by asking attendees to write on small slips of paper the names of Black people who had lost their lives to state violence. They could be people that the attendees knew personally. They could be names of people they had heard or read about in the news. As long as they were Black, and had lost their lives to state violence, their name could be written down. I would read those names during our meditation at the beginning of class. As I passed around slips of paper and explained the instructions again, I was met with bewildered faces. People were visibly hesitant, concerned about what to do if they did not know a name. If they did not know anyone, I suggested, the moments before class began would be a great time to strike up a conversation with another student in the room and ask whose name they had written. This seemed to calm some people, but one White woman asked loudly and coarsely, "Do we have to write a name?" I told her it was voluntary. I do not remember whether or not the woman wrote down a name. But I know that she stayed in class, and I proceeded to teach.

I do not know what the relationship is between the White women yogis who made/offered space for YBL classes and the White woman who asked if she had to write down a name. Maybe one is the exception, and one is the rule? More often than not, Whiteness shows up as the woman who wanted to practice, but not participate in a particular way. Not as the women who shared their resources and essentially *got out* of the way. And maybe that is why I have the reaction that I do, why Black peoples' interactions with White people in similar spaces are often fraught: usually the experiences that people of color have with White people, and in this case White women yogis, are experiences of White people taking up space, without contributing to it. How can people of color be expected to open up their spaces to that kind of behavior, especially when White people have all the spaces already?

When talking to some YBL students, I heard some of my concerns echoed back to me, but I was also pushed to wrestle with some new questions. A queer Latinx woman who attended YBL classes said she did so specifically because of the instructor and the centering of Black people. Because she considers all-Black spaces sacred, she wanted to be sure that it was ok to join the class, so she talked to the instructor about whether or not the space was closed to non-Black people beforehand. A working-class Latina, she was not exposed to yoga growing up. It was not until college that she was introduced to the practice, and she felt fortunate to have previously taken classes primarily with queer students and instructors. That was meaningful for her, because the space felt affirming and accessible. She was clear that, to her, yoga classes would not feel that way if they were filled with White yogis. She would rather not practice with them. Neither would she like to practice with White teachers. She asserted that White people "take over everything." In the same breath, however, she conceded that having White people involved in YBL may make its mission "palatable," or accessible, to White folks, which she felt was necessary. I am still wondering: for whom it is necessary to have White teachers and participants? And it is striking to me that a queer woman of color was explicit about the beauty of all-Black healing spaces, and making sure to seek consent before entering one. Her words suggest to me that, for some people at least, there is an understanding that Black/PoC only spaces are necessary and rare, and must be preserved and protected. White people are a threat to these healing spaces, in that their entitlement to the space makes it uninhabitable for people of color.

When I spoke to one of the White women yogis who took YBL classes, she said she wanted to participate because she wanted to support the mission: centering Black lives. She also said that she has never felt out of place in a yoga class because most classes she has attended are full of White practitioners. Because of this, she understood how a critical mass of White people participating in YBL classes could make others feel unsafe. (Although she did not specify *who* would feel unsafe, People of Color were implied.) This White woman, to me, represents a "particular kind" of White woman: an anti-racist one. She cares about resisting racism and state violence against Black people independently of YBL. Is her relationship to the space the same as the White women practitioners who made space for YBL class? Is her relationship to the space *different* than that of the White woman who balked at writing down a name?

I would like YBL classes to be a space in which people can learn and find joyful community. It is not a given that each person who attends a YBL class will have a personal connection to state violence, or to state violence against Black people. But I do expect that people will not be surprised by the centering of Black people who have lost their lives to state violence if they have found out about the class through advertisements, friends and/or family, or other yogis who have brought them into the space, as the vast majority of attendees have. What is more, if they are resistant to this kind of practice, there are many to choose from that do not feature this theming, this music, this meditation, this insistence on centering Black lives in this way.

YBL class structure

Yoga for Black Lives classes is intentionally structured. All of the music and poetry that I use is created by Black artists from different genres and periods of history. I keep a digital collection of songs on my devices, and hard and digital copies of pieces of writing that I would like to use, and I update them whenever I come across something I would like to add. I have class playlists with songs from only one artist: Nina, Stevie, Aretha, Solange. I have playlists that fit a theme: one that I frequently use in the warmer months opens with Chance the Rapper's *Summer Friends* and closes with Lauryn Hill covering *Feeling Good*. At some YBL classes, I have been able to have musicians come into the space and provide live music. I think that the music, the poetry, and the theming celebrate Black life as much as they mourn Black death.

As people are coming into class, I usually ask them to write down the name of someone Black who lost their life to state violence. I tell them that could be police violence, and most of the names that are written down are of Black people killed by police. But I explain that state violence could be neglect of public

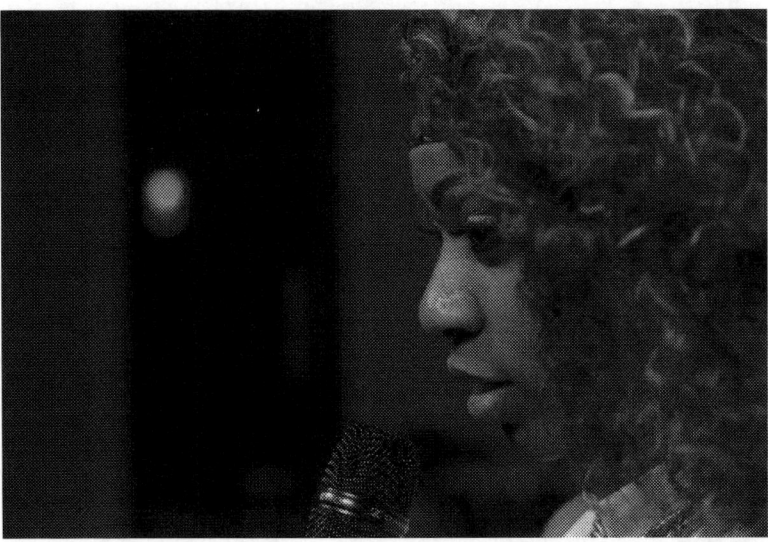

Figure 9.1 Musical theater actress Akilah Sailers has provided live music for YBL classes

resources that leads to illness, like the Flint water crisis, or the mass closing of public schools and overcrowding that furthers a slow intellectual and spiritual death for Black children (Williamson et al.).

When I am ready to begin class, I collect the slips of paper and open the class with breathwork (pranayama). In the silence, I lead a short breathwork practice that is intended to get students to recognize their breath, slow down and lengthen their inhales and exhales (sama vritti). As students sit, focusing on the rhythm of their breath, I read the names they have written down. And after that, I read a poem. As with the music, there are many different Black authors whose work I read aloud for the class. One I find myself reading often is this one by Ross Gay:

> **A Small Needful Fact**
> Is that Eric Garner worked
> for some time for the Parks and Rec.
> Horticultural Department, which means,
> perhaps, that with his very large hands,
> perhaps, in all likelihood,
> he put gently into the earth
> some plants which, most likely,
> some of them, in all likelihood,
> continue to grow, continue
> to do what such plants do, like house
> and feed small and necessary creatures,
> like being pleasant to touch and smell,
> like converting sunlight
> into food, like making it easier
> for us to breathe.

After the poem is finished, I move the class into poses (asana). We may begin, traditionally, with sun or moon salutations, then more standing poses, inversion or backbends, seated poses, and then end with final resting pose, also called corpse pose (savasana). If the class is restorative, we may never leave the floor, only doing five poses over the course of 90 minutes. Whatever the sequence of poses, they correspond with a theme that is underscored by music and poetry. That theme may be precarity, and the sequence is built around a particular inversion that turns the body upside down, or at least brings the heart above the head, and then counters with some grounding poses, helping students explore both feeling unsettled and stable. The theme may be openness, and may utilize a sequence with many heart-openers and expansions, pushing the class to explore the exhilaration and challenges to opening ourselves to life's possibilities. Even as I have asked students to hold the names of those who have lost their lives to state violence, the class is also asking students to explore a range of emotions related to the loss – and celebration – of Black life. During the final resting pose, I often reread the poem with which I opened class. Students are invited to listen to me (or to tune me out), as they feel inclined. The purpose is to have them revisit those words, just as they will revisit their breath and their daily lives after class, getting curious about the effects of the practice on their body, breath, mind, and heart. Do they hear different words in the poem than they did at the beginning of class? Are their breath patterns different? How does it feel for them to be in their body now? And what from this practice do they want to take with them as they move back into the world?

At the beginning and end of each class, I (or another teacher) share with participants the name of the organization or cause to which donations from the class are being given. Sometimes it is a protest, sometimes it is a defense fund, and sometimes it is a bond fund. There is a discussion of the organization and what they are trying to achieve, how they resist state violence against Black people[5].

Settler colonialism and yoga

In addition to being a yoga teacher, I am also a university worker. When I think about the space created in yoga classes, and different relationships people have to the space (Whose is it? Who can use it? How and why?), I think about settler colonialism. And I think about the university as a driver of settler colonialism's progress. At the same time, the university has generated resources for the development of postcolonial and decolonial studies. Universities, as colonial institutions, also produce and contain their decolonial contestation (Paperson). We are reminded that while one of the most important contributions of settler colonial studies has been its offering of the settler-native-slave triad, it is also limited in that it urges us to think of settlers, natives, and slaves as fixed identities as opposed to relations of power concerning land. In the triad, as often described, settlers refer to White people, natives to Indigenous people, and slaves to Black people. While this treatment of the triad interrupts binary understandings of the relations produced by colonialism (oppressor/oppressed, Black/White, colonizer/colonized), it does not account for the complicated (messy) relationships created by the process (King) (Paperson).

The settler-native-slave triad asks us to make things fit, as opposed to letting them show us something. For example, the triad leads us to the question of whether or not Black people become settlers. In the colonial United States, Black people were primarily a tool for acquisition of land. Since they were "freed", they have lived on said land as "free" persons. Black people are not native to the US, so they must be settlers (according to the logic of settler colonialism). But that understanding does not take into account that a defining feature of Blackness is the impossibility of settlement, as the processes of settler colonialism have rendered Black people out of place on land (see: slavery, sharecropping, redlining, gentrification, predatory lending, etc.). This is not to say that some Black people have not been able to engage in settlement, but it is more useful to ask *when* and *how* they have been able to do it, and confront the messy answer, than to lump Black people into an identity category in which they do not belong. What is more, if we think of the slave in the triad not as an identity, but a set of relationships – enslavability, murderability, total fungibility – we can see *when* and *how* Whiteness, anti-Blackness, and indigenous erasure (technologies of settler colonialism) are used in spaces where there are no White, Black, or Native people *per se*.

White YBL participants, then, must navigate some complicated relationships as well. Just as slave and native are not fixed identities, neither is settler. Those who can be considered settlers are those who are able to access Whiteness. Whiteness is property; the right to have rights (Harris). It is normativity, citizenship, and innocence. And yes, it is true that Whiteness is most often accessible to those people who are understood as White, but Whiteness is not available to all White people at all times in the same way (see: White privilege). As with the other triad categories and technologies of settler colonialism, it is important to ask *when* and *how* Whiteness is being employed. As it pertains to Yoga for Black Lives, whether or not White participants can engage in the space would depend on whether, when, and how they access Whiteness, and how that affects Black and PoC participants and their practice.

Instead of asking whether YBL is part of the settler colonial process, a more useful question may be, "*When* and *how* is YBL a part of the settler colonial process, and when and how is it resistant to it?" I have been approaching this question about "what to do with White participants" as if "White" is a fixed identity, as well as "Black" and "Indigenous" and "People of Color." YBL could be more resistant to the process of settler colonialism if I reframe my approach: how do the complicated relationships represented by the settler-native-slave categories show up in YBL? What does that mean for how the project operates and grows? Also, inasmuch as settler colonial spaces carry their contestation within them, YBL is always already resistant. And my task is to identify the spaces of resistance that are already there, refashioning colonizing technologies.

One way in which Yoga for Black Lives undermines the settler colonial project is that it makes us mindful that the process is happening, and that we are a part of it. Any YBL class that takes place in what is known as the United States is likely to take place on stolen land. What is more, it is likely to take place on stolen land that has been settled, which means that some people have been displaced, and that displacement was violent. The cycle of displacement and settlement, and the violence it produces, has likely happened more than once, and is currently happening in some form. When we bring our presence to the reality that we are a part of the settler colonial process, we are also able to see how state violence against Black people is a part of the settler colonial project (Nichols, 2014). How we understand our role(s) in both the destruction and regeneration of Black life, then, is incredibly important. It is my hope that YBL helps contribute to this awareness.

Additionally, to take what can be a version of yoga that pushes us to ignore the colonial foundation upon which it has been built in the west, and shift it to a "version" of the practice that asks us to center and grapple with the ways we are a part of a settler colonial process is an important step in undermining it. Centering Black lives (which, in the settler colonial process, are tools) is reframing what

Blackness is, imbuing it with different meanings. What is Blackness in the YBL space? Blackness cannot just be one thing (death). All aspects of Black life have to be a part of the space. Rhythm, what Black people create, how Black people live; YBL has to be a space where Black people [re]imagine Black life, create community.

At the same time, Yoga for Black Lives *is* part of the settler colonial process. Generally, it is still exclusive in many ways: most people who attend the class are young and physically able-bodied. More women and cis-gendered folks are in the classes than gender non-conforming and trans people, and I know that impacts who feels welcome and included, as my students have mentioned. But crucially, Yoga for Black Lives does not repatriate land. It does not do the fundamental thing that decolonization demands, and in that way it makes use of decolonization as a metaphor (Tuck & Yang). Yet and still, a decolonizing frame has been helpful in that it asks some questions about YBL that I cannot yet answer. Trying to ask the questions in the right way, and work towards responding to them gives me a road map for YBL's future.

Future directions for YBL

In January of 2017, I relocated to Ann Arbor, Michigan. I came to the University of Michigan to take a faculty position in the Program on Intergroup Relations (IGR). IGR is a social justice education program that uses Intergroup Dialogue pedagogy to bring students from various social identity groups (race, gender, class, ethnicity, socioeconomic status, sexual orientation, religion, citizenship status, and others) together to learn about their membership in these groups, how they impact their lives and interactions within systems of oppression, and how they might collaborate across difference to work towards social justice. I was excited to come to Michigan, and I am proud to be a part of the Program. I work with dedicated colleagues and bright students. But moving – away from the place I called home generally, and to a liberal White college-town specifically – changed many aspects of my life. My yoga practice was one of them. Another, I believed, was my relationship to police violence. I remember walking around town during my first weeks of living in Ann Arbor, and questioning my relationship to the police because *I did not see them*. I intended to continue Yoga for Black Lives in Ann Arbor. Yet, my physical practice stalled, and two years passed without me finding a new studio "home," or a yoga community.

In early 2020, the COVID-19 pandemic rearranged just about everyone's relationship to everything, in dramatic ways. I was just beginning to adjust to the new routines of virtual teaching, leaving my home for essentials only, and calibrating the balance between being informed and run-down by world news when my yoga practice re-emerged. The sense that each morning I would face a brand new world urged me to find ways to confront the unknown without expectation. Meditation allows me to practice observing without judgment. When I took a "break" from my yoga practice upon moving in 2017, I believed that I did not possess the mental, emotional, or physical energy to sustain it. I was sad, confused, and disorientated, and thought that my practice would "return" when I no longer felt those emotions. Yoga in our American context has become – in many ways – about reaching goals and obtaining perfection, most easily observed in a physical practice. I could not see that my practice, in some ways, was always with me: in self-study, in breath work, in creating rituals to care for myself, in meditation. Yoga has also been touted as a practice one engages when they want to "feel good," not one we engage – as YBL does – in order to bear witness to what is happening inside of us, and in the world. People may not be attracted to YBL because bearing witness to the pain of state-sanctioned violence against Black people is not something they are ready or willing to do. Others may resist YBL because being reintroduced to that pain can lead to re-traumatization. With this in mind, I am continuing to build YBL as a space that adheres to *ahimsa*[6]: no one is forced to practice this way. Also, YBL offerings must strike a balance between providing opportunities for collective grief and Black joy.

In May 2020, George Floyd was murdered by Minneapolis police, and uprisings against racial injustice broadly – and police violence explicitly – started in the US and spread around the world[7]. Everyone – it seemed – was on the streets in protest, or on the internet in solidarity, or both. The confluence of the pandemic and George Floyd's murder made Black death visible to those who had, up until that point, been ignorant of White supremacy's ability to end Black lives prematurely. The simultaneity of these deaths has again laid bare the impacts of anti-Blackness, and pushed those who deny them to find new justifications for the rampant loss of Black life. Though I had been thinking about re-starting YBL, for some reason I was hesitant to do so when the uprisings began. I am not exactly sure why, except to say that I did not know what the "right" thing to do was. I received an email from the yoga studio director who had made space for the first YBL class, however, and I took it as a sign that the moment was right to begin again, even if I did not quite know where it would lead. I spent much time in the past – and in this chapter – ruminating over the role of White people in YBL following George Floyd's murder. Whiteness responded in many ways: racist reactionism, performative activism, guilt-ridden platitudes. There are also White people who are starting – or continuing – their liberatory work. I decided to trust that this is what the studio owner was doing: continuing her work by using the structure she had to hold space for Yoga for Black Lives.

I asked a young woman graphic designer who had been working with me to revamp and maintain my academic website if she would like to work on YBL's website, and social media presence broadly. She was excited to do so, and now brings her talent in that area to YBL's online presence. Doing that work has pushed her to take accountability for deepening her knowledge around abolition, whiteness, and justice work more broadly. She is a White woman, and her experiences with YBL – the way she's taken responsibility for the content while trying to responsibly locate herself in an organization that is about Black liberation – has prompted me to think more deeply about what it means to "reset" YBL as an accountable community. We do not "heal others," we create a community that can hold healing and hope as part of our ongoing struggle towards justice. Part of what this means, I think, is that YBL cannot "make whiteness be accountable," but it can set up a space where White folks can hold themselves accountable.

YBL classes resumed in late July 2020 and are held regularly, taught by YBL network teachers. The teacher network emerged from need: I do not have the capacity to teach yoga, lead Yoga for Black Lives, and be accountable to my primary university job in equal measure, and I really want to be accountable to each space, not minimally present when life allows. But the creation of a teacher network is also about sharing the work, and realizing that the restoration and regeneration of Black life is a project that requires many gifts and talents. The project benefits – we benefit – when this work is rooted in relationship. We could understand the practice of yoga as attempting to bring ourselves in right relationship to self, others, your conception of god(s), and land/earth. This work is both process and goal. Growing the YBL teacher network, and the YBL team generally, creates a space for those of us involved to work on these relationships and build trust in real time.

There are now six Black, Indigenous, and People of Color (BIPOC) women who teach YBL classes, contribute yoga content for YBL social media, and are generally contributing to the building-out of YBL. I am glad that my hesitation to restart YBL did not prevent me from doing so. The social and political moment called for it, and I think that the classes provide an opportunity for collective grieving and restoration. But reviving YBL has also been life giving. In a time of physical isolation, I am expanding my own – and others' – community. YBL is also allowing us to focus on long-term struggle and process, which is just as much a part of liberation as realizing the world in which we want to live. People in the United States – and the world – have refocused their attention on the Black Lives Matter movement because of the most recent wave of murders of Black people by the police and White vigilantes[8]. But the demands of the movement, and the work of actually carrying them out is a long struggle. Part of that struggle is about creating and making possible self and community care that does not rely on resources external to our communities, because those "resources" are violent themselves. Engaging in this work through YBL is incredibly hopeful to me.

It is not lost on me, however, that the Black Lives Matter movement – and abolition specifically – are not immune to co-optation or dilution. As YBL continues to develop, I have realized that I need to be vigilant about its mission and contribution to movement work. I consider partnerships with studios more deeply; I am more curious about their interests, even as I am excited about them. I find that I am in relationships with more people around YBL, and to some extent I am grateful for those connection because these movements, frankly, need more people to win, but I am also still skeptical. I think often about the woman in my YBL class years ago who did not want to share a name of someone who had lost their life to police violence. I feel the same concern, frustration, and anger when I get the sense that some studios want to "partner" with YBL in an attempt to assuage their guilt, or prove to their few yoga students of color that they are responding appropriately to the movement. As a result, YBL's language around abolition has become more specific on our website and social media, and of course within our network. I want people to understand what YBL is trying to fund and support, and what we are not. Importantly, YBL classes are now offered to specific populations: some are for Black participants only, Black, Indigenous and People of Color (BIPOC) only, and some are open to all. Many participants and all of the YBL teachers have shared positive feedback about this shift, and that leads me to believe that people appreciate the opportunity to choose with whom they would like to share their practice.

I did not know any yogis of color when I arrived in Ann Arbor, but I know more now, and they are connected to YBL. We joyfully brainstorm and daydream about YBL's next steps. What would it look like to hold Yoga for Black Lives workshops? When could that happen? How would YBL shift and change in this new context? What could be possible if we held longer sessions that incorporated breathwork, meditation, asana, some kind of presentation or speaking around state violence against Black people, and some community-building component? These new forms do not have to be bound to any one place. Unfortunately, the processes of settler colonialism are still taking place all over. But people are resisting all over, and Yoga for Black Lives could be a part of that resistance in different localities.

For example, although many Chicagoans – many people across the country – see the guilty verdict rendered to police officer Jason Van Dyke for the 2014 murder of Laquan MacDonald[9] as justice served or a victory, it does not mean that the killings of Black people by the police will end, or that we have entered a new era in which Black people are not fungible. What would it look like for YBL to continue to engage the conversation that MacDonald's death and VanDyke's conviction have re-ignited? What would it look like to frame the killing, mourning, trial, protest, and conviction as parts of an ongoing process of removal (through murder and dispossession) and occupation? What would a yoga class mean then? And what would it look like to engage those with access to Whiteness in an ongoing conversation about YBL, its mission, and settler colonialism (which is both a driver and outcome of state violence against Black people)? Whose responsibility is it to begin and maintain that conversation? How do I incorporate that into YBL's offerings?

During quarantine, I, like many people, have attempted to make sense of what this physical separation means for our ability to understand who and what we are as a nation. Some have argued that the necessity of staying in our homes as we watch the world shift around us has deepened a sense that "we're all in this together." But, in response to COVID-19's disproportionate impact on Black people, and ceaseless police violence, abolitionist Ruth Wilson Gilmore (citing writer M. NourbeSe Philip) reminds us that "if we were all in this together, *we wouldn't be in this together*" (Books, 2020). I am inspired by Black and Indigenous activists who have joined together to make visible the connections between struggles against state violence towards Black people and struggles to disrupt our understanding of our nation's "founders" as anything other than settler-colonizers.

I believe that this time in our nation's history has immense potential to politicize and radicalize people around [de]colonization, White supremacy, and a host of other deeply rooted problems. I also believe that the intent to uproot them will never be as powerful as the political, intellectual, emotional, interpersonal, and spiritual work we actually do to achieve those ends.

These questions give rise to many more, some open-ended, some still closed. Many of the questions are reflective of a hopeful curiosity. Some still hold my cynicism and skepticism. I think that is ok right now. What is most valuable, I think, is that once again, this practice has created space. As I have engaged questions of whether and how we enter the yoga space, and whose space needs protection, I have found new questions with which to wrestle. Words that come to my mind often are those of poet Aracelis Girmay:

Elegy
What to do with this knowledge that our living is not guaranteed?

Perhaps one day you touch the young branch
of something beautiful. & it grows & grows
despite your birthdays & the death certificate,
& it one day shades the heads of something beautiful
or makes itself useful to the nest. Walk out
of your house, then, believing in this.
Nothing else matters.

All above us is the touching
of strangers & parrots,
some of them human,
some of them not human.

Listen to me. I am telling you
a true thing. This is the only kingdom.
The kingdom of touching;
the touches of the disappearing, things.

Notes

1 On July 6, 2016, Philando Castile and his partner Diamond Reynolds were pulled over by police officer Jeronimo Yanez in St. Paul, Minnesota. Yanez asked Castile for his license and registration, and Castile told the officer that he had a firearm in the car. Yanez told Castile not to reach for it and as Castile reached for the license and registration, Yanez shot seven times into the car, fatally wounding Castile. Reynolds captured the aftermath of the shooting on her phone's camera, while her four-year-older

daughter watched from the back seat of the car. Jeronimo Yanez was charged with manslaughter and dangerous discharge of a firearm, but was acquitted on all charges.
2 On July 5, 2016, Alton Sterling was shot dead in Baton Rouge Louisiana. Sterling was approached by two White police officers at a convenience store, who were responding to a report that an armed man was threatening a convenience store customer. The officers apprehended Sterling, and then shot him while trying to control him as he reached for a gun in his pocket. Though the convenient store manager reported that Sterling was not the person who threated the customer, and that he had a gun because people who had been selling items outside the store – as Sterling had – were robbed recently, the officers who shot him were not charged. They were found by the Department of Justice to have acted in a "reasonable and justifiable manner."
3 *Asana* is a Sanskrit word that translates to "seat" in English. In the context of yoga philosophy, asana –or physical poses - are but one of the Eight Limbs of the practice.
4 For 41 days in the summer of 2016, the #LetUsBreathe Collective held the Freedom Square encampment in the Lawndale neighborhood on Chicago's West Side. Launched across the street from Homan Square, a Chicago Police Department "Black site" known for illegal detention and torture, the Freedom Square tent community was created and maintained as a way to imagine a world without police. It featured free stores, food, classes, community events and childcare.
5 Some organizations for which YBL has raised funds: Bresha Meadows' Defense Fund, Chicago Community Bond Fund, Sage Community Health Collective & Assata's Daughters, Brave Space Alliance, Detroit Justice Center, Chicago Freedom School
6 *Ahimsa* is a Sanskrit word that refers to the yogic principle of non-harming.
7 On May 25, 2020, police officers in Minneapolis, Minnesota killed George Floyd. Floyd was arrested for allegedly using counterfeit money for a purchase. During the arrest, Officer Derek Chauvin kneeled on Floyd's neck for approximately 9 minutes while Floyd lay handcuffed face down on the ground. Two other arresting offers, J. Alexander Kueng and Thomas K. Lane, looked on which Floyd repeatedly said he could not breathe. Floyd was unconscious and motionless for the last few minutes Chauvin kneeled on his neck, though Chauvin did not relent. Video of the killing taken by bystanders went viral, sparking national and international uprisings around racial injustice and police violence.
8 In February of 2020, White residents Travis McMichael and his son Gregory McMichael, along with William "Roddie" Bryan, chased and shot Ahmaud Arbery while he jogged through a neighborhood in Brunswick, Georgia. McMichael Sr. and Jr. claimed that they were following Arbery because he fit the description of a robbery suspect in the area. For months after the shooting, no arrests were made, though local police knew of the shooting and it was videotaped. When the video went viral, it sparked calls for accountability and arrests, and exposed the reluctance of Glyn County law enforcement officials to investigate or charge any of the men who killed Arbury. In March of 2020, police entered the home of emergency medical technician Breonna Taylor using a "no-knock" warrant to search the premises because Taylor's boyfriend, Adrian Walker, was suspected of selling drugs. Believing the police to be intruders, Walker shot at the police who returned fire. Breonna Taylor was fatally shot in the crossfire. Taylor's death not only sparked protest, but brought awareness to – and remind many of – the ways that police violence harms black women.
9 On October 20, 2014 17-year-old Laquan MacDonald was killed on the streets of Chicago by police officer Jason Van Dyke. Original police reports stated that MacDonald was acting erratically and wielding a knife towards officers when they fatally shot him. In 2015, dashboard camera footage of the shooting emerged, showing MacDonald walking away from officers when Van Dyke shot him 16 times. Van Dyke was then charged with first-degree murder, and was found guilty of second-degree murder and aggravated battery with a firearm in 2018.

Bibliography

Books, Haymarket. 2020. "Ruth Wilson Gilmore on Covid-19, Decarceration, and Abolition." *Haymarket Books*. April 17. Accessed August 27, 2020. https://www.haymarketbooks.org/blogs/128-ruth-wilson-gilmore-on-covid-19-decarceration-and-abolition.

Gay, Ross. 2015. "A Small Needful Fact." *Split This Rock*. April 30. Accessed 2018. https://␣ww.splitthisrock.org/poetry-database/poem/a-small-needful-fact.

Girmay, Aracelis. 2011. "Elegy." In *Kingdom Anamalia*, by Aracelis Girmay, 132–133. Rochester: BOA Editions.

Harris, Cheryl I. 1993. "Whiteness as Property." *Harvard Law Review* 106(8): 1707–1791.

Kaushik-Brown, Roopa. 2016. "Toward Yoga as Property." In *Yoga, the Body, and Embodied Social Change: An Intersectional Feminist Analysis*, by Beth Berila, Melanie Klein and Chelsea Jackson-Roberts, 67–89. Lanham: Lexington Books.

King, Tiffany. 2014. "Labor's Aphasia: Toward Antiblackness as Constituative to Settler Colonialism." *Decolonization: Indigeneity, Education & Society* 10. https://decolonization.wordpress.com/2014/06/10/labors-aphasia-toward-antiblackness-as-constitutive-to-settler-colonialism/.

Nichols, Robert. 2014. "The Colonialism of Incarceration." *Radical Philosophy Review* 17(2): 49–67.

Page, Enoch. 2016. "Enclosing Yoga as White Public Space." In *Yoga, the Body, and Embodied Social Change*, by Beth Klein, Melanie Berila and Chelsea Jackson-Roberts, 41–66. Lanham: Lexington Books.

Paperson, La. 2017. *A Third University Is Possible*. Minneapolis: University of Minnesota Press.

Tuck, Eve and K. Wayne Yang. 2012. "Decolonization Is Not a Metaphor." *Decolonization: Indigeneity, Education & Society* 1(1): 1–40.

Williamson, Vanessa et al. 2018. *Black Lives Matter: Race, State Violence and Representation in the United States*. https://www.brookings.edu/events/Black-lives-matter-race-state-violence-and-representation-in-the-united-states.

Chapter 10

Hozho Yoga
Indigenous movements illuminating human and more-than-human interconnections

Tria Blu Wakpa

In a sepia-toned film, titled *Hozho Yoga* (2017), Haley Laughter, a Diné (Navajo) woman, practices yoga on Diné lands with grace and precision. Laughter is a yoga teacher and founder of Hozho Total Wellness, an organization committed to bringing yoga to Native people. Hózhó, as Laughter explains, is a Diné philosophy "meaning walking in beauty and harmony and well-being, so in equilibrium with our mental, physical, emotional, and spiritual well-being and the way that we interact with other people and the way that we define ourselves as indigenous people and our connection between mother earth and our creator and the different elements and the universe. [In this way], Diné philosophy is pretty much what yogic philosophy is" (Laughter 2020). The visually stunning, wide-shot film features Laughter's feminine and fit figure, full length in the foreground, and beyond her in the distance, tsézhiin 'íí 'áhí ("black rocks protruding up" or Bennett Peak), a mountain, jutting, rising, and sloping against a cloudy, but sunlit sky in what is often referred to as Newcomb, New Mexico. Laughter's white, collared blouse, with dark blotches, resembles cowhide, and almost recalls Diné regalia, but instead of being tucked into a full-length skirt, is knotted at the waist. Her hair is tied in a tsiiyéé or Diné bun, and she wears the Diné-style of moccasins; dark suede covers her feet, and strips of white elk skin and cowhide leather wrap up her calves. Diné ways of knowing view "every strand of hair [as] connected to a star" (Laughter 2020). Moccasins, which are inextricable from Diné identity, connect them to Mother Earth and Father Sky, and the process of making moccasins itself illustrates Hózhó.[1]

In these ways and many others, *Hozho Yoga* clarifies the interconnections among human and more-than-humans (such as nonhuman animals, air, land, water, sky, and the universe) and the mind, body, and spirit – understandings which are central to Diné and yoga philosophies. Indeed, one of Laughter's intentions in creating the video, which was directed by Robin Silverfox, was to "visually connect the land with yoga" and Diné people and practices, and portray herself as "one with the elements, earth, mountains, and air" (Laughter 2020). A black leotard reveals Laughter's bare legs, which in the sepia-colored film are nearly identical to the tone of the mountain. "Night Owl," an experimental, electronic song by Broke For Free plays, but the almost thunderous sound of the wind remains audible; human and more-than-human chords combine ("Broke For Free – Night Owl"). In profile in Mountain Pose, Laughter is already in motion when the film cuts to her, stretching her arms above her head, bringing her palms together in prayer. Mind, body, and spirit unite. She too is a mountain, sacred to the Diné people, rooted to and rising from the land. Then, Laughter steps forward into Warrior Three, lowering her torso parallel to the earth while lifting her back leg (Figure 10.1). The woman warrior balances. She is in equilibrium with the elements that surround her. Her arms, extended to either side, lift upward, opening her chest, creating a bird's breast. She transforms into a soaring eagle with white tailfeathers, thereby referencing a very sacred bird to the Diné and many other Native nations (Morales). As Laughter shared with me, "The eagle is one of the most sacred birds in Navajo/Diné culture…It's the bird that flies the highest, is the strongest, most powerful, resilient bird that we have. We use it for ceremony, and it's in the creation stories also" (Laughter 2020). Laughter's extended back leg momentarily lifts slightly higher, allowing her to glide closer to the earth.[2]

Today in the U.S., there is a growing interest in yoga among Native Americans. Given the vast diversity of Native peoples who primarily live in urban areas, and the ways that settler-colonial discourses often exclude them from narratives and statistics (Tuck and Yang 12, 23), it is challenging to delineate exactly when Native people began to practice yoga. However, Laughter told me that when she first began posting representations of herself practicing yoga on HEALTHY ACTIVE NATIVES!!!!, a Facebook group for Native people which in August 2020 has over 76,000 members ("HEALTHY ACTIVE NATIVES!!!!"), she was the only Native person she was aware of who was practicing or teaching yoga.

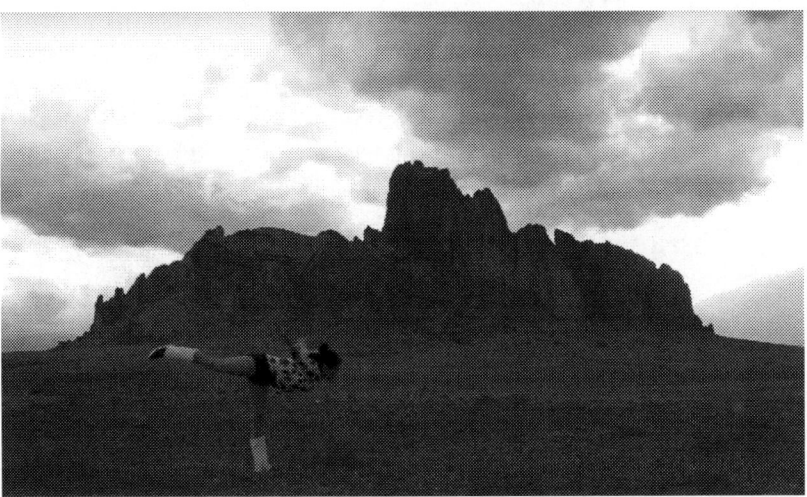

Figure 10.1 Haley Laughter, in Warrior Three, transforming into a soaring eagle with white tailfeathers

In a way, this also corresponds with my own experiences. A woman of Filipina, European, and tribally-unenrolled Native ancestries who has practiced yoga for 25 years and taught for 11, I first began offering yoga classes to Lakota people on the Rosebud Reservation (in what is often referred to as South Dakota) in Summer 2011 as a means of enacting reciprocity while doing research for my dissertation. To my knowledge and based on the interactions I had with Lakota people, at the time no one else was teaching the practice on the Rosebud Reservation.[3]

In the contemporary moment, nearly a decade later, Native people practicing and teaching yoga are much more visible on social media and in mainstream depictions. Articles that I have located highlighting Native yoga teachers are mostly dated on or around 2018. In addition to illustrating how Native people are often omitted from settler-colonial discourses, this relatively recent date also may reflect the ways that U.S. settler-colonial discourses have often portrayed yoga as exclusively for fit and flexible White bodies with class privilege. This (mis)perception may discourage some Native people from practicing yoga.[4] Indeed, one of Laughter's intentions in creating *Hozho Yoga* was to encourage more Indigenous people to practice yoga, which is a way of defying such U.S. settler-colonial narratives surrounding yoga.

Although contemporary representations of yoga practitioners and teachers in "nature" abound on the partition of Turtle Island often referred to as the U.S., again these depictions often do not feature Native people. Scholars have also critiqued the Eurocentric construct of nature, which – unlike Indigenous epistemologies – dichotomizes human and more-than-human persons (Inoue and Moreira). Although a comment on the *Hozho Yoga* video refers to Laughter's surroundings as a "gorgeous backdrop" (Natalie Rose), which reifies anthropocentric worldviews of humans on a stage created by land (Mattingly), I argue that Laughter's yoga practice decenters human dominance. Not only is Laughter in audible and visible relationship with more-than-human elements in the film, but also, the shot is composed so that Laughter is much smaller than the mountain behind her (Mattingly).

The eclipsing of Native people from yoga discourses and representations is perhaps expected given that in general they are often excluded from settler-colonial narratives and/or frequently rendered to the past. As citizens of Native nations with inherent sovereignty, Native people interfere with the aim of settler colonialism, which is for non-Native people to make their homes on Native lands (Tuck and Yang 6). For this reason, settler colonialism operates to "destroy and disappear" Native people who have resisted and continue to resist this genocidal structure through a multitude of means, including by practicing yoga (Tuck and Yang 6). Some Native people view yoga as a way to alleviate the adverse health effects that ongoing colonization continues to inflict, allowing them to enrich their Indigenous knowledges and identities (Middletent; Blu Wakpa, "Yoga Brings You Back to Who You Are" 4, 11). Because settler colonialism has sought to control Native people's bodies and practices – including through removal and relocation and attempting to regulate their movements and disconnect them from

Indigenous ways of knowing – Native people (re)claiming Indigenous kinetic connection on Native lands is an important tactic of "survivance."[5]

Although yoga and Diné philosophies emerge out of completely different sociohistorical contexts, they also share similarities as Indigenous epistemologies (Miller 19, 25). Yoga and Diné ways of knowing often acknowledge and enact relationships among humans and more-than-humans. The late esteemed yoga teacher and practitioner, B.K.S. Iyengar writes, "Whilst performing asanas, the yogi's body assumes many forms resembling a variety of creatures. His mind is trained not to despise any creature, for he knows that throughout the whole gamut of creation, from the lowliest insect to the most perfect sage, there breathes the same Universal Spirit, which assumes innumerable forms" (42). Similarly, as Michelle Kahn-John (Diné) and Mary Koithan articulate, the Diné philosophy of Hózhó, which is foundational to Diné life, "requires conscious awareness of the collective and interconnected relationships between self and others. Others are broadly defined and include the universal whole: (1) the elements of nature, including animals and insects; (2) the Creator; (3) the Diné holy people; (4) spirits; (5) Mother Earth; (6) Father Sky; and (7) the distinct characteristics and cycles within nature and the universe, such as seasons, night, day, sun, moon, stars, time" (Kahn-John and Koithan 27). In contrast, settler-colonial logics dichotomize humans and more-than-humans and hierarchize humans above all other beings.

Given the ways that settler-colonial constructs and discourses have detrimentally affected Native humans and more-than-humans and caused the current climate crisis, it is vital to highlight Native representations and innovations. Native cultural productions can enact counter logics and narratives that offer possibilities for transformation and innovation beyond the settler-colonial imaginary. This essay centers analysis of the film, *Hozho Yoga*, and concludes by bringing another film, *Hot Hooghan Yoga*, into the discussion. The two cultural productions, which feature Laughter, were posted to the Hozho Total Wellness YouTube channel in February 2017 and April 2019, respectively. In some ways a striking departure from the formally choreographed *Hozho Yoga*, *Hot Hooghan Yoga* depicts a scene from a yoga class that Laughter teaches to seven Diné women in a Hogan, the historical and in some cases enduring home for Diné people, which they continue to use for everyday living as well as ceremonies. Through her work with Hozho Total Wellness – including the events that she has organized, the media attention that she has garnered, and the social media presence that she has cultivated – Laughter is a well-known figure within Native American yoga circles and beyond. I juxtapose the two films because despite their differences, they both demonstrate the powerful and vital ways that Laughter fuses yoga and Diné cultural practices. The titles of both the films also foreground how the Diné are innovating their cultural identities and practices through yoga.

In my examination of these videos, I employ a "choreographic analysis" or close readings of bodies and movements, which is a primary methodology in Dance studies as well as a critical intervention that the academic field makes. Because of Cartesian dualism – which notably contrasts with yoga and Diné understandings of the body as a holistic entity – other fields often overlook the knowledge inherent in and evidenced through movement forms. Eurocentric epistemologies also construct the written word as superior to other forms of knowledge production, so writing about movement practices is a way to articulate the vital understandings that bodies carry, innovate, and transmit. It is important to emphasize that scholarship is always subjective; at the same time, analysis that imposes a Eurocentric lens to discussing Indigenous bodies and movements is problematic and violent. Also, as Dance studies scholar Kate Mattingly noted, "movement practices also cannot be adequately analyzed without taking into consideration the identities of practitioners; in other words, bodies and their movement practices are mutually constitutive. Laughter endows the asanas with Diné/Navajo symbolism as the asanas transform her own mental/emotional/physical wellbeing" (Mattingly).

Accordingly, in this essay, I use pan-Native and Diné, tribally-specific lenses to speculate about what the yoga poses Laughter performs enact and signify, which draws on the broader efforts of Dance studies to see the body as capable of conveying meaning through movement (Foster). Based on previous research that I have done and my over three decades of experience as a martial artist, I know that Indigenous peoples have drawn on more-than-human, kinetic knowledge – and in particular, more-than-human, kinetic animal knowledge – to develop and strengthen their movement modalities, and these understandings inform my close readings. Within the broader field of Dance studies, Indigenous epistemologies therefore inspire me to speculate about what relationships the poses articulate and how they signify. Similar to the ways that movement practices cannot be separated from cultural specificities, in the context of Diné women and their dreams, John Dadosky writes Diné "belief and practices regarding dream accounts reflects the heart of their 'ethos' as a people" (18). Drawing on cultural knowledge to interpret the symbols in a person's dream – much like deciphering the meaning in poses and sequencing – can be a way of self-reflecting, deepening understandings, generating new knowledges, and even comprehending what the future holds. Through the process of writing this essay, I have gained greater knowledge about how yoga poses exemplify Indigenous epistemologies and enact Indigenous connections among humans and more-than-humans.

I also use decolonizing methodologies in this essay, holistically centering Laughter's body and movements along with her words and intentions.[6] To further my analysis, I draw on two interviews that I did with Laughter. In the first, which we did in 2018, Laughter articulated connections between yoga and Diné philosophies and how yoga has helped her to strengthen her identity as a Diné woman despite U.S. assimilation policies and practices aimed at undermining Native peoples, practices, and their sovereignties. In the second, which we did in 2020, after she read an initial draft of this essay, I mostly asked her questions about Diné philosophy, and her answers and insights helped me to strengthen aspects of this analysis. Some scholars whom I have interacted with (mis)understand engaging with the people I am writing about as detrimental to the research I am doing. Yet, these concerns, which often (mis)take research as objective and position the researcher as the sole expert, are not only misguided, but also harmful as they reify unequal power dynamics by hierarchizing the researcher above practitioners. In Dance studies, such assumptions are especially ironic given that a primary premise of the field is that bodies and movements contain and create knowledge. In contrast, I understand both Laughter and myself as experts, and her contributions have unquestionably enhanced this essay.

I argue that in the videos, Laughter blends yoga and her Diné cultural practices in ways that challenge settler colonialism by making visible Native people and practices in the contemporary moment and their enduring interconnectedness with more-than-human relatives and holistic understandings of the mind, body, and spirit. Although as I have articulated, Native American and Indigenous South Asian philosophies recognize the interconnectedness among humans and more-than-humans and the inextricability of mind, body, spirit, so as not to collapse the vast diversity of Indigenous worldviews, this chapter focuses on how a choreographic reading of yoga practices in *Hozho Yoga* and *Hot Hooghan Yoga* convey the Diné philosophy of Hózhó. Along with "honoring all life," Hózhó philosophies underscore "developing pride of one's mind, body, soul [and] spirit" (Laughter 2020). A close reading of Laughter's body, poses, transitions, and sequencing also provides insight into why Diné and other Native people – whose tribal nations also have epistemologies which emphasize human and more-than-human respect and reciprocity and mind, body, spirit connection – might draw on yoga as a way to strengthen their Native identities.

Given the fluidity of movement forms and social structures – such as race and gender – *Hozho Yoga* and *Hot Hooghan Yoga* could also be interpreted as reinforcing settler-colonial (mis)understandings of Native women. For example, the leotard and Diné regalia that Laughter wears in *Hozho Yoga* could be (mis) construed as simultaneously sexualizing and exotifying her. The precision of her practice could be (mis)taken for her desiring and/or requiring discipline through practices that have non-Diné origins. Her demonstration of yoga – in lieu of a Diné practice – could be (mis)interpreted as her being assimilated and "inauthentically" Native. The solo performance in the sepia-colored film could be (mis) read as Laughter being the "last" Native woman of her tribe, fulfilling the settler-colonial trope of the "vanishing Indian" (Huhndorf 19). Even Laughter's association with "nature" risks reinforcing stereotypes of Native people. These possible and problematic readings highlight the inescapable, systemic binds that Native people – and other nondominant groups, such as women – necessarily navigate. However, rather than centering settler-colonial stereotypes, this chapter emphasizes Laughter and other Diné women's ongoing resistance to oppressive structural forces through yoga.

Hozho Yoga

By moving through a sequence of yoga poses named for and modeled after human and more-than-human beings, Laughter makes visible their interrelationships and the interconnectedness of mind, body, and spirit while challenging settler-colonial logics and narratives. Arguably, a non-Native person performing a similar yoga sequence could also create these connections; however, as a Diné person on Diné lands, Laughter's very presence is an act of resistance. Through yoga, she makes visible contemporary Diné people and communicates how Diné ways of knowing and moving endure and innovate, which challenges settler-colonial narratives of Indigenous peoples and practices as static and/or extinct. From Warrior Three – a sacred eagle gliding parallel to the earth, as I earlier described – Laughter lowers her back leg, so she is in Mountain Pose once again. Yoga, pan-Native, and Diné discourses construct a warrior as a spiritually developed person – and not necessarily one who engages in physical fighting (Peltier 103). As Jennifer Nez Denetdale, an acclaimed Diné scholar and the first Diné person to earn a Ph.D. in History, writes, "To be a warrior means to be compassionate and loving and to defend Dinétah" (51). Likewise, Laughter told me that in Diné understandings:

> the warrior is a leader. The warrior is somebody who thinks of their people and who has great discipline and the ability to stay focused…They're about the community and leadership. And I feel like with yoga, it's the same discipline. [Being a warrior is] abstaining from things that hurt you and putting your mind, your focus into learning and knowledge, staying humble, and recognizing your connection to mother earth, the sky, and your creator. (Laughter 2020)

Although the warrior may be gendered male in some Diné understandings, Laughter emphasized, "a man or a woman can be a warrior…in Navajo/Diné culture, we are a matriarchal society. So, it's the women who are in charge" (Laughter 2020). Laughter briefly brings her hands together in prayer above her heart center, so her fingertips are eye-level. In contemporary yoga, Diné, and Eurocentric understandings, a person's hands in prayer also connote spirituality.

In Laughter's vision then, perhaps her prayer is her body, her humanness, and the more-than-human elements that surround her. Once again, her arms quickly sweep above her head into prayer, and she comes into Forward Bend. Her fingers rest momentarily on the earth before she lowers the palms of her hands, reminiscent of the way that a more-than-human animal might paw the ground. This position, as dance scholar Sammy Roth observes, is reminiscent of "rolling through the feet (toe, ball, heel) when landing jumps, articulating through each joint to allow for the most cushioning and stable base, as well as preparing for a potential rebound into another spring" (Roth). Similarly, resilience, including the ability to bounce back, has been an important tactic of Native survivance given the genocidal structure of settler colonialism (Vizenor 1). Throughout her sequence, Laughter does not use a yoga mat, which is an intermediary with the ground and could symbolize commercialism; instead, she literally connects her body with the earth (Musial).[7] From Forward Bend, she steps one foot back and then the other into Downward Facing Dog. Laughter places her palms on the rocky surface of the ground, which cannot be comfortable unless one has trained and toughened their skin, communicating that connecting with the earth can at times be challenging. As she did with her fingers, Laughter finds footing with her toes first, followed by her heels. In Downward Facing Dog, she presses her chest towards her thighs. She is a human, shape shifting from a more-than-human animal ready to pounce to a rooted entity.

The features of the Diné lands on which Laughter practices contribute to and deepen the connections that she makes among humans and more-than-humans through yoga. With her grounded heels and sloping back in Downward Facing Dog, Laughter resembles the mountain behind her (Figure 10.2). In the interview I did with her, Laughter explicitly told me, "[Diné people] believe the body is Mother Earth" (3). She also told me, "Yoga is an expression of who I am, connected to the elements and the earth, in a place that I come from…or being a part of the land" (4).[8] As she transitions into Plank Pose, there is a slight halt in her movement, so she appears to take the shape of another mountain, but with a slightly different formation. Mother Earth is in Laughter's sight during these poses. Laughter then lowers into Chaturanga, also sometimes referred to as Crocodile Pose, and sweeps her heart forward into Upward Facing Dog, changing her view from the earth beneath her to the land far beyond. Although crocodiles are not indigenous to Diné lands, many lizards are, including the horned toad ("Shicheii"). Many Diné people refer to the horned toad as "grandpa," "which is a name that comes from cultural stories" and illustrates the interconnections among humans and more-than-humans in Diné understandings ("Shicheii"). Laughter presses back into Downward Facing Dog[9] and draws her left knee slightly forward – like a more-than-human animal readying

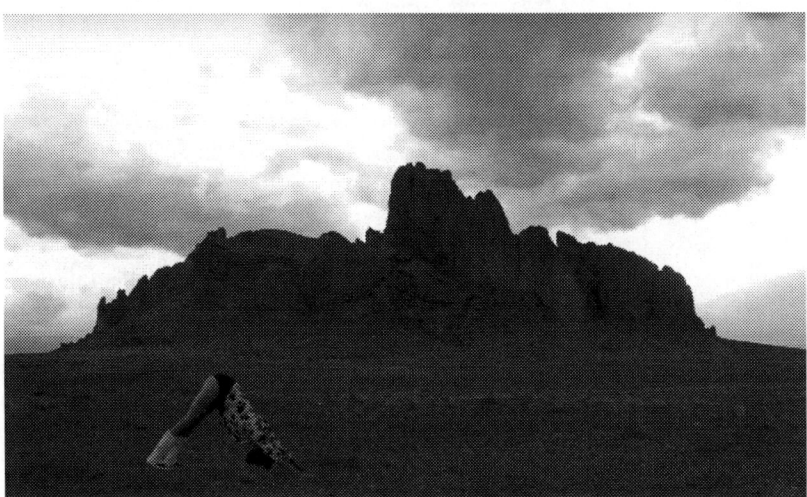

Figure 10.2 Laughter connecting her palms and feet with the earth in Downward Facing Dog

to run – before then extending her leg upward. She bends her knee a bit and "ever so slightly repositions her right hand under her heart" before flipping her Downward Facing Dog (Figure 10.3), so she is supine to the sky (Roth). Laughter's micro movements evidence the consciousness of her practice; "this and other little adjustments point to a deep attunement to anatomical alignment" (Roth). Lifting her left arm level with her heart center, she then gradually raises it higher, emphasizing the mountain behind her, Father Sky, and beyond.

From a Diné perspective, the relationships among human and more-than-humans which Laughter illustrates through her movements are reciprocal and spiritual. The sound of the wind is audible once again, and Laughter pauses momentarily as the wind ruffles her blouse, visually clarifying the more-than-human's continued presence. As Laughter articulated in our 2018 interview, humans are connected to the wind. She stated, "Air is our breath, the breath of life. It is also the way that we conduct ourselves, communicate, and speak to others. The words we choose, or our prayer" (3). In this initial interview, Laughter also described concluding the yoga classes that she teaches with a song or prayer. She said:

> In the end, what I do for [my students] is I sing them a song, and I tell them creation stories, how the song was created. And then I talk to them about how it was created. And I talk to them about how it vibrates from the inside out and goes all the way up into the sky, into the universe and heavens, and it becomes a prayer or an offering. And the song vibrates all the way, and it creates equilibrium, hózhó, it creates balance. (3)

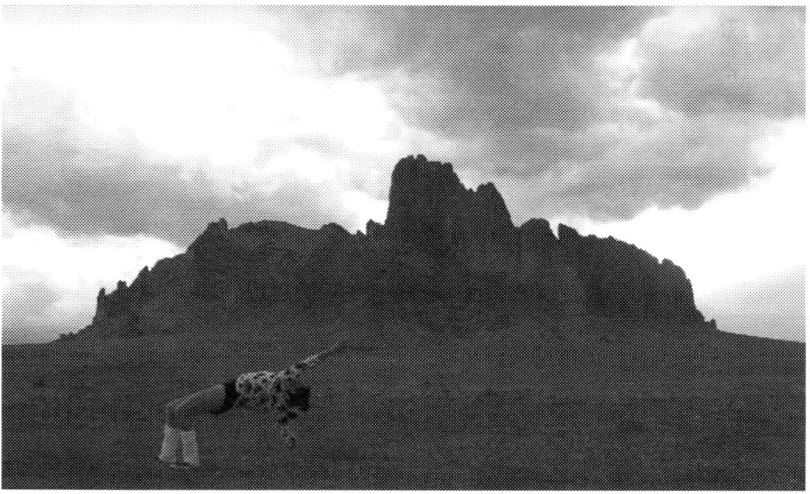

Figure 10.3 After flipping her Downward Facing Dog, Laughter lifts and arcs her left arm, gesturing to the more-than-humans surrounding her

In the film, the wind itself is a song in harmony with the music.

Laughter's yoga sequence also highlights Hózhó principles of balance and harmony. She transitions back into Downward Facing Dog, her left leg lifting skyward. Hardly hesitating, she sweeps her foot forward into Low Lunge, her hands framing her left foot. "For a brief but full moment, Laughter settles in this position before lifting into Warrior Two; this pause allows her stabilize and find her equilibrium before continuing on" (Roth). As she transitions into Warrior Two, her left arm rises while her right arm sweeps in a half circle from beside her foot to the sky and then lowers. The circling motion of her right hand resembles the movement of the sun as it rises each day in the east and sets in the west. For Diné and other Native peoples, circles are significant and sacred. Laughter also told me that circles represent the Hogan (2020) – again, the traditional Diné home – which is constructed in the shape of a circle (Thompson 14). The front door of a Hogan also faces east, the direction in which the sun rises (Thompson 14). Laughter further reflected that for the Diné, circles represent the four sacred colors and four sacred mountains that delineate the Diné homelands as well as cycles of life (2020). "Everything happens in cycles. [In our lives,] we come to a full circle. We give life. You're born; you live life; and then there's death…And there's different stages within [the] life that you have. You're a baby; then you're an adolescent; then you're an adult, and then [you become] an elder" (Laughter 2020).

The variation of the movement of Laughter's left and right hand to achieve the same position of the arms – extended, shoulder-height with palms facing downward – also suggests that there is more than one way to achieve balance. Indeed, "Hózhó is built on positive certainties of the innate capacity of each individual to achieve wholeness, happiness, health, balance, harmony, and ultimate wellbeing through attentive conscious practice of the Hózhó attributes" (Kahn-John and Koithan 27). This position connotes balance not only because both arms extended is a typical way for people to steady themselves, but also because Laughter's arms are parallel to and in balance with Mother Earth and Father Sky. As she transitions into Warrior Two, Laughter's gaze remains earthbound. Then, for the first time in the film, Laughter lifts her gaze to meet the viewer's. Her return of the viewer's gaze also creates balance by challenging or at least acknowledging that she is more than a passive object. Her face remains calm as she flips her palms skyward, which is yet another way of creating balance, as previously her palms faced the earth. Through the two different positions of her hands, "Laughter also enacts reciprocity through an energetic exchange, as some yoga teachers share that palms down during a seated meditation grounds a practitioner's energy into the earth, whereas palms up allows a person to receive energy from the space" (Roth).

Arms still extended, Laughter brings her hands into prayer above her head, underscoring the sacredness of balance and harmony and of Hózhó and other Diné worldviews, which U.S. settler colonialism has often targeted. She draws her hands to her heart center and bends her knee, lowering more deeply into Warrior Two, until her thigh is parallel to the earth. It is as if her moving prayer has given her physical strength to intensify the pose. From her hands in prayer in Warrior Two, Laughter extends her arms, transitioning into Exalted Warrior. Her right hand rests just below the back of her right knee while her left hand first extends towards the earth and then sweeps to the sky. She pauses momentarily, allowing the wind to ripple the white sheep skin string of her tsiiyéé (the Diné hairstyle, and as I will explain, ceremonial practice) before moving into Extended Side Angle Pose. As Laughter transitions, "her arms stay balanced in a straight line, teetering simultaneously with her torso," illustrating the effort and concentration that achieving balance can sometimes require (Roth). Her left fingertips connect with the earth, and she turns her gaze upward to her raised, right hand, and beyond it, Father Sky. In transitioning from Exalted Warrior to Extended Side Angle – shifting her left fingers from reaching towards the sky to literally connecting with the earth – Laughter reifies the harmonious relationship between Father Sky, Mother Earth, and human beings when one is in a state of Hózhó. The left side of the body is also where a human's heart, one of the most vital organs, is located.

The tsiiyéé is itself a conscious practice that exemplifies Diné worldviews. As Amanda Blackhorse writes, "the tsiiyéé is worn by men and women...Each strand, the yarn that is used, and the way in which it is wrapped has much purpose. It is sacred to the Diné, it is more than a tradition – it's a form of prayer and a spiritual practice." In our follow-up interview, Laughter also explained to me that like yoga, the tsiiyéé exemplifies knowledge and discipline. She told me that for the Diné, hair:

> represents your knowledge, the way that you live, and your identity. By pulling your hair back and making it nice, it shows discipline and it shows that you know who you are. It shows that you plan...In more modern times, of course, we wear our hair down, but in a traditional ceremony you should have it up. They say when a woman has her hair waving everywhere, her thoughts are all scattered or when she's cutting her hair, she's not disciplined. And so, it's also a representation of who you are...the discipline that you have within yourself, and the beauty you have within yourself, also modesty and healthy thoughts about taking care of yourself, your land, your people, your family.

Here, Laughter's description of the tsiiyéé echoes Kahn-John and Koithan's discussion of Hózhó as "conscious awareness of the collective and interconnected relationships between self and others" (27). The attention directed to developing consciousness is another link between yoga and Diné understandings. Notably, through her organization, Hozho Total Wellness, Laughter aims to "help Indigenous people heal through the conscious physical movements of yoga" (Middletent). Yet, wearing one's hair in a tsiiyéé remains an ongoing act of resistance, which challenges settler-colonial norms. As Blackhorse describes, in February 2016, a referee forbid Diné and non-Diné young women, high school basketball players, from wearing their hair in a tsiiyéé during a game, "because it violated the Arizona Interscholastic Association rule book regarding 'hair control devices.'" This incident demonstrates the enduring ways that settler-colonial logics and institutions attempt to control Native bodies and practices.

Laughter then shifts the direction that she is facing, further delineating the connections between different human and more-than-human entities. Rather than depict Laughter repeating the same yoga poses on her opposite side, the film transitions to the same wide-shot, but superimposes Laughter in Mountain Pose as the image of her in Extended Side Angle fades. Portraying Laughter doing the poses on both sides would show balance, but perhaps not be as aesthetically interesting. The fade suggests that time has elapsed for Laughter to complete the sequence on the opposite side, which is how yoga is typically practiced to achieve balance in the body. Dance scholar Sammy Roth also notes that "as the film fades in, the line that Laughter's right arm makes as it disappears is exactly aligned with the center line of her body, again signaling equilibrium and balance. The use of fading in and editing the repetition of the postures throughout the sequence, albeit with different facings, hints at the non-linearity of time and the cyclical nature of life" (Roth). In Mountain Pose, Laughter is already in motion. She lowers her arms, which appear to have been extended above her head – perhaps in prayer – to her sides. Although this is the same action that Laughter performed at the opening of the film, when she faces the viewer, the motion – which begins slightly above the shoulders – suggests a large bird slowly lowering its wings. Similar to the way that Laughter's Downward Facing Dog and Plank earlier in the film are reminiscent of the mountain behind her, her Mountain Pose in motion and facing the viewer suggests another more-than-human being. As if to underscore Mountain Pose as bird-like, Laughter then transitions into Eagle Pose (Figure 10.4).[10] Before

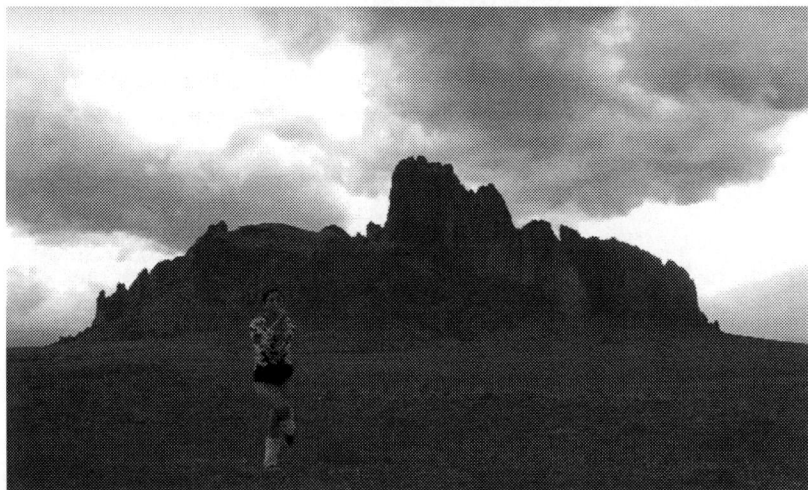

Figure 10.4 In Eagle Pose, Laughter's wrapping of her arms and legs resemble bean tendrils climbing corn stalks

her extended arms reach her body, Laughter lifts her right leg, snaking it around her left. Her right arm wraps beneath her left with the left elbow nestled into the crease of the right, and her arms twist again, so her palms meet. The blade edge of her left hand centered before her face creates the illusion of an eagle's beak. But her twisted legs and arms connote other more-than-human entities, such as snakes and vines.

In a Diné, culturally-relevant reading, Laughter's wrapping of her legs and arms in Eagle Pose could also suggest bean tendrils climbing corn stalks in a Three Sisters Garden. As Laughter discussed, for the Diné, corn is connected to the human body – specifically, the spine – and also ceremonial practices. She stated:

> The Navajo people have always had corn, and we believe that we came from corn and that it's part of the spine too. So, for instance, the base of our spine is like corn. Corn is rooted into the ground; our legs are rooted into the ground. Our legs are roots and the base of the spine is where [the corn plant] sprouts up. Everything grows from the bottom up, all the way up to the cervical spine, and then right there's your head, your mind. That's where your thinking is. And the tádídíín, the corn pollen, is what we use to pray with, to acknowledge the holy people with…And so, the connection would be [human bodies are] like the corn stalks, roots, legs, ground, then the spine comes up. [Where] there's the corn stalk [is] our rib cage, and our arms are the corn husks, and then it gets all the way up into our mind. And that's where the tádídíín touches also. When we pray, we touch our head with it. We put it on our head, our tongue and we make a path for ourselves.

In our 2018 interview, Laughter also discussed corn as being very sacred to the Diné and a staple of their diet (Blu Wakpa, "Yoga Brings You Back to Who You Are" 9). She told me then that an elder had revealed his knowledge about the interconnections between human bodies and corn plants after watching her do backbends (Blu Wakpa, "Yoga Brings You Back to Who You Are" 9). Laughter discussed drawing on this Diné teaching to create a "mediation around corn" for Diné women elders who were weavers by asking them to imagine their spine as a cornstalk (Blu Wakpa, "Yoga Brings You Back to Who You Are" 9). The elders thanked and complimented Laughter, telling her that her guided meditation "'just brings me back home. Brings you back to the memory of having corn, and how we came from the corn, and how sacred it is, and how our body [is] sacred and how it connects" (Blu Wakpa, "Yoga Brings You Back to Who You Are" 9). The elders' comments illustrate how yoga can be activated as a Diné culturally-relevant practice that furthers interconnectedness between human and more-than-human relatives.

Composed of corn, beans, and squash, the Three Sisters Garden exemplifies plant and human interrelationships and balance. As Melissa Kruse-Peeples writes, "For many Native American communities, three seeds – corn, beans, and squash represent the most important crops. When planted together, the Three Sisters work together to help one another thrive and survive...[T]hese crops complement each other in the garden as well as nutritionally." Along with the Haudenosaunee and Hopi, Kruse-Peeples specifically mentions the Diné in her discussion of the Three Sisters Garden. The author writes, although:

> [t]he tradition of calling these crops the 'Three Sisters' originated with the Haudenosaunee...[i]n the Southwest, there are traditions of planting the Sisters together as well as in separate fields. In dry farmed areas like Hopi and Navajo nation, the Sisters are planted in separate areas of fields with wide plant spacing to maximize limited water. In areas with adequate water the Sisters can be planted together in close proximity to get the companion planting benefits in the same cycle.

In other words, there is not one way to plant the Sisters. However, to best support the Sisters' growth, one must account for and act in accordance with the environment. Similarly, achieving Hózhó does not follow a prescribed path. "Hózhó reflects the process, the path, or journey by which an individual strives toward and attains this state of wellness. Thus, translating the complex meaning of Hózhó without reducing its expansive meaning is difficult" (Kahn-John and Koithan 25). Along with yoga and the tsiiyéé, gardening is another conscious practice that has the potential to promote wellness and strengthen human relationships to more-than-humans. As Kerry Frances Thompson writes, "For Navajos, planting, hunting, gathering, and raising sheep are all part of complex relationships between the people, the Sun, the earth, the Holy People, and the rest of Creation" (151). Understanding yoga as enacting Hózhó, as Laughter does, also demonstrates how Diné worldviews are dynamic and possess the potential to indigenize non-Diné movement practices; again, this combats settler-colonial (mis)representations of Native people, practices, and knowledges as relegated to the past. Additionally, the ability for Native people to indigenize movement practices has allowed them to thwart settler-colonial aims in critical ways that contribute to Native presents and futurities (Blu Wakpa, *Native American Embodiment in Educational and Carceral Contexts* vi).

Laughter's yoga sequence continues to underscore human and plant connections and harmony. From Eagle, Laughter transitions again into Mountain Pose. She steps her left foot out a little wider than shoulder width and takes Garland Pose. Although prayer is perhaps the most common hand position for Garland Pose, Laughter brings her arms into Eagle once again. Instead of suggesting corn and beans intertwined, her pose is shorter and wider, like squash. The film abruptly cuts, but again to the same wide shot with Laughter where she was before. Laughter is in a different variation of Garland Pose; yet, she still resembles a plant, with her feet together and heels lifted, but knees pointing out in opposite directions, like leaves. Her hands are extended in prayer above her head, as if she is growing towards the sun. Laughter's gaze, which is initially directed to the earth, shifts to the viewer as she draws her hands in prayer to the crown of her head, emphasizing human and plant relationships through the physical connection that she makes (Figure 10.5). For the Diné, the crown of the head is another link that connects them to human and more-than-human relatives. Laughter shared with me that unlike many Native peoples, the Diné typically do not wear eagle feathers – a symbol of community-bestowed honor – in their hair. Instead, she stated that the Diné "are told through the creation stories and through our elders the reason why is because we have an invisible eagle feather connected to the crown of our head when we are born. And so, wherever we go, we have an eagle feather with us [representing]… our identity and our connection to creation and to our creator and our sacredness, the sacredness within us." Laughter pauses with her wrists resting on the crown of her head for five seconds, so far, her longest duration of holding a pose in the film. The shape of her palms and wrists touching also suggests an eagle feather extending from the crown of her head skyward and her Diné/Native identity. Similarly, in Indigenous sign language, a person makes the sign for Native person, tribe, or nation by raising their index finger at the top of the head, indicating an eagle feather (Seton, Scott, and Powers). Like a plant, Laughter perhaps appears unmoving, but she is at work in her stillness.

Taking the interconnections among humans and plants further, Laughter next transitions into Headstand, which is often done with the crown as the only part of the head touching the earth. The invisible eagle feather Laughter wears that connects her to the creator, also literally connects her to the earth. Once again, the film cuts to her in this new pose, but maintains the same wide shot with Laughter

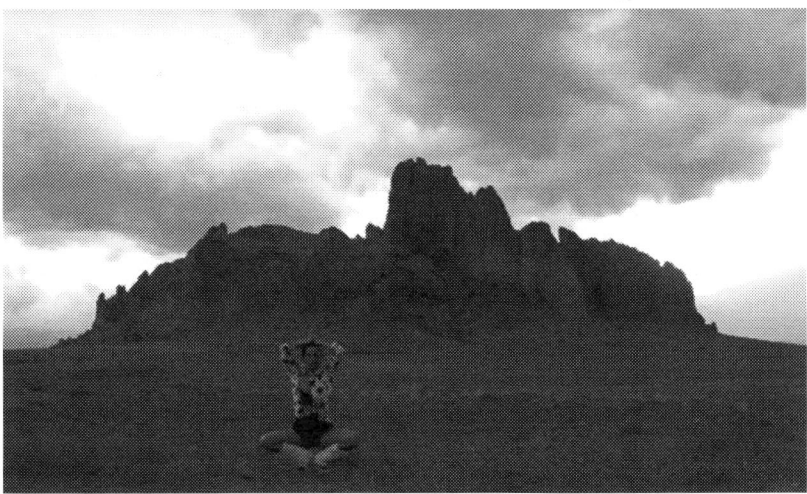

Figure 10.5 In Garland Pose, Laughter's hands in prayer at the crown of her head suggest an eagle feather and her Diné/Native identity

on the land not far from where she was before. Laughter is in profile view and already upside down. With her hands cradling her head and elbows and her knees still bent, she is almost the perfect opposite of her previous Garland pose. For humans, the head holds the brain – which like the heart – is one of the most critical parts of the body. However, for plants, the roots are most integral. By connecting the crown of her head with the earth in a way that is analogous to a plant's roots, Laughter creates another variation of a plant-like pose, highlighting human and more-than-human interconnections.

In Headstand, Laughter makes visible how the Hózhó philosophy of maintaining harmonious relationships with one's environment through respect and reciprocity is a practice and a process. For nearly a minute and a half, Laughter maintains Headstand, which is longer than she holds any other pose in the film. In Headstand, Laughter is also as yet the most centered in the frame. Both the duration with which Laughter holds the pose and her positioning in the frame emphasize the importance of Headstand within the sequence that she performs. With her left leg still bent, Laughter extends her right. The movement is slightly hesitant, and the left leg rises to meet the right before the right fully extends, perfectly reminiscent of seedlings growing and sprouting in a stop motion film. With both legs fully extended in Headstand, Laughter's body wavers slightly, making visible the effort it takes to maintain this challenging pose in general and perhaps with the wind blowing in particular; again, this illustrates the sometimes struggle of maintaining balance with the elements and in one's life. Yet despite the challenge of doing Headstand on the rocky earth amid the at times audible wind, Laughter remains in equanimity and balance.

Although Hózhó represents balance as a utopian state, dance scholar Brenda Dixon Gottschild has also emphasized the value of "keep[ing] ourselves off center in order to stay on target." The example that Gottschild provides to illustrate her point is Headstand. She writes: "Reversals/inversions can be invaluable in offering alternative approaches…[i]n the same sense that the hatha yoga headstand is performed not only to physically stimulate circulation to the brain but also to psychically offer the practitioner the experience of seeing the world in chaos – upside down – and to find one's center off center." (Gottschild 172). Because the structure of settler colonialism causes "chaos" by attempting to assimilate Indigenous peoples to a new world order that adversely affects their relationships with one another and more-than-humans, movement practices that teach people to find equanimity and (re)establish relationships are valuable. For example, yoga teachers often encourage students who lose their balance and fall out of a pose to remain composed and attempt the challenge again and/or rest in Child's Pose. This is valuable training that can help people to cope with the frustration, injustice, and violence that settler colonialism causes. Moreover, as settler-colonial discourses often attempt to obscure systemic oppressions – at times by blaming individuals for their supposed deficiencies – "[r]eversals/inversions" can strengthen people's critical thinking skills to expose false rhetoric, which is often the first step in working towards social change.

In Headstand, Laughter bends her right leg into a variation of Tree pose, which again resembles the leaf-like Garland Pose she previously performed (Figure 10.6). She extends both legs, and her body sways slightly like a plant blowing in the wind. Slowly she begins to lower her legs, pausing with them slightly above a 90-degree angle from the earth. This pose, still upside down, resembles Laughter's earlier Downward Facing Dog, which appeared both like a large, more-than-human animal and the mountain behind her. Laughter's sequence of poses and their similarities to other poses that she has performed suggests the inextricable connections among human and more-than-human persons, which settler-colonial discourses often overlook. By doing the same pose upside down or from a different direction, Laughter asks the viewer to consider how a change in perspective might shift and/or deepen one's consciousness and understanding. She lifts her legs once more, then lowers them into an upside-down Garland Pose; again, transforming into a plant. Her left leg briskly extends skyward.[11]

The final poses in the film emphasize human responsibility to Mother Earth and Father Sky as integral to Diné spirituality and the Hózhó principle of "walking in beauty" (Laughter 2020). As the image of Laughter in Headstand fades, the film portrays her in profile, positioning herself for Dancer's Pose, still centered in the same wide-shot. Yet, after the fade, "the clouds are in a different location, conveying not only the passing of time, but also that these more-than-humans move along with Laughter" (Roth). Dancer's Pose requires tremendous balance – not only as a person stands on one leg, but also as they steadily kick their elevated leg into their hand to open the shoulder and chest on that side. With energy and intention, Laughter reaches forward with her left hand – again, the heart side – and her arm is parallel to the earth and sky. In yoga descriptions, the kicking of the foot

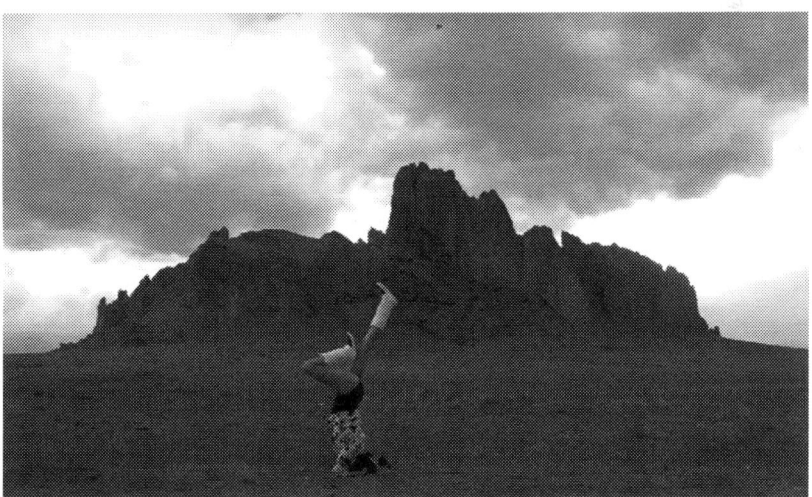

Figure 10.6 Laughter appears like a plant in upside-down Garland Pose

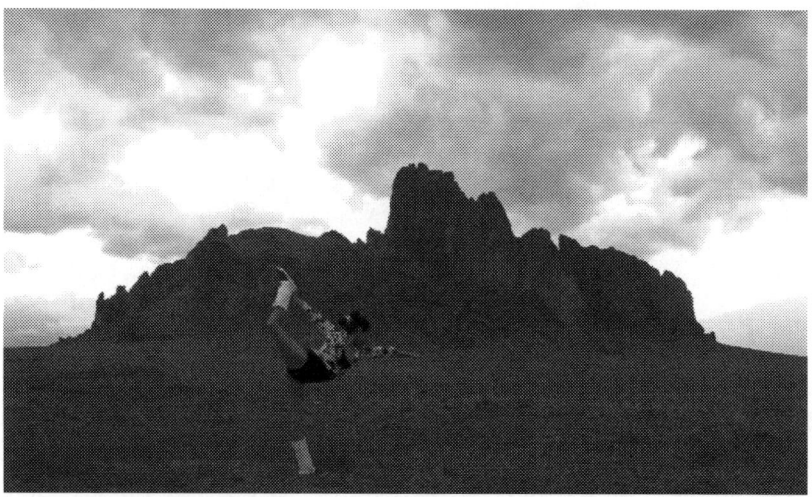

Figure 10.7 Laughter "opening her heart" in Dancer's Pose

into one's hand in Dancer's Pose is sometimes referred to as "opening the heart," which can convey spiritual change and growth (Figure 10.7). Steadily and with focus, Laughter eases out of the pose as she came into it. This image of Laughter fades as she emerges facing the viewer in the center of the wide-shot. Standing, she brings her right leg into Tree Pose with her foot in the Half-Lotus variation. She brings her hands to prayer, slightly above her heart center. She seems to take a deep breath, and reaches her hands, still in prayer, to the sky. Immediately, she opens them as if in gratitude to the sky, but also simultaneously gesturing to the grandness of the mountain behind her. Laughter brings her hands to prayer at heart center, again connoting spirituality. With her right leg still in Tree Pose and her foot in the Half-Lotus variation, she bends her left knee, lowering her hips, and bringing her right shin parallel to the earth in a hip stretch. Laughter then places her hands on the earth, also as if in thanks. As Laughter sets her hands on the earth, this image of her quickly fades, transposed with another image of her in the same shot. She braces her hands behind her, helping to support her body weight while she prepares for Toe Standing Pose, which demands exceptional balance. Laughter brings her left hand to heart center followed by her right; as soon as her hands briefly touch, the film fades.

Conclusion: *Hot Hooghan Yoga*

This essay conducts a close reading of *Hozho Yoga* to delineate how Laughter's yoga practice on Diné lands illustrates the Diné philosophy of Hózhó, including the interconnections among human and more-than-humans and the inextricability of the mind, body, and spirit. Laughter's presence and practice challenge settler-colonial discourses by illuminating Diné people's ongoing and conscious connection to the land, including their reciprocal and spiritual relationships with more-than-human relatives and their revitalization and innovation of their practices through yoga. For Laughter, yoga has been a powerful tool to (re)connect with her Diné identity, which settler colonialism had estranged her from. As she expressed in 2018, "Yoga's where I found my identity, and it's where I found who I was. Yoga brings you back to who you are" (Blu Wakpa, "Yoga Brings You Back to Who You Are" 12).

As Kate Mattingly notes, "Native people practicing and teaching yoga is also a tactic of resistance to the genocidal structure of settler colonialism because yoga is based in the ideas of balance, well-being equanimity; yoga is literally a life force (pranayama) that sustains people" (Mattingly). Laughter continues to leverage yoga in new ways that support Native people's resistance to settler colonialism. In our 2018 interview, she told me:

> I have a vision, Tria, and vision starts with Navajo of course. But I have this vision of a hogan-shaped yoga studio that is heated by sweat lodge rocks. It's a place where people come for meditation, for yoga, and a place where they come for teacher training, where they come conference, whatever. This is the vision that I have. Somehow, it's going to happen. I'm manifesting it. It will be a place for our people to heal, and it will go not only for this reservation, but all reservations will have their own place of mediation, their own place of healing. Teachers with Indigenous Yoga Instructors Association, with Hózhó Total Wellness, can go and teach. (11)

Hot Hooghan Yoga depicts the realization of Laughter's vision, which notably centers Diné women, whom the racialized and gendered structure of settler colonialism not only marginalize, but also mark for death and disappearance (Simpson). The short video shows Laughter teaching a class to seven Diné women practicing yoga together in a Hogan. A crackling fire burns in the structure's center, audible even with Laughter's instructions and a song by the Native group, Harmony Nights. The film opens with the women in Extended Side Angle. Although only Laughter's upper body is evident in the shot, the energy and intention in her extended arm are evident. The women whom Laughter teaches straddle yoga mats and wear yoga pants, t-shirts, and shorts; they are clearly Native women in the contemporary day. Some of the women seem more comfortable in the poses than others, suggesting that there are regular practitioners and relative newcomers and that more Native people are becoming yoga practitioners. Laughter asks the women to momentarily extend their front leg, then bend their knee to come into Warrior Two. One Diné woman, wearing a red bandana, takes Warrior II, a pink yoga mat with Native-designs between her feet, again evidencing how Diné and other Native people are indigenizing yoga. She too extends her arms with energy, intention, and vision, characteristics that have allowed Diné people to perpetuate and innovate their cultural practices despite the persuasive and pervasiveness of settler colonialism. She flips the palm of her extended arm from facing Mother Earth to Father Sky. Consciously, she reaches forward into Extended Side Angle. Laughter is just beginning to give another instruction when the video abruptly cuts (Figure 10.8).

Yet, as Susan Foster, whose work is essential in Dance studies, articulates, even when the ephemeral ends, it persists ("Choreographing History," 5). After our second interview in which Laughter beautifully told me the Diné creation story of how the eagle and canary unite to carry the first song from the heavens to the Diné people, she called me back (Laughter 2020). Laughter had shared the creation story with me as a way to illustrate the "correlations among vibration, movement, yoga, dance, music, and sound." But there was something she had left unsaid, which needed to be spoken. Laughter continued, "Movement, sound, vibration is what we use in ceremony to create Hózhó or equilibrium balance. When the medicine man sings and you sing with him all night or when it's chants,

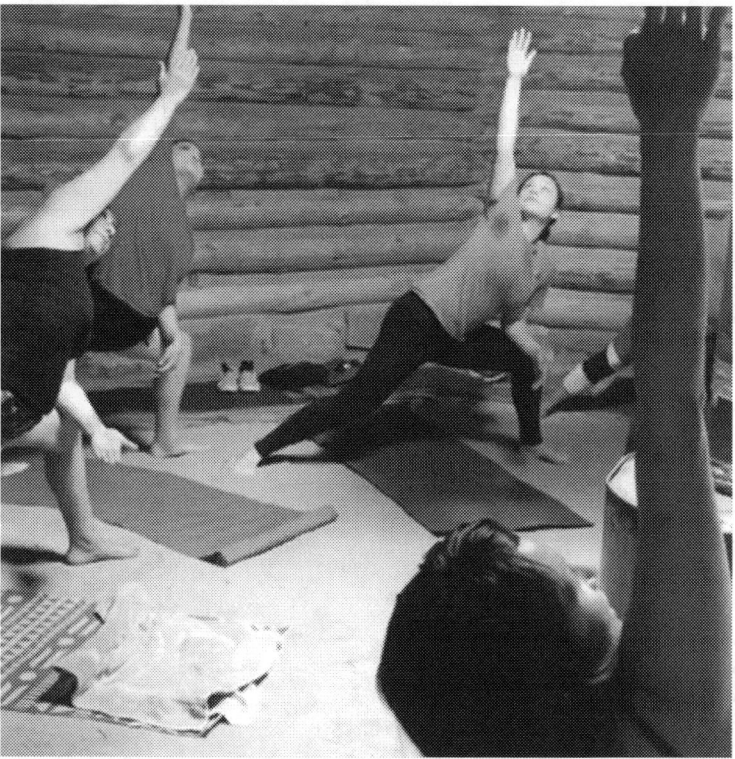

Figure 10.8 Laughter realizing one of her visions by teaching yoga to Native people in a Hogan

it's music, the vibration creates equilibrium, like earth, all through our bodies and that goes all the way up to the creator, to the heavens." As the knowledge that Laughter added illustrates, like Dance studies, Indigenous epistemologies instruct us that even when the ephemeral ends, it persists, in some cases, extending beyond what is visible or knowable – at least to humans. Yet, Indigenous epistemologies also draw our attention to the ways that the ephemeral persists beyond human forms and understandings to that of more-than-human animals, air, land, water, sky, and the universe, to which we are connected and from which we have much to learn.

Acknowledgments:

I acknowledge and thank the Gabrielino/Tongva Tribe and the Fernandeño Tataviam Band of Mission Indians on whose lands I resided and worked as a guest while writing this chapter. I could not have written this paper without the knowledge, expertise, and generosity of Haley Laughter. For their support strengthening this work, I am grateful to: Sammy Roth, Susan Foster, Cara Hagan, Kate Mattingly, and Jennifer Musial. I dedicate this chapter to my first yoga teacher, my mother, Laurie Andrews.

Notes

1. Citing a Diné woman interviewed in the 1990s, Laura Jane Moore writes, moccasins "'were first worn by the holy people and reflect our culture and our identity as Diné...It is by a Navajo's moccasin the Holy People recognize that a person is Diné...Moreover, the construction of the moccasins is critical because the sole 'represents mother earth' and the top, which is 'dyed red to represent the rainbow...is father sky.' The sinew that ties together the sole and the top represents lightning and thus the 'union of mother earth and father sky [which] brings forth all life.' As when a Navajo weaves, the process of making moccasins expresses hozho, harmony between nature and the supernatural, and the power of thought" (30).
2. Dance scholar, Sammy Roth notes, "As Laughter steps into Warrior Three, her arms arc from the sky to point directly in front of her before sweeping down, out to the sides, and up to create this bird-like position. When linked with the subsequent lift of her back leg and extension of the ankle, these initial transitions extend her energy circularly from sky to earth and back to the sky using her whole body" (Roth).
3. Yet, I am cognizant that Native and non-Native people frequently travel to and from the Rosebud Reservation, so it is very possible that someone was practicing and teaching yoga there prior to me. At the same time, many Lakota people on the Rosebud Reservation whom I have interacted with were familiar with yoga through mainstream media even if they did not practice it themselves.
4. For instance, Laughter stated that when she first began posting images of herself practicing yoga to HEALTHY ACTIVE NATIVES!!!!, a prominent Native person involved in the group told her, "'Haley, I'm sorry to tell you this, but I don't think that Natives really like yoga,'" which Laughter told me "inspired [her] to push harder" (Laughter 2020).
5. Native studies scholar, Gerald Vizenor, describes survivance as "an active sense of presence over absence, deracination, and oblivion; survivance is the continuance of stories, not a mere reaction, however pertinent" (1).

6 A term coined by Linda Tuhiwai Smith, decolonizing methodologies recognizes and refutes the hierarchal power dynamics of Eurocentric, supposedly "objective," academic research and seeks to do ethical and reciprocal work that is useful to Indigenous communities.
7 In a comment on this manuscript, Jennifer Musial also noted, "Without [a yoga mat or towel], it's more like stripped down or raw yoga." Musial's description reminded me of how Laughter discussed what it means to "decolonize yoga" in our 2018 interview (Blu Wakpa, "Yoga Brings You Back to Who You Are" 8). The concept of "decolonizing yoga" is often fraught. In a U.S. context, when yoga discourses center Native peoples, Indigenous South Asian and South Asian practitioners, origins, and influences on the practice are often overlooked; in contrast, when narratives focus on Indigenous South Asian and South Asian experts, origins, and influences, Native peoples and sovereignties are often omitted (Blu Wakpa, "Decolonizing Yoga?" 1). In our interview, Laughter stated, "Coming back to the basics begins with us inside, and being proud of who we are and knowing our culture, and knowing these different aspects that make us who we are. When you take it to the broader aspect of people speaking to decolonizing yoga, what I've read a lot about is taking it back to the true form of yoga, and to decolonize the aspect, once again, of a lot of dancing and music and making it appealing, but just going back to the basics of the original practice, which would be meditation while moving. Hatha yoga. Or the different aspects of the yamas, the way of life, basically. As far as decolonizing yoga, for me as an Indigenous woman, as a Diné woman, I would say that it would be being able to offer and being able to give our students, our teachers, an authentic yoga practice with the basics while incorporating the basics of indigenous philosophy. The basics like reconnecting with breath and the cultural teachings that our grandparents carried with them. It is important to know where we come from, where yoga comes from, and even though yoga is not a practice indigenous to the U.S., our ancestors also had holistic practices that colonization has targeted, and so yoga is like coming home, a way of reconnecting with our ancestors and our original ways of life. Again, the basics. I think we get so wound up in the details of things. Making it simple is better than complicating it." Laughter's lack of the yoga mat could indicate an aesthetic choice; however, as this excerpt evidences, it is also indicative of how she understands decolonizing yoga.
8 In the previously published interview, Laughter states that she is from Shiprock. However, she clarified that her paternal family is from Tall Mountain, Arizona, and her maternal family is from Chichiltah, New Mexico.
9 As Sammy Roth notices, Laughter "begins this movement from her toes, which ripples up the rest of her spine" (Roth). This articulation evidences the interconnections of different "parts" of the body.
10 Sammy Roth observes, "Throughout this balancing pose, Laughter makes micro-adjustments in her core and by pressing her arms and legs against each other. There is negotiation between her many parts to create a balanced whole" (Roth).
11 As Sammy Roth describes, "When Laughter initially performs the upside-down Garland Pose, her toes point toward the left edge of the tallest mountain behind her. Then, as she extends her leg, her toes draw an imaginary line to the top of the mountain" (Roth). Through this trajectory, Laughter's moving, human form draws attention to the different features of the fixed and massive more-than-human, towering behind her.

Works cited

Blackhorse, Amanda. "Blackhorse: Diné Tsiiyéé? [Hair Bun] Is Power." *Indian Country Today*, February 2016, https://indiancountrytoday.com/archive/blackhorse-diné-tsiiyéé-hair-bun-is-power-yeyYO4tB-kOqsIzdu4bIbQ. Accessed 26 March 2020.

Blu Wakpa, Tria. *Native American Embodiment in Educational and Carceral Contexts: Fixing, Eclipsing, and Liberating.* PhD dissertation. UC Berkeley, 2017.

Blu Wakpa, Tria. "Decolonizing Yoga? and (Un) Settling Social Justice." *Race and Yoga* vol. 3, no. 1, 2018, pp. i–xix.

Blu Wakpa, Tria. "Yoga Brings You Back to Who You Are: A Conversation Featuring Haley Laughter." *Race and Yoga* vol. 3, no. 1, 2018. https://escholarship.org/uc/item/3dz8g5k8.

Dadosky, John. "Three Diné Women on the Navajo Approach to Dreams." *Anthropology of Consciousness* vol. 10, no. 1, 1999, pp. 16–27.

Foster, Susan Leigh. "Choreographing History." *Choreographing History*, edited by Susan Leigh Foster, Bloomington: Indiana University Press, 1995, pp. 3–21.

Gottschild, Brenda Dixon. "Some Thoughts on Choreographing History." *Meaning in Motion*, edited by Jane Desmond, Durham: Duke University Press, 1997, pp. 167–77.

"Healthy Active Natives!!!." *Facebook*, https://www.facebook.com/groups/Healthyactivenatives/. Accessed 11 May 2020.

"Hot Hooghan Yoga." *YouTube*, uploaded by Indigenous Yoga Channel by Hozho Total Wellness, 25 April, 2019. www.youtube.com/watch?time_continue=2&v=inP7La5fhGs.

"Hozho Yoga." *YouTube*, uploaded by Indigenous Yoga Channel By Hozho Total Wellness, 27 February 2017. www.youtube.com/watch?v=7zGhI83tEnE.

Huhndorf, Shari M. *Going Native: Indians in the American Cultural Imagination.* Ithaca: Cornell University Press, 2001.

Inoue, Cristina Yumie Aoki, and Paula Franco Moreira. "Many Worlds, Many Nature(s), One Planet: Indigenous Knowledge in the Anthropocene." *Revista Brasileira de Política Internacional* vol. 59, no. 2, 2016, pp. 1–19.

Iyengar, B.K.S. *Light on Yoga.* New York: Schocken Books, 1979.

Kahn-John, Michelle, and Mary Koithan. "Living in Health, Harmony, and Beauty: The Diné (Navajo) Hózhó Wellness Philosophy." *Global Advances in Health and Medicine* vol. 4, no. 15, May 2015, pp. 24–30, doi:10.7453/gahmj.2015.044.

Kruse-Peeples, Melissa. "How to Grow a Three Sisters Garden." *Native Seeds/SEARCH*, 27 May 2016, www.nativeseeds.org/blogs/blog-news/how-to-grow-a-three-sisters-garden. Accessed 26 March 2020.

Laughter, Haley. Personal Interview. 16 April 2020.

Mattingly, Kate. Comments on Paper. 4 April 2020.

Middletent, Kansas. "Be Indigenous Yoga Inspired: Haley's Healing Journey" *Native Hope*, https://blog.nativehope.org/be-indigenous-yoga-inspired-haleys-healing-journey. Accessed March 18, 2020.

Miller, Amara. *Yoga R/Evolution: Deconstructing the 'Authentic' Yoga Body.* PhD dissertation. University of California, Davis, 2018.

Moore, Laura Jane. "Elle Meets the President: Weaving Navajo Culture and Commerce in the Southwestern Tourist Industry." *Frontiers: A Journal of Women Studies* vol. 22, no. 1, 2001, pp. 21–44. https://www.jstor.org/stable/3347066.

Morales, Laurel. "Eagle Feathers: Sacred to Navajos, Protected by U.S." *Arizona Public Media*, June 2015, https://news.azpm.org/s/31531-eagle-feathers-sacred-to-navajos-protected-by-government/. Accessed 30 March 2020.

Musial, Jennifer. Comments on Paper. 25 April 2020.

Natalie Rose. "Comment on "Hozho Yoga." *Youtube*, uploaded by Indigenous Yoga Channel by Hozho Total Wellness, 27 February 2017. https://www.youtube.com/watch?v=7zGhI83tEnE&lc=UgjcIjbgKMhgoHgCoAEC.

Navajo Wotd. https://navajowotd.com/word/naashoii/

Nez Denetdale, Jennifer. "A Biographical Account of Manuelito: Noble Savage, Patriotic Warrior, and American Citizen." *Reclaiming Diné History: The Legacies of Navajo Chief Manuelito and Juanita*, University of Arizona Press, 2007, pp. 51–86. *JSTOR*, www.jstor.org/stable/j.ctt181hxxf.7. Accessed 31 March 2020.

Night Owl. "Broke for Free." *YouTube,* uploaded by Broke For Free, 9 January 2011, https://www.youtube.com/watch?v=9oKl99PEbHw.

Peltier, Leonard. *Prison Writings: My Life Is My Sun Dance*. Edited by Harvey Arden. New York, St. Martin's Press, 1999.

Roth, Sammy. Comments on Paper. 27 August 2020.

Seton, Ernest Thompson, Hugh Lenox Scott, and Lillian Delger Powers. *Sign Talk; a Universal Signal Code, Without Apparatus, for Use in the Army, Navy, Camping, Hunting, and Daily Life*. New York: Doubleday, Page & Company, 1918.

"Shicheii." *NavajoWOTD.com*, https://navajowotd.com/word/shicheii/. Accessed 13 May 2020.

Simpson, Audra. "The State Is a Man: Theresa Spence, Loretta Saunders and the Gender of Settler Sovereignty." *Theory & Event* vol. 19, no. 4, 2016. *Project MUSE* muse.jhu.edu/article/633280.

Smith, Linda Tuhiwai. *Decolonizing Methodologies: Research and Indigenous Peoples*, 2nd ed. London, UK: Zed Books, 2012.

Thompson, Kerry Frances. *Alkidaa' da Hooghanee (They Used to Live Here): An Archeological Study of Late Nineteenth and Early Twentieth Century Navajo Hogan Households and Federal Indian Policy*. PhD Dissertation. University of Arizona, 2009.

Tuck, Eve, and K. Wayne Yang. "Decolonization Is Not a Metaphor." *Decolonization: Indigeneity, Education & Society* vol. 1, no. 1, 2012. pp. 1–40.

Vizenor, Gerald. "Aesthetics of Survivance: Literary Theory and Practice." *Survivance: Narratives of Native Presence*, edited by Gerald Vizenor, Lincoln: University of Nebraska Press, 2008, pp. 1–24.

Chapter 11

Yoga asana and the performance of gender in American exercise

Cara Hagan

Introduction

The body as conceptualized in Puritanical America has always been a site fraught with rigid expectation. Throughout history, men and women have been taught to fit into prescribed roles that govern the use of their bodies. As bodies exist in motion for much of our lives, the body in motion often acts as a litmus test for the performance of gender. For women, the expectation to exude an idealized femininity is part of an obligation for being granted access to societal acceptance. This means that while popular ways of moving may shift over time, the underlying impetus for popular movement remains the same. Cultivating dichotomies between the sexes and manufacturing the archetypal woman-in-motion serves to bolster the patriarchy and reinforce myopic notions of women's place in society. In this dichotomy, there exists little room for nuanced or gender non-conforming bodily expressions. Thus, women's wellness in America has been a battleground for conflicting theories of how to approach exercise in concert with social and spiritual pursuits since the 19th century. While this story includes attempts and triumphs at subverting the American tendency toward White, able-bodied, heteronormative conceptions of gender, many of the oppressive ideologies articulated in the 19th century are at work today. Postural yoga – with its history in the United States beginning just before the turn of the 20th century – is a site of such gendered performance. As a decidedly feminized (though not always feminist) practice in America, yoga is not exempt from perpetuating harmful conceptions of the feminine, embodied.

In this chapter, I take up the notion and experience of gender through the lens of "fitness" as understood in an American context. Though not entirely divorced from spirituality (at times, fitness and spirituality have been bedfellows on the path to self-improvement), the world of fitness, the wellness industry, and the commodification of lifestyle separate from spiritual pursuits need to be understood if one is to fully appreciate the trajectory of yoga in the United States and its participation in upholding a physicalized dualism. As it exists today, the landscape of American fitness exists to reinforce a culture of individualism where one's efforts – and their subsequent results – are signs of not only desirability, but also morality, intelligence, and patriotism. Since structural inequity and the supremacy of visual culture are carried out by White society, this means that most often these traits are reserved for only certain sects of society while others strive, and often fail, to meet these standards. These mechanisms for embodied hegemonies were put in place long ago, and a walk along their journeys helps us to understand contemporary manifestations of their legacies, from Madonna to the "Naked Athena."[1]

In response to the dualistic discourse presented in the first half of this chapter, this piece culminates in a brief exploration of the ways yogic philosophy and practice include areas of slippage that allow for a more inclusive gender experience. A set of guiding questions and a small handful of readily applicable practices offer nuanced alternatives to the norms that persist in American society, while providing possible avenues into a more accepting and affirming future of yoga in America.

A journey through history

Prior to, and throughout the 1800s, the prevailing philosophy regarding men's and women's bodies was that they are inherently different, with men's bodies being superior to women's bodies in terms of strength and intelligence. As a result, women in the middle and upper classes in America were taught to overplay their supposed weakness so that they could remain under the care and protection of men who, following the rise of industrialization, sought to embody "manly, ideal men"[2] through the cultivation of strenuous exercise practices. The first mention of women's exercise in Western mass media came in the form of an influential essay by French philosopher Jean Jacques Rousseau titled, *Emile, or Treatise on Education* (1762). Circulated widely throughout the Western world, Rousseau encouraged "pleasant, moderate, and healthy exercise" for women, and extolled the "value of manual labour and bodily exercise for strengthening the health and constitution" for men. These differences were recommended not just because Rousseau believed that physical activity helped people to be in touch with the natural tendencies and rhythms of human experience, but for the avoidance of producing a "degenerate race," lest "children [be] made tender before birth by the softness of their parents" (Rousseau, 1762). Although Rousseau's essay appeared before an articulated philosophy of eugenics became commonplace in American society, his ideas were in alignment with what would come to be called, *positive eugenics*, or the cultivation of desirable traits in people through purposeful reproduction. *Positive eugenics* is not to be confused with *negative eugenics*, the system of eliminating undesirable human traits through practices like forced sterilization (which is still in practice today[3]). It should, however, be understood that both forms of eugenic practice are problematic. The philosophy and practice of eugenics went hand-in-hand with a widespread belief in *Social Darwinism*, a notion coined by British philosopher Herbert Spencer in the 19th century that espoused "survival of the fittest" among the human population (Singleton, 2007).

This meant that those who were powerful were that way because they were inherently better humans. This belief was used to justify slavery, colonialism, racism, sexism, and various forms of social and political conservatism. Both the eugenics movement and Social Darwinism influenced how people used their bodies in the 19th and early 20th centuries.

In her book, *Physical Culture and the Body Beautiful: Purposive Exercise in the Lives of American Women 1800-1875*, Dr. Jan Todd describes the emergence of oppositional ideas to those held by men like Rousseau. Women (and men) whose politics were in alignment with the soon-to-emerge Women's Suffrage movement, encouraged women and girls to take up exercise with more rigor and in more variety than those proposed in the writings of Rousseau and his proponents. One woman of note is British writer Mary Wollstonecraft, and her essay, *A Vindication of the Rights of Woman* (1793). Her work not only directly challenges many of the ideas written in Rousseau's essay, but also proposes a form of physicality in women that is inspired by the highly detailed, kinetically expressive depictions of the female body in the Greek statuary of the Hellenistic period:

> I know it will be said that woman would be "unsexed" by acquiring strength of body and mind, and that beauty – soft bewitching beauty! – would no longer adorn the daughters of men. I think, on the contrary, that we would then see dignified beauty and true grace, arising from many powerful physical and moral causes. It wouldn't be relaxed beauty or the graces of helplessness; but rather the beauty and grace that appears to make us respect the human body as a majestic structure that is fit to receive a noble inhabitant, in the relics of antiquity. (Wollstonecraft and Brody, 2020)

It is important to mention that in her endorsement of the bodies as seen in Greek statuary, Wollstonecraft perpetuates a *different*, though equally *impossible* bodily ideal for women as articulated by her male contemporaries. Artists in the Hellenistic period were judged not on how well they represented their models in metal or stone, rather on how well they corrected their inherent imperfections with regard to proportion and symmetry (Osborne, 1986). Though her writing couples opinions on how women should use their bodies and the importance of formal education for girls and women, her essay upheld notions of an accepted femininity of the time. In its commitment to a universal and "transitory love" (nurturing), monogamous marriage (domesticity, motherhood, and the societal preference for married women over single ones), bodily grace (feminine bodily indicators), and public display of virtue and fidelity to God (piety), Wollstonecraft's work walks a line between radicalism and acceptance that allowed her ideas to take hold in well-to-do society in the form of a burgeoning physical education movement for girls and women in the 1800s.

As schools for girls and stand-alone gymnasiums in New England began to emerge in the early 1800s, so did routine physical practice for the girls in attendance at those schools and gymnasiums. At first criticized for offering physical education to girls and young women, these establishments soon became the sites of a short-lived trend in women practicing European-style gymnastics. Exercise luminaries of the time, like husband and wife J.A. Beaujeu and Madame Beaujeu-Hawley, were among the first to monetize exercise. Having opened a women's gymnasium in Dublin in 1824, with subsequent gymnasiums opened in Boston and New York, the Beaujeus "recommended during the 1820s that women participate in exercises remarkably similar…to those described by men. Furthermore… women's participation in this earlier exercise movement tended to transcend female submissiveness" (Todd, 1998). Chin-ups, dips, ladder-climbing and more were taught to women as a means of achieving strength and beauty. Furthermore, women were encouraged to partake in these strenuous exercises as a way to prepare for emergencies that may arise in a woman's life that would require her to run, climb, or otherwise exert herself.

Unfortunately, the gymnastics trend only lasted until about 1830. By then, many came to criticize the women's gymnastics movement, citing the masculinization of women and the possibility of severe injury to not only their joints and muscles, but to their reproductive organs. While the physical culture in the 1830s for men would evolve to include pursuits such as weightlifting and body building, for women, the movement would result in the widespread practice of calisthenics, a much more subdued form of exercise. In fact, many of the exercises produced little to no effect at all on the muscle tone, flexibility, and cardiovascular improvement of the body. As Todd puts it:

> Where Beaujeu and Fowle had argued for utilitarian robustness, the devotees of calisthenics favored a more ethereal model of beauty and fitness. Calisthenics proponents also generally adhered to the new, upper-class cult of femininity and embraced the idea that women should be slender, willowy, and pliant. (Todd, 1998)

The desire for women to be thin intensified in the decades following and by the turn of the century, fat shaming was part and parcel of the physical culture movement as it was deployed thorough print media and subsequently, radio and the screen. Silent film actress Amelia Summerville was quoted in an 1895 newspaper article saying, "I can only urge all fat women to try dieting, as it brings its own reward. An oversupply of flesh is so much in the way, and one feels so clumsy, and so like a house!" (Enid Daily Wave, 1895). Likewise, an advertisement for a weight loss supplement ran the entirety of the year 1916 in the Muskogee Times Democrat saying, "people who are overburdened with superfluous fat know all too well the discomfort and ridicule that over-stout people have to bear" (Muskogee Times Democrat, 1916). These articles and advertisements were almost always accompanied by a photograph or drawing of an example of accepted womanhood, in both body and fashion. Thinness was not only a sign of beauty, it was a sign of American exceptionalism. The export of images of beautiful American bodies was, and still is, part of the American hegemonic project.

By now, you understand that any consideration for the physical education and purposeful exercise of girls and women in the antebellum era and in the decades following the civil war did not apply to poor women, immigrant women, and women of color. In fact, Black women especially were hardly considered women at all as they did not often have access to many of the necessities for achieving "true womanhood."[4] For example, female slaves were denied their right to motherhood through chattel slavery (though they gave birth, their children could be sold), their "purity" was subject to the whims of their masters, and their bodies were engaged in the rugged work of agriculture, domestic work, and other such pursuits. Free Black women and immigrant women often attended to the children of wealthy White women, and worked as domestics, or as factory workers. Their very existence in the American context went against every tenet of "true womanhood" set forth by dominant culture at the time.

While there is scant written about Blackness and physical culture and/or fitness prior to the 21st century, that doesn't mean women of color were not influenced by and did not participate in physical culture. In fact, many Black people worked to gain a foothold in American society by morality signaling through fashion and physical culture. In her 2017 survey of Black women and physical culture in the early 1900s, Ava Purkiss summarizes the relationship of Black women to notions of health and wellness in the early 20th century. Citing the need for Black women to distance themselves from histories of the sexualization of their bodies and the rotund mammy stereotypes found in mass media, Black women engaged in physical culture to comply with an acceptable body politic of the time. As in the White community, this pursuit was multilayered and class-based. Purkiss explains:

> The single-minded focus by many elite African Americans on attempting to fit themselves into nineteenth-century ideologies of ladyhood was motivated in large part by a desire to replace dominant cultural assertions of the group as primarily understood through their bodily associations with sex and rape with narratives that proved them to be middle class and, as a result, pious, chaste, modern, and worthy of attaining the supposed advantages of membership in the cult of domesticity. (Purkiss, 2017)

There is evidence too, that like White women of the time, Black women used meditation and other contemplative techniques to address their fitness and wellbeing. Black author and educator Alice Dunbar-Nelson, "exercised and meditated regularly" in the early decades of the 20th century (Purkiss, 2017).

As yoga had come to the United States around 1893 with the arrival and subsequent fame of Vivekananda following his appearance at the Chicago World's Columbian Exposition, American women became the primary audience for the practice. "Women of unusual culture and refinement" (The Evening World, 1911) were said to be those who were drawn to yoga, at times attracting criticism that the practice would lure them away from the call of familial womanhood (Hearst, 1908). Newspapers like the "Women's Page" inside the Mercury newspaper of

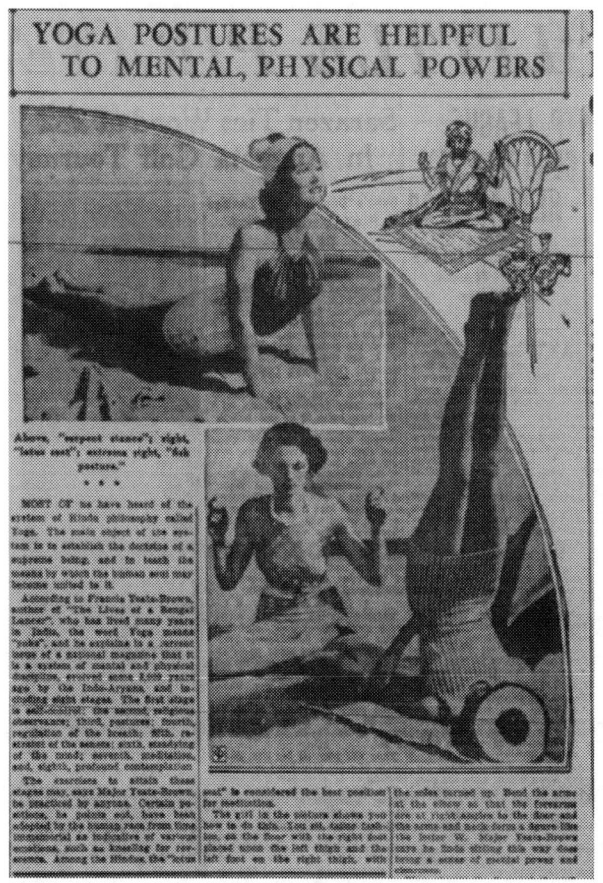

Figure 11.1 Clipping from "The Women's Page" of the *Mercury* newspaper, 1935.

Pottstown, Pennsylvania, a suburb of Philadelphia, where Dunbar-Nelson Lived, boasted stories about yoga practice ("*Yoga Postures are Helpful to Mental, Physical Powers*") (Figure 11.1). Aside from the male teachers – mostly Indian men hoping to rectify an image of Indian effeteness in the wake of British colonialism – White women in fashionable wear and visually pleasing poses were photographed alongside these articles. White men are conspicuously absent.

As eluded to earlier in this essay, the physical culture movement of the 19th and early 20th centuries was a nationalistic one, especially where the philosophy of White women's bodies and their ability to birth numerous and healthy babies was concerned. Reproductive health scholar Christa Craven writes:

> At the turn of the 20th century, the eugenic movement was becoming increasingly concerned with the fifty percent decline in birthrate among white women

from 1800 to 1900 – from 7.04 to 3.56. Influenced by the eugenic sentiments developing in Germany at the time, United States nationalists suggested that strategic population control efforts could contribute to the propagation of the "white race." (Craven, 2011)

As the 20th century wore on, the debate over what kinds of exercise served women's ultimate purpose or masculinized women, continued through public discourse and through the teachings of female physical educators in American universities. Notable women of the academy instructed scores of young women on how best to use their bodies with respect to the perceived differences between men and women.

It was because of the movement for Muscular Christianity, that Columbia University professor Josephine Rathbone had the opportunity to study yoga and physical education in India in the 1930s for the purpose of deepening her ability to offer yoga as part of her "Methods of Relaxation" course. Muscular Christianity promoted a rugged masculinity punctuated by physical training as an aspect of religious and nationalistic duty. Missionaries from United States colleges, in particular, Springfield College in Missouri (where Rathbone's husband, Peter V. Karpovich was employed as a professor of physiology), traveled abroad to establish YMCA branches as sites for their physical and spiritual work. Because of the exchanges that occurred during these missions, yoga became part of the physical training administered for young people at the Indian YMCAs and one of the reasons yoga is offered at many American YMCAs today. Rathbone's own work was aimed at addressing "Americanitis," a condition brought on by increasing industrialization and resultant nervousness. Following her travels to India, Rathbone brought yoga guru Bishnu Charan Ghosh (who was by all accounts, a eugenicist and staunch Indian nationalist) to her class to share yoga poses with her students. Though her work was groundbreaking in that it advocated for a balance between exertion and rest in physical education no matter one's gender, Rathbone held rather conservative beliefs. She was adamantly anti-women's rights and vocally homophobic, most especially in regard to lesbians. Although she adhered to accepted gender norms of the time, she was not immune to bodily scrutiny and suspicion of her work. One such TIME Magazine article characterized Rathbone and her class this way: "Dr Josephine L. Rathbone, a stocky, cheerful little woman worries about people who worry…She puts her pupils through a course in learning how to control their muscles, cultivating the will to relax" (Vertinsky, 2014). Rathbone taught until 1959.

A professor at Howard University from 1925 to 1967, Maryrose Allen was one of the most recognized Black physical education professionals in the mid-20th century. Teaching at a time when White students were four times more likely to enter college than Black students (Verbrugge, 1997), Allen taught a small section of middle-class Black society, but had a profound effect on physical culture in Black communities, nonetheless. It is said that by 1953, 80% of the female gym teachers working in Black public schools in Washington, DC were Allen's students (Verbrugge, 1997). Like Rathbone and other contemporaries in physical culture and education between the 1920s and 1960s, Allen was a believer in, and advocated for different approaches to exercise for women and men. Like practitioners and philosophers before her, Allen believed that women should be the embodiment of beauty, virtue, and grace, the sacred site of motherhood. Compacted by the realities of race relations in American during her tenure, Allen encouraged her students to see physical culture as part of a holistic approach to respectability and social mobility in a White world. Access to mainstream society was the goal for many HBCU students and their mentors. Martha H. Verbrugge explains in her work, *Active Bodies: A history of Women's Physical Education in 20th Century America*:

> By schooling Howard undergraduates in white, middle-class morality, Allen opted for the common path of normalization. In the same way, contemporary black intellectuals and activists portrayed African American women as feminine and virtuous, historically black schools instructed female students about grooming and decorum, black nurses and teachers adopted the rules of respectability, and black beauty pageants and commercial cosmetics sometimes absorbed white norms of attractiveness and charm. Normalization implied that because white and black women shared the same qualities, they must be equal. (Verbrugge, 2012)

Maryrose Allen's legacy is still felt at Howard University and beyond. The institution remains a strong advocate of women's health and wellness and boasts a robust roster of physical education opportunities.

Now that a brief journey through the world of 19th- and early 20th-century exercise has been explored, how do the themes of femininity articulated by philosophers, teachers, and practitioners appear in 21st-century manifestations of exercise and yoga practice? How are these notions challenged and ultimately put to bed? Beginning with an exploration of how White women's bodies in motion reify 19th-century conceptions of gender performance in postural yoga, the second half of this essay ultimately brings us to examine how we may choose different ways of considering our moving bodies through a critical lens.

Old ideas re-packaged

On her 2004 "Re-Invention" tour, Madonna started the performance of her famous 1990 song, "Vogue" with a series of yoga poses (full wheel and headstand among them) in between whispers of the famous lyric, "strike a pose." While Madonna dons a golden corset, a pair of black booty shorts and fishnets, her backup dancers are in contemporary revisions of 18th-century Rococo garb and, as the song suggests, move in ways indicative of voguing, a dance style derived from queer people of color in the ballroom scene of the 1970s and 1980s. This complicated mash-up of cultures represents a hyper-performative manifestation of a cis-gender heterosexual femininity. Madonna, who has been a part of the pop music scene since the early 1980s, has embodied various definitions of femininity over her more than 40-year career, from spunky tease, to mature sex symbol. She has reinvented herself numerous times in an effort to stay relevant in the music industry, that is to say, pertinent to crowds spending money on her albums and merchandise. Her 2004 tour came on the heels of such a transformation, where her previous, sexy-and-somewhat-socially-conscious persona of the 90s gave way to a more spiritual one, brought on by the birth of her daughter. In a 1998 interview with Oprah Winfrey, Madonna expressed her worry at getting "a fat ass" during pregnancy, and how she was introduced to Astanga yoga as a way to exercise. "I'm gym-free!" she exclaims, to raucous applause from the audience (Madonna, 1998). Madonna continued to capitalize on the exponential popularization of yoga in the public eye with her 2000 movie, *The Next Best Thing*. In the film she plays Abby, a Los Angeles yoga teacher who becomes pregnant by her gay best friend, Robert, played by Rupert Everett. In the film, Madonna shows her yoga once more and performs the trope of heterosexual-woman-with-ticking-biological-clock.

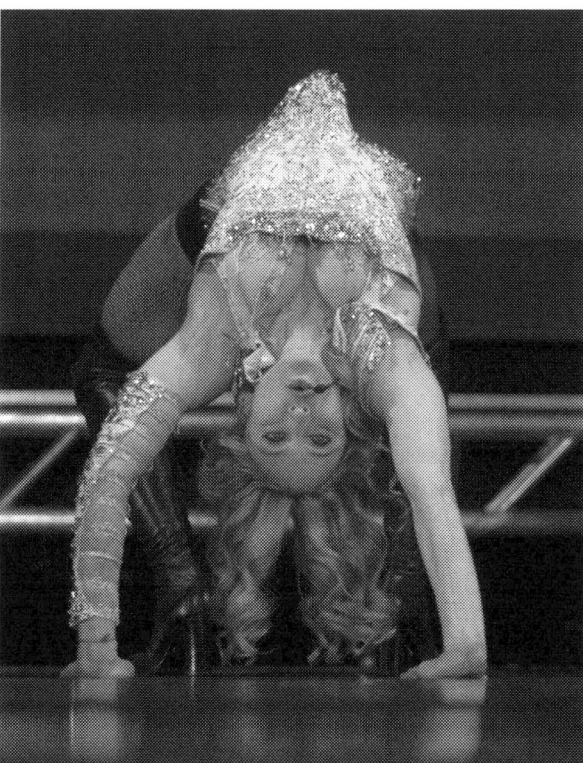

Figure 11.2 Madonna performs "Vogue" on her "Re-Invention tour in 2004. Getty Images.

As demonstrated by the 19th-century ethos of exercise related to women's bodies, Madonna's eschewing of fatness, her pivot to a public-facing spirituality, and the importance of that transition in the observance of the birth of her biological daughter should come as no surprise. Madonna's asana-as-performance, her corseted voguing, her dismissal of the gym, her portrayal of a woman with an urgent desire for children, her adoption of yoga as a path to self-improvement, all contribute to the American hegemonic project. Madonna's music, commentary, and imagery continue to influence perceptions about the American woman and her body, across the world.

Since Madonna's hay day, many other female pop artists and actresses have harnessed yoga in public as a way of communicating their commitment to wellness and to the maintenance of a visible, kinesthetic femininity. One example includes singer Janelle Monáe and the music video for her 2015 single, *Yoga*. With her video, Monáe bucks visual-kinetic norms and claps back at the histories of respectability politics as they relate to the bodies of Black women as "a queer Black woman" (Spanos, 2018) making reference to and performing yoga on a popular platform. Even so, both the song and the video can be read as ableist, heteronormative, appropriative representations of the practice as commonly experienced in the United States. Though the video features a multicultural cast, Monáe and her castmates can be interpreted as cis-gender, thin, and able-bodied, as they perform intermediate and advanced yoga poses and dance moves in bright red leggings and matching stiletto heels (Monae, 2015). Like that of many celebrities, Janelle Monáe's work is constantly being scrutinized and analyzed. While many yoga purists and culture police have condemned the video for its cultural insensitivity, others, like queer and feminist scholar Rebecca Kumar, view the song and the video as an expression of reclamation:

> As black female pop stars translate South Asian culture into different racialized contexts, they challenge the color line by incorporating black women into yoga and Hindu iconography – which have been policed by both the dominant white culture and anti-Black South Asians, respectively. As a result, their work resists forms of white supremacy that negatively impact non-black women of color, too. Finally, black goddess politics de-essentializes India's nativistic and nationalist versions of Hinduism, which tend to be misogynistic and anti-black. (Kumar, 2018.)

Other examples of White female celebrities harnessing the power of yoga as public performance include Taylor Swift and her 2016 appearance on the Jimmy Fallon Show, where she discusses her love for yoga and jokingly claims to have invented a pose, *Pegacornasana*. Actress Kate Hudson continues to interact with the yoga industrial complex through her own yoga and athletic wear company called, *Fabletics*, established in 2013. The company was worth $300 million dollars as of 2018 (Forbes, 2018).

Where White women's bodies are concerned, one need not be a celebrity to participate in the use of the body as a site of assumed safety and socio-cultural power. In the summer of 2020, the sacredness of the White female body in motion was put on display during the protests in Portland, Oregon for Black Lives Matter. Protests erupted across the world following the murder of George Floyd in May of 2020. In the overwhelmingly White, affluent city of Portland, the protests continued for more than 50 straight days. On the night of July 18, the "Naked Athena," (Figure 11.2) wearing only a face mask and beanie hat, sauntered out in front of federal law enforcement and proceeded to perform what have been interpreted as yoga poses, among other types of movement. Though pepper bullets were shot near her feet, she was not seriously hurt during the confrontation. Rather than mar her body, law enforcement sought only to scare her. During the incident, White men put their own bodies between her and the police, reifying the history of White men coming to the aid and protection of White womanhood. Had she been fat, Black, trans, or read anything other than young, thin, and White, she would have been in imminent danger of bodily harm or even death as the history of violence against women and non-binary people in the United States shows us. Although it came out that the woman is a White-passing woman of color, and that her "tree pose" in particular may have been a response to experiencing a minor injury in her foot, in this instance, perceptions matter. The Naked Athena's performance garnered wide praise from people citing the power of her vagina, likening her to a host of vulva-bearing goddesses including Lajja Gauri and Sheela Na-Gig.[5]

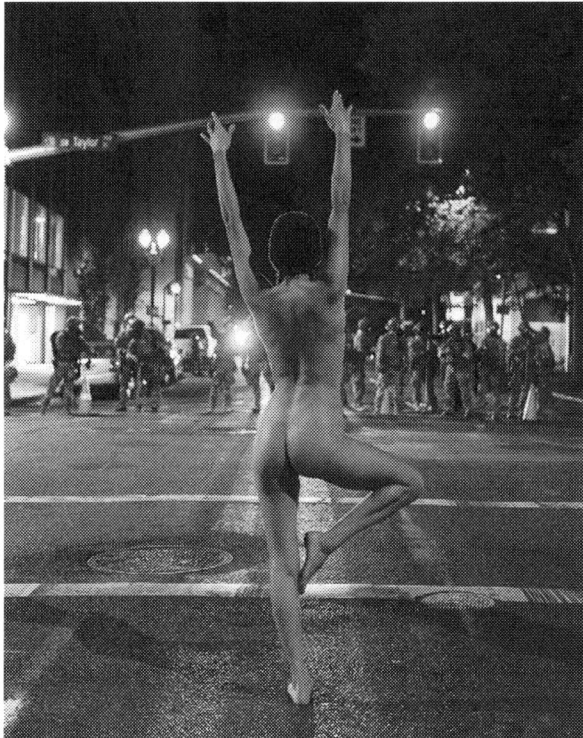

Figure 11.3 The Naked Athena, Portland, Oregon, 2020.

Reclaiming yoga as a site for expanded definitions of gender

Given the history and contemporary events explored in this chapter, how do we disrupt our ongoing attachment to harmful dualistic ideas imposed upon the body in motion? Where can we experience the unfixed, or non-binary in yoga practice? Where do queer aesthetics appear in yoga philosophy and why is this important? How do we reference or employ those ideas in yoga asana and our broader experience of yoga in America? And how does a practice versed in the historical nuances of gender and contemporary manifestations of yoga offer more inclusive interpretations of yoga asana for a society that is more attuned to the spectrum of gendered experiences and identities?

Where yoga was historically practiced by men and is generally expressed in terms of masculine and feminine opposites (Surya Namaskar/Chandra Namaskar, Pingala Nadi/ Ida Nadi, heating/cooling), there exist important areas of blurred gender lines in various mythologies related to yoga.

A good place to begin in disrupting the binaries along which American and the wider Western perception of movement operate is recognizing that yoga is a composite spirituality and practice, one that encompasses parts of Hindu, Jain, Buddhist, and Sufi philosophies and cultures in various amounts (Mallinson, Singleton, 2017). In this way, we can begin to think of yoga as an unfixed concept where we in the West have accepted some, but not all parts and possibilities of the practice. Like the construction of gender in the West, the construction of yoga practice in the West has been one of omission (facilitated by a host of mechanisms, among them Indian nationalism and American capitalism), where the most palatable and vendible parts have been preserved while those that cannot be readily appropriated in this way have been left to fall to the wayside and even shunned.

We need not look further than the yogic writings most referenced in the West to find actual recognition of gender-fluidity and possibilities for a more expanded consideration of bodies in motion. A most salient example is that of the Mahabarata. This epic poem tells the story of two factions of the same family, the Pandavas and Kauravas, who are engaged in a war to become the rulers of the kingdom of Hastinapura. The central character, Arjuna, is one of the five Pandavas brothers, and the story ultimately follows his journey through trials and tribulations in pursuit of triumph over the Kauravas. In a section of the story nearing the end of the tale, Arjuna is cursed to become a member of the "third gender" – a eunuch – for one year following his rejection of Urvashi's (a celestial maiden in the kingdom of Indra, king of heaven) romantic advances. During this period of Arjuna's transition, he resists bodily legibility as Brihannala, "a son or daughter without parents" who teaches dancing and music to palace maidens in the kingdom of Virat, where he and his brothers are in exile (Dharma, 1999).

The prince [Bhuminjaya] looked at Brihannala. Although a eunuch, he was huge-bodied and appeared to possess great power. His arms, covered with bangles and bracelets, seemed like decorated serpents, and his shoulders, draped with white silk, were as broad as a palace door. Having faith in Sairindhri's words, Bhuminjaya said, 'O Brihannala, whatever you may be, drive my chariot today. (Dharma, 1999).

Brihannala's physicality can be read here in a variety of ways. As a non-binary entity who engages in both traditionally feminine (dance) and masculine (charioteering) movement, they demonstrate that a mixture of movement modalities in a single body is possible. In Brihannala's physicality as someone "resembling an elephant" with a "deep voice that [echoes] around the court," while also "walking with the gait of a broad-hipped woman," they demonstrate physical juxtapositions that challenge 19th-century bodily sensibility as dictated by traditionalists and eugenicists with regard to size, gait, and vocal modulation. And although Arjuna's journey from man to eunuch and back again is problematic in that Arjuna's foray into transness was a temporary disguise, the fact that Arjuna/Brihannala experience their gender as transitory means that in a metaphorical sense, gender can be experienced as an unfixed concept, like yoga itself.

Other examples of this unfixed state of being include myths related to the lunar god Chandra. Originally a female deity according to some sources, Chandra is more generally depicted as a male deity who is the quintessence of male beauty. It is said by some that the depiction of Chandra as a male is due to patriarchy in Hindu culture (Teich, 2013). Chandra's providence over things like fertility already suggests a fluidity of roles related to gender, as fertility is more generally ascribed to female-identified deities. One story in particular that shines a light on the queer presence in Chandra's mythology is that of Chandra's affair with Tara, a star goddess. Their child, Budh (Mercury), was cursed to be androgynous by Brihaspati (Jupiter), Tara's husband. Upon becoming an adult, Budh searched for a partner who was like them, and found Ila, "a prince who entered an enchanted grove and turned into a woman" (Pattanaik, Rulli, 2019). Though Budh sought to end their own curse by appealing to Shiva and Shakti, the story goes that it was only partially mitigated: when the moon is waxing, Budh is male; when the moon is waning, Budh is female. The physical manifestation of Chandra in yoga practice embraces the fluidity found throughout the mythology as it is inherently "half (ardhachandrasana)." There is no "full moon pose." It is often experienced as a pose where one constantly waivers as they pursue balance, and stretches in all directions, simultaneously (Pattanaik, Rulli, 2019).

Taking the theme of balance further, there exists another aspect of Hindu mythology that foregrounds ambiguity in gender expression. Ardhanarishvara, a composite manifestation of Shiva and Parvati, is the equal embodiment of both male and female in one, androgynous body (Figure 11.3). Ardhanarishvara literally means "the Lord (isvara) who is half (ardha) woman (nari)" (Seid, 2004). Shiva and Parvati are lovers, and their physical union represents the negation of duality in the supreme being, transcending gender. Often posing or dancing in iconography, Ardhanarishvara is seen with their weight in the left hip (feminine side) meant to accentuate that part of the body, which necessitates a curve in the spine that can be read as a more feminine expression of movement on the right side (masculine side), too. At the same time, three of Ardhanarishvara's four arms are motioning strongly toward the sky, with just one arm, the left front arm, relaxed easily toward the ground. This could be read by some as a more masculine styling of the arms, overall. Possessing a fully-developed breast on the left side and no breast on the right side, flowing locks of hair on the right side and hair tied up on the left side, one could read this styling of Ardhanarishvara as a cross-mixture of feminine and masculine qualities. As there exist variations in representations of Ardhanarishvara across time and geography, readings of the deity have the potential to encompass a variety of meanings.

Interesting to note is that the emergence of Ardhanarishvara in Sanskrit literature is preceded by a cadre of one-breasted goddesses, many of whom did away with one of their breasts by choice. Remarkably, the goddess Kannaki from the pre-medieval literary work, the *Shilappatikaram*, describes how she became so. After her husband was beheaded under suspicion that he stole an anklet from the queen of Pandya where they were residing, Kannaki rips off her left breast (most

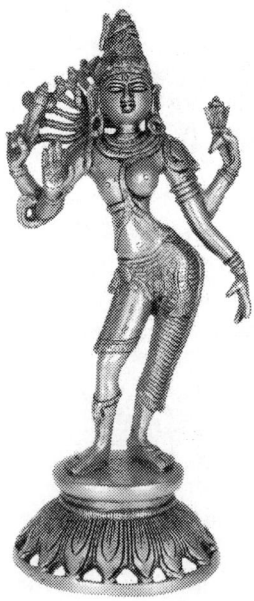

Figure 11.4 Ardhanarishvara

often thought of as the side of the feminine) and "cast it on the city which was burnt to ashes." Thereafter, with only her right breast (retaining feminine qualities on the side most often thought of as male), she becomes the goddess of chastity (Kalidos, 1991). Given the way in which the one-breasted deity has its roots in goddess figures and the way in which Parvati gives of herself to meld with Shiva, some scholars feel that the term "Lord" Ardhanarishvara is a misnomer:

> Logically speaking, it is a female deity who gives her half to a male or and accommodates the Male Principle within Herself to make out a composite Hermaphrodite or Androgyne. So, the assumption of agamic texts like the *Karanagama*[6] in viewing Ardhanarishvara as a male form is basically wrong. (Kalidos, 1991)

Though it cannot be overlooked that androgyny and/or transness is often the result of a curse throughout these mythologies – which points to patriarchal cultural conceptions of bodily legibility and morality throughout history – these examples demonstrate the presence, the problems, and the possibilities presented by their existence. Now that we have a foundation upon which to build a more aware and inclusive yogic experience, here are a handful of ways the work can be taken up in more depth:

- Be mindful when participating in the yoga fashion industry. Large companies like Lululemon, for example, have histories of harmful marketing campaigns and inherent philosophies that discourage people outside of the White, cis-gender, able-bodied, thin paradigm to participate in the lifestyle they purport to sell through their clothing. Research to find and invest in local companies and independent artists whose textile work honors bodily difference, the earth, and the well-being of their clientele.
- Learn the histories of yoga that disrupt the status quo. For example, where White women have historically used yoga as a way to "relax," "workout," or "improve (a marker of the eugenic movement)," Black women have a history of using yoga as a liberatory tool. As an example, Erica Huggins of the Black Panthers talks about how she taught herself to meditate as a way to cope while imprisoned from 1969 to 1971 (Huggins, 2020).
- Actively disrupt the perpetuation of "yoga porn" on social media. Search any social media platform and you'll find hordes of young, thin, cis-gender, White women doing any number of challenging, visually stunning poses: Eka Pada Rajakapoasana, or One-Legged King Pigeon Pose, advanced variations of Natarajasana, or Lord of the Dance Pose, various iterations of Hanumanasana, or Monkey Pose, and the list goes on. What many of these visual presentations of asana do is perform the female ideal explored earlier in this chapter: "slender, willowy, and pliant," and ultimately, sexually desirable from a White male perspective. Instead, work to show a variety of bodies and poses on social media, in a variety of settings. The more would-be

practitioners see themselves depicted on social media, the more likely they may be to practice and participate in yoga community.
- Actively disrupt dualistic language and actions in your practice and/or teaching. When you first learned to do warrior II, for example, what were you told? Was there a decidedly masculine aspect to the description of its physicality and energies? How did you approach your practice of the pose based on your impression of the pose? It is important to become aware of how a pose actually feels, and how it is working with your body, to find all of its gendered nuance.
- Don't let conventions of gender infiltrate your relationship with your body in your asana practice. Do you force yourself into difficult poses because it proves you are strong (manly, according to the philosophies and ideas explored in this essay) or flexible (feminine, according to the philosophies and ideas explored in this essay)? Do you desire to perform certain practices that may be harmful to your body because it may be perceived by others to say something about your bodily identity?
- Get clear about why you're practicing yoga. Is it to be more beautiful, physically? And if so, whose notions of beauty are you trying to achieve? Are you practicing to become mentally clear? To engage in self-study? To learn more about another culture? Your reasons for practicing are no one's business but your own, but clarity for yourself will help you to approach your practice, the places you show up, and the ways you show up in those spaces, with honesty.

Yoga Asana as part of the landscape of American exercise isn't going anywhere soon. Our perceptions and definitions of gender, however, are in a state of flux. If we can come to our mats with an intention to have a more multifaceted experience of ourselves and honor that same journey of those in our yoga communities, we can co-create a more inclusive experience of yoga for every body.

Notes

1. Identified only as "Jen" in the media, the woman who walked out in front of federal officers during a Black Lives Matter protest in Portland, Oregon in July, 2020, is known colloquially as, the "Naked Athena."
2. A term used in the 19th century to describe ultimate masculinity.
3. In September of 2020, it came to light that unnecessary hysterectomies were being performed on migrant women in ICE detention centers.
4. Like the terms, "manly men" and "manly, ideal men," which were used to describe the virility men sought in 19th and early 20th century Western culture, "the cult of true womanhood" was a term used in the 19th and early 20th century to describe a feminine ideal which extolled the virtues of domesticity, piety and submissiveness as hallmarks of the ideal woman.
5. Lajja Gauri is an Indian fertility goddess, while Sheela Na-Gigs are pseudo-erotic stone carvings of women holding their vaginas open found on Norman churches throughout Europe. The twittersphere erupted in the hours and days following the July 18 event, with many hailing the woman as a "goddess" and "divine feminine warrior."
6. The Karanagama refers to one of the 28 Śaivāgamas, a collection of post-Vedic Hindu religious scriptures.

Sources

"2004 Madonna Reinvention Tour." *YouTube*, 2010. https://www.youtube.com/watch?v=QOzDcw82q70.

"Amelia Summerville, Once She Was Fat, Now She's A Trilby." *Enid Daily Wave*. August 17, 1895.

Craven, Christa. "Histories of Struggle Activism for Reproductive Healthcare since the 1800s." Essay. In *Pushing for Midwives: Reproductive Rights in a Consumer Era*, 24–39. Philadelphia, PA: Temple University Press, 2011.

Dharma, Krishna. *Mahabarata: The Greatest Spiritual Epic of All Time*, Torchlight Publishing, 1999.

The Evening World. "More Than 5000 Women in New York Are Followers of Swami Abhedananda." *The Evening World*, 7 Sept. 1911, 4–4.

Hearst News Service. "Lured by Mystic Teaching." *The Pittsburgh Press*, May 3, 1908.

"How to Reduce Your Weight." *Muskogee Times Democrat*, October 12, 1916.

Huggins, Erica. "Bio: Ericka Huggins Official Website." *Erickahuggins*, http://www.erickahuggins.com/bio.

Kalidos, Raju. "Ardhanari in Early South Indian Cult and Art." *Proceedings of the Indian History Congress* 52 (1991): 1037–1043.

Kumar, Rebecca. "'Let Yo Booty Do That Yoga': Black Goddess Politics." S&F Online 14, no. 3 (2018): 9–21.

Ladd, Brittain. "Kate Hudson Wants Fabletics To Rule The World." *Forbes Magazine*, July 13, 2018. https://www.forbes.com/sites/brittainladd/2018/07/12/kate-hudson-wants-to-rule-the-world/.

Madonna. "Oprah Winfrey Show." Episode. Chicago, IL, May 29, 1998.

Mallinson, James, and Mark Singleton. *Roots of Yoga*. London: Penguin Classics, 2017.

Monae, Jonelle. "Yoga." *VEVO*, 2015. https://www.youtube.com/watch?v=0OkB6p_FZAw.

The Next Best Thing. Film. Paramount, 2000.

Osborne, Harold. "Symmetry As An Aesthetic Factor." *Symmetry*, 1986, 77–82. https://doi.org/10.1016/b978-0-08-033986-3.50011-2.

Pattanaik, Devdutt, and Matthew Rulli. "Ardha-Chandrasana." Essay. In *Yoga Mythology: 64 Asanas and Their Stories*. Uttar Pradesh: HarperCollins Publishers, 2019, P. 61–66.

Pence, Agnes M. "Yoga Postures Are Helpful to Mental, Physical Powers." *The Mercury*, April 8, 1935, sec. Women's Page.

Purkiss, Ava. "'Beauty Secrets: Fight Fat': Black Women's Aesthetics, Exercise, and Fat Stigma, 1900–1930s." *Journal of Women's History* 29, no. 2 (2017): 14–37. https://doi.org/10.1353/jowh.2017.0019.

Rousseau, Jean-Jacques. *Emile, or Treatise on Education*, 1762.

Seid, Betty. "The Lord Who Is Half Woman (Ardhanarishvara)." *Art Institute of Chicago Museum Studies* 31, no. 1 (2004), pp. 48–49+95.

Singleton, Mark. "Yoga, Eugenics, and Spiritual Darwinism in the Early Twentieth Century." *International Journal of Hindu Studies* 11, no. 2 (2007): 125–146. https://doi.org/10.1007/s11407-007-9043-7.

Spanos, Brittany. "Janelle Monáe Frees Herself.". *Rolling Stone*, June 25, 2018. https://www.rollingstone.com/music/music-features/janelle-monae-frees-herself-629204/.

Teich, Howard. "Chandra Moon // The Lunar Deity." *Solar Lunar*, 25 Feb. 2013, http://solarlunar.com/chandra-moon-god/.

Todd, Jan. *Physical Culture and the Body Beautiful: Purposive Exercise in the Lives of American Women, 1800–1870*. Macon, GA: Mercer University Press, 1998.

Verbrugge, Martha H. "Gender, Race, and Equity." Essay. In *Active Bodies: A History of Women's Physical Education in Twentieth-Century America*. New York: Oxford University Press, 2012, P. 273–304.

Vertinsky, Patricia. "Oga Comes to American Physical Education: Josephine Rathbone and Corrective Physical Education." *Journal of Sport History* 41, no. 2 (2014): 287–311.

Wollstonecraft, Mary, and Miriam Brody. *A Vindication of the Rights of Woman*. London: Penguin Classics, 2020.

Chapter 12

Embodying liminality through yoga
An autoethnography exploring the spaces between

Sanaz Yaghmai

Introduction

The United Nations High Commissioner for Refugees (UNHCR) is the United Nations agency which protects and supports forcibly displaced populations and refugees. As defined by the UNHCR, a refugee is a forcibly displaced migrant who "has a well-founded fear of persecution for reasons of race, religion, nationality, political opinion or membership in a particular social group" (UN Refugees). They are at risk of human rights violations and either their government cannot/will not protect them or may be the body persecuting them (Amnesty; United Nations General Assembly).

In early 2019, I moved from Los Angeles to Greece and spent six months volunteering at the Malakasa Open Refugee Camp north of Athens. The camp is home to roughly 2,600 refugees predominantly from Afghanistan, as well as Syria, Iraq, and Pakistan, and 98% of the residents speak *Farsi* or *Dari*, two dialects of the Iranian language. Being an Iranian-American, Farsi is also my native language. Through a collaboration with the non-governmental organization (NGO) Refugym I was granted access to facilitate trauma-informed yoga healing circles as part of the Refugym team. Refugym is a grassroots, refugee-led organization offering sports and exercise programming. The founder, Brittany Pummel, recruits camp residents who have a background or desire in teaching sports/exercise classes and supports them in getting a class added to their weekly sports programming. I felt this was the perfect NGO to introduce this healing circle because of their commitment to creating sustainable programming. Ideally, my goal was to find a local refugee to mentor and support towards taking over the yoga healing circle.

I facilitated 80 hours of classes with women, a brief series for men, a children's "yoga and creative expression" class, and I offered interpretation services (Farsi to English) for a few NGOs. In addition, I led two trauma-informed care trainings for humanitarian aid workers in the city of Athens. Finally, in November of 2019 another collaboration opportunity arose with the NGO *OMPowerment Project*. Together we offered a week-long trauma-informed yoga leadership training for the Afghan women refugees.

This chapter offers the reader a glimpse into my experience connecting with Afghan refugees. I begin with the refugee experience and make my way into highlighting aspects of my personal story which led me down the path of yoga. I then address aspects of my sociopolitical history that overlap with that of the refugee experience. We transition into my experience facilitating classes at camp and end with a few case studies. Consent has been received by all case study participants and some names have been changed for anonymity.

Scattered throughout the chapter is the invitation to pause and return awareness back to the present state. Can you notice how the words land in your body? I invite you to notice the space between sensations and thought, without judgment. It is in the spaces "in between" where we make meaning, in the liminal, from the Latin word *limen* or "threshold." Finally, I invite you to always listen to your body and take care of yourself.

The refugee experience in 2020

According to the UNHCR's global statistical database, as of 2018, 25 people are forced to flee every minute. As of June 2019, the world's highest levels of displacement were reported, with a staggering 70.8 million people forcibly displaced as a result of persecution, violence, conflict, and human rights violations (UNHCR, 2004). More than two-thirds of the asylum seekers come from five countries, with Syria and Afghanistan being the top two countries of origin. According to the Asylum Information Database (AIDA) of the European Council on Refugees, as of 2016, Greece began to see an unprecedented rise in asylum seekers entering the islands. Currently, in 2020, the number of asylum seekers in Greece is 50,000+, compared to just 3,300 in 2015, over half of whom are women and children (International Rescue; AIDA).

Typically, those fleeing Middle East and South Asian countries head toward Europe by way of human smugglers via land and sea. They make their way into Turkey then sail across the Aegean Sea in overcrowded rubber dinghies and enter European lands by way of Greece or Italy. According to the United Nations Office on Drugs and Crime (2011), "migrant smuggling by sea is the most dangerous type of smuggling for the migrants concerned" (8). The tragedies crossing that Aegean strip of the Mediterranean are record breaking, revealing a higher death rate than any other border crossing in the world; on average five people a day, an alarming 19,000 have been reported dead or missing since 2013, and an estimated half are children (FRA 2020; Meierotto & Fragkias 2017; Ansa 2019).

Unfortunately, European nations are fortifying their border control policies and further jeopardizing the maritime journey, by implementing pushbacks:

> Push-backs are a set of state measures by which refugees and migrants are forced back over a border – generally immediately after they crossed it – without consideration of their individual circumstances and without any

possibility to apply for asylum or to put forward arguments against the measures taken.

— European Center for Constitutional and Human Rights.

This tactic has been used for years and currently there are reports of it being used in the U.K., France, Croatia, and Italy, to name a few. Governments throughout the EU are knowingly violating the *"prohibition of collective expulsion*" laws stipulated in the European Convention on Human Rights. It is also an illegal act which breaches international law set forth by the 1951 Refugee Convention.

Independent reporting from grassroots organizations in Greece are in contact with some of the recent victims of these crimes. There are numerous cellphone videos showing ships designed for life saving, with masked and armed men aboard, firing shots and intercepting refugee dinghies, transferring them into life rafts, pulling them toward Turkey waters and abandoning them in the open sea. Spiegel International, a German-based investigative journalism company, obtained footage from a 30-year-old Palestinian man, Naim, taken in May 2020. The Spiegel team conducted a joint investigation with Lighthouse Reports and Report Mainz, interviewing numerous eyewitnesses, forensically analyzing videos, and comparing them with geodata. Spiegel International reported that Naim's footage was the first to confirm that the masked men are beyond doubt aboard a Greek Coast Guard vessel. They reported "masked men, almost certainly Greek border control officials, regularly attack refugee boats in the area" (Christides and Lüdke 2020). A Turkish Coast Guard vessel arrived after the refugees had been left several hours floating in the open sea.

> Men in white protective equipment helped the refugees off the lifeboat and took their temperatures. Naim then had to remain in quarantine for more than two weeks - in a nasty camp full of filth and mosquitoes, he says. Naim is now allowed to move freely in Turkey, but still feels trapped. He says: "I can't go forward and I can't go back". (Christides and Lüdke 2020)

Pause. Notice.

On July 16, 2020, Human Rights Watch published an article updating readers on the on pushback efforts:

> Greek law enforcement officers have summarily returned asylum seekers and migrants at the land and sea borders with Turkey during the COVID-19 lockdown. The officers in some cases used violence against asylum seekers, including some who were deep inside Greek territory, and often confiscated and destroyed the migrants' belongings.

Lighthouse Reports (2020) stated that state actors are further exacerbating the situation by exploiting the Covid-19 crisis, casting the asylum seekers as Covid-19 vectors as their argument for amplifying their punitive measures, and abandoning asylum laws stipulated in the European Convention on Human Rights. The director of International Rescue Committee (IRC), Imogen Sudbery, put out a statement on March 3, 2020, stating:

> It is shameful that people seeking safety and protection, arrive on Europe's shores only to be threatened by the European forces to whom they are looking for safety. It is clear that vulnerable people are being used as pawns in a bigger political context, caught up in escalating relations between actors involved in the Syria conflict.

If the families are lucky enough to make it to land, they are met with further human rights violations and increasing tensions. The situation is Greece is reaching a breaking point and today we are seeing both asylum seekers and humanitarian aid workers on the Greek islands of Lesbos, Samos, and Chios, being targeted by local populations. The islands' reception centere are severely unequipped and currently functioning at six times their capacity (International Rescue). The AIDA Greece report declared:

> Reception facilities on the islands remain substandard and may reach the threshold of inhuman and degrading treatment…Overcrowding, lack of basic services, including medical care, limited sanitary facilities, and violence and lack of security poses significant protection risks. The mental health of the applicants on the islands is reported aggravating.

According to the American Psychiatric Association, it is said that "about one out of three asylum seekers and refugees experience high rates of depression, anxiety, and post-traumatic stress disorders" (3). When refugees are met with prolonged stays in dangerous, unhygienic conditions, and compounded with insecure immigration status and limitations on work and education it gravely impacts their mental health (American Psychiatric Association).

On March 1, 2020, the National Security Council of Greece made the decision to suspend access to the asylum system, with no legal basis, and imprison undocumented people who cross the border (Human Rights Watch). The following day, Human Rights Watch reported on social media footage that revealed a Syrian man from Aleppo being killed by Greek authorities with a rubber bullet, while crossing into Greece.

> Human Rights Watch has been unable to verify the facts concerning this particular incident. However, Greek forces appear to have used excessive or disproportionate force, including teargas, as women, men, and children from Syria, Iran, Afghanistan, and other countries have gone to the border hoping to cross into Greece.

Pause. Notice.

Staci K. Haines, author of *The Politics of Trauma* (2019), writes, "Trauma is an experience, series of experiences, and/or impacts from social conditions, that break or betray our inherent need for *safety, belonging, and dignity*" (Haines 2019). The safety, sense of belonging, and dignity of refugee families is often stripped away before they decide to flee. It is likely the reason they risk their life, in search of a sense of safety among a community who value and respect their existence.

Where there is trauma, there is resilience. They coexist. We must acknowledge the collective resilience attached to the phenomenon of the refugee identity. The word *refugee* is not to be mistaken as an identity. As we work to understand the refugee experience it is important that we acknowledge the word is a sociopolitical phenomenon which highlights their liminal existence, between *what once was* and *what will be*. The identity has a profound consequence on one's health and wellbeing, resulting in a host of challenges from depression, PTSD, anxiety, insomnia, alcohol abuse, and suicidal ideation, to name a few (Anagnostopoulos 2017, 1).

Families, often with small children, await their fate, in this liminal state. With exposure to unfathomable challenges from traumas, past and present, they adapt, persevere, and survive with limited to no resources. They love and care for one another creating a home in this liminal space, one which often continues to be fraught with danger. Their home, a waiting room of sorts, embedded with uncertainty and fear. They live in the threshold between a life of chaos and *potential* freedom. The hope for freedom, resilience, and community keeps them afloat.

When looking at the lives of the Afghan community at the camp, from pre-migration to a life on the move, their experiences were laden with traumatic stress, both individually and collectively. The families I met had fled their homes for many reasons, all of which fall under at least one of the following categories: political, religious, social, national persecution, and/or gender-based violence/threats. They chose the treacherous journey through the waters because it was their only form of survival. When you have lost all sense of safety, when your environment continually robs you of your dignity, and threatens your daily existence, your soul's inherent response is to seek safety.

In the poem *Home*, Warsan Shire, the award-winning Somali writer, educator, and poet vividly captures the unimaginable scenarios causing someone to flee. Below is some of Shire's noted prose, from "*Home*", often stamped across poster boards at protests. Her words have become a rallying call for refugee advocates today (Kuo 2017).

> no one leaves home unless
> home is the mouth of a shark
> you only run for the border
> when you see the whole city running as well

> your neighbors running faster than you
> breath bloody in their throats
> the boy you went to school with
> who kissed you dizzy behind the old tin factory
> is holding a gun bigger than his body
> you only leave home
> when home won't let you stay.
>
> You have to understand,
> that no one puts their children in a boat unless the water is safer than the land
>
> (Shire, lines 1-11, 24-25).

On several occasions during our yoga healing circles at least one woman would briefly mention her horrific experience on the boat. It was undoubtedly a predominant shared traumatic experience among the community. Every time one would begin talking about their experience, I could sense the energy of the room shift. It felt taboo, it was not to be spoken of. Always followed by a brief moment of silence another woman would offer soothing words, "You are safe now," "That time has passed and it will never happen again," "You are here with us."[1] Almost every time I felt my heart sink as my tears welled up. The asana practice after those heavy moments was deeply restorative.

Pause. Notice.

What led me to yoga

I was introduced to yoga by way of my divorce. Societal messaging around how a 30-year old Iranian woman *should* be living had seeped into my belief system and weighed heavily on my self-worth. Therapy and Kundalini yoga allowed me to delve into self-inquiry, or *svadhyaya* in Sanskrit. I was able to unravel and dismantle thought patterns, or *samskaras*, that had shaped my identity, allowing me to make more conscious choices. New information discovered in therapy was processed viscerally through Kundalini yoga practice, which led to "aha" moments during yoga that were explored in therapy. I had embodied a beautiful dance between the two healing modalities.

In time, I began to experience what it means to practice yoga off the mat. I began examining the role systemic structures play in governing my direct life experiences and I became more conscious of the collective impact. Being a therapist, I wanted to support individuals and communities who are not accounted for and represented when these systems were created. I decided to take on a clinical psychologist position at a maximum-security prison at the California Department of Corrections and Rehabilitation (CDCR).

The inmate population is deeply embedded in a system of oppression within the prison industrial complex. As reported by a non-partisan criminal justice think tank, *The Council on Criminal Justice,* Black people are incarcerated at a rate 5.1

times higher than White people and Hispanic people 1.6 times higher than White people (Sabol et al. 2019). It was important that I place myself within this system and connect with those behind prison walls, to listen, hold space, and remind them they are not forgotten.

As I began to establish my footing and understand the hierarchy at play I began to notice the deafening culture of silence. There was an unspoken expectation to look the other way, to only pay attention to issues pertaining to your scope of practice, and to never report grievances with correctional officers. However, staying silent went against every fiber of my being. After consulting with a co-worker and supervisor I decided to submit a memo to the Investigative Services Unit at CDCR reporting alleged illegal activity between correctional officers and inmates.

Ten days after submitting the memo, while walking through the prison yard, I was attacked by an inmate. He ran towards me from behind. I heard footsteps approaching and turned around but it was too late. He punched me directly in the face. My head hit the concrete wall behind me and he continued punching with both fists while I crouched on the ground until officers arrived.

Could the attack be related to the memo? It was too much to process at that time. The attack instilled a multilayered experience of fear, mistrust, and paranoia. I grappled with conflicting emotions. I wanted to go back, but my body would not allow it. I was diagnosed with PTSD and started therapy again and a few months later I decided that it was time to return to a consistent yoga practice.

Pause. Notice.

I began with trauma-informed yoga training and as I delved into the intersection of trauma and yoga I felt my body come alive again. I had spent almost a decade in graduate school and not once had we discussed the power of incorporating the body and movement in healing trauma. I began to experience an integration of mind, body, and spirit. The attack had me questioning my career path, the significance of my voice, and my ability to use it. Yoga reminded me that I can liberate myself from my suffering by practicing to let go of dichotomous thinking; capable or incapable, worthy or unworthy, the trauma had instilled immense self-doubt. I was reminded to bring loving-awareness in between the dichotomy, to embrace the existence of a liminal space. I practiced noticing the ebbs and flows of emotions, feelings, and triggers without judgment. I learned that the *spaces in between* is where pain unravels.

Months later I began a 200-hour Hatha yoga teacher training journey through *The Tree*, in South Los Angeles. They are a non-profit organization offering donation-based yoga, workshops, and community wellness gathering into Black and Brown communities. Both yoga trainings had addressed topics around social justice through yoga which further piqued my interest. I gained additional training through the *Off The Mat, Into The World* organization which bridges yoga and social activism. It was then that I noticed that my social and financial privileges had granted me access to endless yoga teachings and trauma healing. Western capitalistic culture has stripped the ancient healing practice from its roots. At $15 to $18 per class yoga is marketed as a practice for the financially privileged, therefore, making it inaccessible to marginalized communities. I chose to leverage my privilege and share the same teachings that had profoundly supported my healing.

I decided to commit to the practice of *Karma yoga*, performing action as selfless service without an attachment to results (Satchidananda 2014). I had been following the refugee crisis emerging in Europe since the rise of the Syrian civil war in 2015, and decided to volunteer in a refugee community and facilitate yoga healing circles.

The circle of hope, a trauma informed yoga healing circle

Developed by Catherine Ashton, founder of the nonprofit organization *Yoga to Transform Trauma*, the *Circle of Hope* offers practitioners a framework blending traditional support groups and yoga. Through self-inquiry, observation of thoughts, and sensations we deepen our self-awareness while cultivating connections through storytelling. Through a structured sharing circle format rooted in community guidelines, ritual, movement, and the Yamas and Niyamas (Adele 2009) the healing circle invites practitioners to continually return to, notice, and examine their present state.

The research on yoga in the refugee community is fairly limited; however, practices found to be most effective for the treatment of trauma are those which enhance self-awareness and self-regulation while continuously bringing the individual back into the present moment, such as yoga (van der Kolk 2015; Caplan 2018; Gard 2014). As a trauma-informed facilitator my goal is to honor the unique lived experiences of trauma. Therefore, I am less focused on mastering alignment and more on inviting students to notice and move in ways that feel safe, to choose when they want a challenge, and to rest when they need. This means returning inward to assess their present state, noticing the moments in between, and choosing the path forward. I am a guide while they examine and redefine their relationship with their mind, body, and spirit. Trauma lands differently in all bodies. They are the expert of their body and experience. My intention is to co-create spaces which cultivate that which trauma robbed, *safety*, *belonging*, and *dignity* (Haines 2019).

Pause. Notice.

The insider-outsider role

When situating myself within the refugee community, it is important that I acknowledge the nuances of my identity and role. First and foremost, I was entering as an outsider and I was particularly conscious of my privilege and "otherness" being another volunteer in the humanitarian aid system. But there's more beyond the boundary which separates me from them. The aim here is to notice where the boundaries blur. In *The Space Between*, Dwyer and Buckle (2009) explore the strengths and challenges researchers hold in their roles as insider *or* outsider, encouraging researchers to step away from a dichotomous perspective and embrace occupying spaces which honor the complexities of the human experience. It is in the acknowledgment of the space "in between," the liminal space, where the complexity and totality of the human experience can be examined (Dwyer 2009).

In addition to the salient sensation of being an outsider, literally, I also carried a more subtle *felt-knowing* of being an insider. There was familiarity, I felt close to home, in fact I felt a sense of family. Iran and Afghanistan are neighboring countries with shared traditions, culture, and the ancient, poetic language of Farsi. In addition, I am an Iranian immigrant, born to immigrant parents who fled Iran in 1980 due to the Iran–Iraq war. In this section I provide a glimpse into my parent's historical context, highlighting the shared complexities of war, while revealing how mere luck is sometimes what determines one's fate.

Fleeing Iran

My parents left their homeland of Iran in 1980 after facing socio-political unrest from the Isamic Revolution and the Iran–Iraq war. The years preceding the revolution of 1979, the King (or "*Shah*"), Mohammad Reza Pahlavi, had been establishing rich ties with the Western world. This led to an uprising of a pro-democratic and radical leftist movement in 1977 that was seeking to tame the autocracy (Axworthy 2013). The supreme leader of the clergy (or "*emam*"), Ayatollah Khomeini heeded the uprising and by December of 1979, a national referendum vote approved a new theocratic republic. Khomeini became the Supreme Leader of the newly established *Islamic Republic of Iran*.

The destabilization of power was seen as an opportunity for war, the United States backed Iraq and started a horrific war in 1980 which lasted eight years. A few years prior, my parents had married and had their first child, my sister, in 1978. So, not only had the Islamic revolution brought about significant socio-cultural shifts that were raising their concerns, but the civil unrest of war had amplified that fear. Government issued exit permits created barriers to leave the country, the war was underway, and given that my father was a physician there was a high likelihood that he would be drafted to serve on the frontlines.

My parents began looking for a way out and fortunately my father was granted a service passport to exit the country and work at the Iranian Hospital in neighboring United Arab Emirates, an eight-year-old nation in the desert along the southern shore of the Persian Gulf. Other family members, however, weren't as lucky. Some of our family and friends were forced to flee the country using backdoor tactics, human smugglers helped them make their way across borders as refugees in Europe. The Iran–Iraq war lasted eight years (1980–1989) with an estimated combined total of 1,000,000 + Iranian and Iraqi casualties.

In hindsight, as I write this essay and reflect on our shared historical contexts, I am also experiencing a sense of collective grief over the loss of cultural identity. My parents experienced a cultural trauma that immensely impacted their consciousness and created fundamental shifts in their identity (Mobasher 2006). They had hoped to move back one day, but four decades later the people of Iran are still suffering. Today, Iran is described as "a repressive, autocratic regime run in the interests of a narrow clique that systematically denies political freedoms and natural rights to the Iranian people" (Axworthy 2013). The pain and grief are particularly visible in my father when he talks about life in Iran. After spending time in the refugee camps my heart has been opened to the shared collective cultural trauma that resides in all our bodies.

Refugees fleeing Afghanistan

During the Iran–Iraq war, the Soviet Invasion was taking place in neighboring Afghanistan from 1979 to 1989. Iranian rebel groups were also among the allied forces supporting the Afghan soldiers. During the Soviet Invasion approximately five million Afghan civilians fled to the neighboring countries of Pakistan or Iran (Associated Press). In the camp I came to find out that many of the women had fled to Iran as children, with their parents, and upon starting families of their own, and escalating tensions between its people, they were forced to flee to Europe to provide a more safe and dignified life for their children. One study revealed that Afghan refugees in Iran face a host of human rights violations such as:

> forced deportation, denial of education rights, lack of employment opportunities, forced labour, lack of access to healthcare, denial of right to liberty, no freedom of movement, forced family separation, regular physical abuses, mistreatment in detention and deportation centres, and forced recruitment to fight in Syria. (Arian 2017)

Alan Taylor, from *The Atlantic* writes, "in the brutal nine-year conflict, an estimated one million civilians were killed…Civil war raged after the withdrawal, setting the stage for the Taliban's takeover of the country in 1996" (2014). Afghanistan was fraught with civil unrest only to be further exacerbated by the U.S. and its allies after the September 11 attacks by al-Qaeda in 2001.

> As other countries joined the war, the Taliban were quickly removed from power. But they didn't just disappear – their influence grew back and they dug in…In 2018, the BBC found the Taliban was openly active across 70% of Afghanistan. The U.S. and their allies have struggled to end deadly attacks by the Taliban. (BBC News)

A recent report in Amnesty International declared that the year of 2018 "documented the *highest ever recorded* civilian deaths, including the highest ever recorded *number of children* killed in the conflict" (2019). To further compound the situation, the de-escalation in Ukraine has amplified the conflict in Afghanistan and as of June 2019 the Global Peace Index ranked Afghanistan as the least peaceful country in the world, replacing Syria. Over the last four decades approximately 2.5 million Afghans have been registered as refugees around the world, the second highest displaced population after Syrians, with Iran being the number one host country (Amnesty, 2019).

Pause. Notice.

Holding space in-between

Upon entering the camp, I had felt an immediate connection to my ancestral roots. I have been fortunate enough to continually visit Iran since childhood and during my last trip in 2014 I spent time in the village of *Khour*, homeland to my ancestors. The camp residents reminded me of the people of *Khour*, which made for a pleasant and comforting welcome. Even the accent of the *Khour* community greatly resembles that of the Afghan accent of Iranian language, *Dari*.

I experienced an internal battle as I learned about the Iranians' mistreatment of Afghan refugees during my time in the camp. I was always treated with utmost respect and hospitality; they embraced me as one of their own. However, personally, navigating this space between being associated with their oppressor, added some complexity to the experience of my role in the camp. It added a heaviness to my situational identity; there was a subtle essence of shame and guilt that arose. Every so often I noticed it enter my body. I acknowledged its presence as it slowly dissipated to the background of my experiences.

In Dwyer and Buckle's (2019) article I identified with their definition of the "*insider-outsider*" role, "this hyphen acts as a third space, a space between, a space of paradox, ambiguity, and ambivalence, as well as conjunction and disjunction" (60). Described as a situational space where similarities are honored, differences acknowledged, and ambiguity welcomed (Dwyer 2019). Navigating my interpersonal relationships in the camp through this lens allowed for a rich and complex personal journey of self-inquiry.

Qualitative field studies show participants are more inclined to share stories when there is an assumption of understanding and shared distinctiveness between subjects and researcher (Dwyer 2019). I was often told that being an Iranian female volunteering in the camp was a welcomed surprise: "It's easy to speak from the heart", one woman said. Another shared "As soon as I heard we have an Iranian volunteer, I had to come to your class, I don't even know what yoga is." Similar sentiments were expressed often, all of which enhanced my experience of community. When there is comfort and familiarity there is greater opportunity to cultivate community and co-create safety. In turn, there is more room to tend to the spirit and nurture one another.

Yoga in the refugee community

The Malakasa camp is housed on an old military base and has a high barbed wire fence around its perimeter. It is 40km away from Athens, which is accessible by train and with a station 800m from the camp. The nearest hospital is in the city of Athens, yet according to the multiple accounts it takes an ambulance five to eight hours to arrive no matter the emergency. The residents who have been officially registered with the UNHCR are given their refugee identification card and a steel shipping container in which to reside. The approximate dimensions are 22 × 8 × 8 ft, they are typically divided into two rooms, and include a bathroom and kitchen. Those who are unregistered and awaiting the processing of their refugee identification papers are given camping tents, with access to portable toilets. There were roughly 2,000 registered and 600 unregistered families during my time there.

It was mid-April 2019 when I began volunteering. I spent the first week going door-to-door introducing myself to the community and announcing the upcoming *Circle of Hope* series. I described the class as a combination of physical practice and group dialogue to build upon the relationship between mind and body while bringing our awareness into the present. There was some skepticism, curiosity, and a few expressions of excitement. Those who knew of the practice described it as a tool for "finding inner peace," many of whom voiced that all refugee camps are in dire need of such teachings. A sense of affirmation washed over me that week, I was feeling eager, nervous, and curious to begin the work.

My work at the camp was my introduction to speaking the language of yoga in Farsi. It was a little nerve wracking because my Farsi is far from perfect and I knew I would struggle with words. I shared my struggle with the women and asked them to correct my mistakes and help me out when I am struggling with finding the right word. They commended me for trying and always encouraged and cheered me on. After our first class, I was in awe of the power shared language holds towards building community. Coming from such similar cultures *and* sharing the same language allowed for a memorable exchange of banter and laughter. It also allowed for intimate and meaningful conversation that would not have been possible had I needed an interpreter. In addition, to be immersed in the poetic language of Farsi within the yoga healing space I felt I was being reintroduced to my roots through a new lens. The words landed differently, the poetry was *felt*, igniting an ancestral reverence.

The class

Throughout my time facilitating the healing circle the number of participants fluctuated, from one to ten women/girls, between 16 and 60+ years old and, during the one-month men's series there were one to five men/boys, between 18 and 45 years of age. Almost everyone I met in the camp identified as Muslim and most women always wore a headscarf. Sometimes a few would remove theirs during our asana practice. Each class had a different topic for self-inquiry with the shared thread of self-care, self-compassion, and community empowerment. My priority was to adapt and allow for topics to unfold naturally while maintaining the circle format along with its ritual. The rituals and consistency set a foundation which cultivated familiarity and connectedness. From placing items in the center of the circle (e.g., a candle, flowers, a shawl draped around them), to the ritual of collective breathing, the agreement to speak one at a time, and the choice to participate or sit back and observe.

Over the course of six months we tapped into various topics: joy vs. despair, hope and faith, safety, community care, love, anger vs. ease, strength, inner child, boundaries, body image, and selflessness. In each class we discussed what the topic means to them and explored the visceral experiences and emotional states they evoke. We engaged in quiet self-reflection, discussed the impermanence of emotions, and the gift of the present moment. We used breath, imagery, and grounding practices to promote self-regulation while cultivating a sense of familiarity and comfort. During asana I would remind them of the choice to practice awareness of the physical body, the space around them, the placement of hands and feet, the breath, and to rest whenever they need. Always inviting self-awareness through various avenues. The intent was to cultivate an environment which practices compassionate self-reflection over judgment and self-criticism.

The participants often sought my advice, referring to me as "*ostâd*," meaning expert or professional. I used these moments as an opportunity to invite them inward (*svadhyaya*), and to look to the wisdom of their community. Many used dichotomous valuing of the self. For example, being a "bad" mother or wife, feeling "not enough" as a daughter, or being a "bad" husband. The invitation always returned to self-compassionate inquiry. We considered what it would look like to honor our feelings while distancing ourselves from labels of "good" vs. "bad". We spoke of our sensations and emotions being messengers inviting us to reflect on our moment-to-moment experiences, to notice their transient nature.

In addition, I acknowledged the extreme circumstance of their reality and reminded them that showing up for themselves and doing their best *is always enough*. These were times where my outsider role would take the lead as I made it clear that I have no expertise of their life and personal struggles. I also believe that centering the individual as the expert is a vital practice of trauma-informed cultural sensitivity, as it respects their unique lived experience. Returning to the concept of svadhyaya, although there were times where I was teaching them new concepts, I reminded them that they are their best teachers and the answers they are seeking can be found through the wisdom of their body, individually and collectively.

To co-create a sense of community, it was important to allow myself to embody the practices of the circle. So, in addition to being the facilitator I was always a participant. Traditional healing wisdom of indigenous sharing circles requires that "all participants, including the facilitator, are viewed as equal and information, spirituality, and emotionality are shared" (Lavallée 2009, 29). I embraced the circle as part of my self-exploration and healing journey. Some days I was more vulnerable than others, sharing deep self-reflections, hopes, and inner battles. I always flowed alongside them during the asana practice and contrary to the advice of Western academia in psychology, I never held back my tears. During the asana it was important that I model variations and normalize what a novice yoga practitioner may consider an "imperfection" or "incapability." For example, cushioning my knees or choosing to rest in the middle of a posture, or perhaps keeping my eyes open during a meditation. Whether we were talking about self-worth, feelings of despair, or if we were falling out of balance from tree pose, the theme of normalizing experiences and embracing the gray area was weaved throughout the series.

Little moments

Many of our classes hold a special place in my heart. One day we had nine women show up, one of whom was breastfeeding her baby throughout the class. She participated in the group share and watched us flow while continuing to breastfeed. There were also young children playing off to the side of the circle. Although the presence of children was a normal occurrence, the breastfeeding mother was a pleasant surprise. Her presence filled the room with a powerful and nurturing energy. There is something so sacred when women come together to care for themselves and one another. On this day, the magic left an indelible imprint in my heart.

Another memorable class occurred during the Holy Month of Ramadan, a time where Muslims practice worship through fasting from sunrise to sunset. Women continued to show up to our 11:30am class despite their fasting. There were typically one or two women in each class who chose to rest and observe the asana practice. They found refuge on the mat, sitting or lying down, some closed their eyes in a meditative state, some watched us flow. One woman shared, "Even though I am not moving with the group, I can feel your energy, it is so calming." Another expressed that watching and breathing with us made her feel like she was also moving. The delicate exchange of energy flowed through us all, as their presence in stillness was also grounding for those in motion. Somatic practitioner and therapist Resmaa Menakem writes "our bodies guide and follow other bodies; a settled nervous system encourages other nervous systems to settle. This is why a calm, settled presence can create room for a multitude of possibilities, and become the foundation for changing the world" (Menakem 2019, 186). Moments like this remind me of the profound ways in which a safe space can impact one's body and spirit.

Pause. Notice.

Case studies

Below you will find a deeper look into the subjective experience of the yoga healing circle and its teachings in their own words.

Zahra

Zahra is a 38-year-old female, residing with her husband and four children. Her husband was a news reporter in Afghanistan. They fled the country due to threats of persecution related to her husband's profession.

It was my first day of teaching class, the yoga mats were laid out in a circle, I was setting up the centerpiece with some flowers and a candle as the first participant walked through the door. A woman with a toddler by her side and his arms wrapped around her leg. We exchanged pleasantries and she asked if her son could attend class. "He gets very distressed if I am not by his side at all times." Of course, I welcomed his presence and encouraged the women to do whatever it is they may need to feel comfortable and safe in this space.

Five women showed up that day. The topic was centered around identifying our strengths. We explored the meaning of grounding and resourcing, practiced intentional breathing and noticed present sensations. Curious and engaged throughout, Zahra shared self-reflections, asked questions, and flowed through the asana, all while tending to her son who was sitting ever-so-quietly on her mat, observing. She encouraged him to participate. It was heartwarming to witness. After class, she stayed back and asked to speak in private.

Courageously, she shared her recent struggles around her mental health. Seeking support and guidance she prefaced the conversation by stating that she used to see a psychiatrist for depression. Holding back tears, Zahra expressed her current struggles. "I haven't been feeling well recently, my spirit is weak." Exhibiting feelings of sadness, she expressed an increase in feelings of agitation and irritability, and was grappling with a lack of motivation. She was struggling to find the will to tend to both her and her family's needs. A wife and mother to three teenagers and a toddler, Zahra was clearly aware that she was at a threshold. She ended by expressing her gratitude for the class and made a commitment to attend every class. I commended her for courageously showing up, boldly speaking her truth, and committing to this practice.

Zahra was first to show up on day 2, and of course with her son by her side. He seemed eager to participate, so Zahra and I agreed that it is best he use his own mat moving forward. His participation brought me such joy. And so, it continued, every week, twice a week, for the first three months. Zahra and her son immersed themselves in their practice. Her presence was calm, her practice disciplined. In no time her son learned the routine of the 90-minute class, from the language to the breath and asana practices, he quietly and eagerly soaked it all in.

Three months in, I had to temporarily leave Greece due to visa restrictions and return three months later. As my departure approached, I reached out to Zahra to see if she would like to take over my role as facilitator. She was hesitant but eager. We set up a few meetings to discuss the process and answer any questions she may have. Her confidence overshadowed her doubt in no time. This was a natural next step, she had transmuted her pain and suffering into agency and resilience. She stepped into the role and officially joined the Refugym volunteer team as the yoga instructor. While I was gone, I remained in contact and supported her through exchanging ideas and themes for each class. Upon my return in November she was ready to delve deeper into yoga and participate in the *OMPowerment* Trauma-Informed Yoga Leadership Training.

In one of our talks she discussed one of the key teachings she's taken away from her experience of the class, the impermanence of emotional states:

> When this class came into my life I was amid emotional turmoil, I was in a really terrible state. I needed some help. I had heard about yoga's impact on

> mental health, so I knew I had to come to this class…After just one class, and after our talks, I felt calmer and knew I had to return, I wanted to immerse myself into the practice and get the maximum benefit…We experience all sorts of stressors, especially as refugees living in this camp, both children and adults, the challenges are endless, and I feel that yoga can help us in accessing a state of calm while we work our way through these challenges…The plight of refugees is truly detrimental to one's mental health and I think it would greatly benefit each and every one of them to begin the practice of yoga.
>
> The most important teachings I learned through the yoga class took place during the discussions in the first half. I learned that no feeling, no sensation is permanent, whether they are "good" or "bad," and therefore we shouldn't take them too seriously. Before, when I was feeling upset or experiencing challenges, I felt as though the feeling would last forever. Despite rationally knowing that it will go away, I did not know how to separate myself from it. After our discussions in class, it began to really sink in…of course, my feelings will change, nothing is permanent, whether it's joy or sadness or anything else, they will all pass.

The Yama, *aparigraha* (non-attachment), seemed to be unfolding. Upon identifying the impermanence of all emotional states, she experiences greater ease to let them go, and remain calm, and in the present.

> When my mind is preoccupied, when I am outside of my body and there is chaos in my surroundings, I come back to the tools of yoga. I separate my mind and body from the discomfort around me. I create a safe and calm space in my mind to reconnect with calm. It has taught me that in situations, my inner peace and my thoughts are most important…and in order to create a calm environment, and bring others peace I must first and foremost focus on myself

Here, Zahra describes her process of *pratyahara*, withdrawing from the external stimuli and focusing on the self, enhancing inner awareness while quieting the external world.

Today, as the world is adapting to a new way of life with the Covid-19 pandemic, the camp was under lockdown for well over a month. Once the camp went into lockdown she began leading her own version of the yoga healing circle with her family of five. Almost every day, they would sit around the kitchen table in their small space and she would begin with a guided meditation. Then each family member, including the toddler, was given the opportunity to speak, uninterrupted, for up to 10 minutes. She would close the circle with some gentle postures and light stretching. I am in awe of her, as an Afghan woman, a mother, and a human being residing in a refugee camp amidst Greece's unprecedented refugee crisis.

Being the team leader that she is, Zahra has agreed to volunteer her time and create content for Refugym's YouTube website[2]. Today she is creating audio recordings with guided meditations and yoga teachings, making the practices accessible to Farsi-speakers.

Javad

Javad is a 42-year-old male, residing with his wife and four children. He is Zahra's husband. He was a news reporter in Afghanistan.

During the men's healing circle there were some meaningful self-reflective conversations around the mind-body interplay. One day we were discerning between the visceral sensations of calm and distress; where do they land in the body, how do they feel, and manifest? Distress was described by some as tension in the head and chest, a racing heart, tension throughout the legs, increased sweating, heat in the head and abdomen region. Calm was typically described as a lightness, or an expansion, a weight being lifted off the soul. The shared experiences of bodily sensations appeared to be a comforting surprise among the men, they knew they were not alone.

As we were wrapping up the sharing circle and preparing to transition to the asana, I noticed a shift in the energy of the room. The "aha" moments and shared experiences had cultivated a comfort and ease among our group, bodies were more relaxed, there were more smiles and head nods of acknowledgment.

Javad further described his distress manifesting as anger or sometimes yelling. He shared a desire to regain control of his actions and better navigate the more challenging emotions. After the class Javad approached me and expressed curiosity around our initial grounding practice, "How did it happen so fast?", he asked. "A sense of calm came in so quickly as I brought my attention to my breath and focused on the rise and fall of my body…that was really helpful". I offered a brief overview of the physiology between the heart, lungs and brain in relation to the nervous system and it led to further self-reflection into the mind-body interplay.

On another day, Javad stayed back and while we were packing, he asked if he could speak with me in private. He graciously thanked me for the class and shared why he made the decision to begin this yoga class.

> My wife has been coming to you for the last few weeks and I wanted to personally thank you for helping her. It's evident that she has been greatly impacted by your classes…Her demeanor has changed, her spirit is calm… and I must admit, at first I didn't believe in yoga and the things she, and others would say about it. But after seeing how it has impacted her in such a short amount of time it piqued my curiosity. And without a doubt, after just one class, and especially after holding this pose [demonstrates "thread the needle"/ Urdhva Mukha Pasasana] and taking a few breaths I felt a release of tension in parts of my body that I didn't know existed…I am a believer now.

At the end of the class he stayed seated on the mat and shared his thoughts about his experience. He expressed that a lot of men have a misconception around yoga and its role in a man's life.

> Men need yoga. A lot of men I know think yoga is not for them. But being here has made me see that it will help us transmute our aggression and violent thoughts into energies that support us in understanding our feelings, energies that make room for growth and healing...Men in refugee camps need a space like this to gather, share and connect because right now we are so disconnected from one another, myself included...We need to find a way to bring more of this into the lives of the men in these communities.

Months after our time together I reached out to ask about his thoughts around the practice of yoga. He replied:

> Even though we only had a few sessions together it had a great impact on me. Yoga captured my attention, it made me realize that we, as refugees, are particularly preoccupied with so many things and in a constant state of worry. We worry about our status, we worry about the uncertainty and progression of our journey, we worry about the war (in Afghanistan), we worry about bread. We are always in a state of worry. Any event that occurs in any part of the world, we fear the repercussions may influence our circumstances. So, we try to remain aware of all events happening globally, because they impact our lives. But through yoga, my attention was redirected on to myself. I noticed that I started to look inward, into my mind, my body, my soul and I saw that first and foremost, this body needs attention. There are different parts to my body, and they need oxygen, they need movement, my thoughts need nourishment. I think the greatest impact and lesson I've learned is that it brings our attention inward. I see Yoga as a tool which enhances my ability to see myself more clearly. And slowly, it directs me to a place of calm, a calmness of mind and spirit.

Javad initially experienced yoga by witnessing its impact on his wife, Zahra. He decided to look beyond his preconceived notions and embody the practice. Through a commitment to truthfulness, the second Yama, known as *satya*, and courageous receptivity to critical self-inquiry. He chose to get curious and expand into new truths, to gain new perspectives and let go of old thought patterns which no longer served him. This is yoga.

Exploring the mind-body interplay and looking into feelings of anger, he chose to delve further into critical self-reflection while delving into other of the eight-limbs. For example, the practice of quieting external distractions, focused concentration, and heightened breath/sensory awareness led to greater insight into the innate abilities of his body. From accessing self-regulation through movement with breath and by deepening his interoceptive and proprioceptive practices, he was awakened to the gateway between mind and body. Javad discovered that his body is an instrument which can be used to both release and transmute physical or emotional pain. Ultimately, this led him to return to class, and advocate for more yoga healing circles within his community.

Pause. Notice.

Yusra

Yusra is a 48-year-old Afghan female, residing in a container with six of her eight children. Yusra fled Afghanistan with her parents at the age of eight during the soviet war. They sought refuge in Iran, living as refugees. Her husband left her a few years ago. Her children were facing extreme harassment and violence due to their socioeconomic status and race. Determined to create a better life she and her eight children fled Iran.

A first-time participant, she introduced herself to the circle towards the end of the class, "I am 47 years old, I have eight children in my life and this is the first time I am speaking my truth." She continued and shared her pain, worry, and fears while expressing her appreciation for this community. She expressed gratitude to the women and encouraged them to continue to show up, as she did

After a few weeks experiencing her gentle presence in class I sat down with her to hear her experience of the class.

> I had never heard of yoga before, I was seeing a psychologist, here in the camp, and he suggested I try it out because I was not doing well. After a few classes with you my psychologist told me that he noticed a drastic shift…I used to go to my therapy sessions and cry the whole time, it was like I had a lump in my throat, and it was very hard to utter a word. My tears would just fall…I did not know this lump existed until you asked us to pay attention to our bodies. I stopped crying after three or four classes with you. I can comfortably speak to the psychologist, I can share my struggles, I talk things through, and I believe that the lump dissipated because of yoga.

Here we see the impact of yoga on releasing stagnant energies in the body. When she was working with a Greek male psychologist and interpreter, she was unable to talk. And by offering a safe environment to tune inward, practice conscious breathwork, and discover some movement, she was able to find some grounding and space to allow her nervous system to settle. The yoga space allowed her survival brain to rest and bring the neocortex back into play, granting her the access to comfortably speak unspoken stories. At the same time, she was continuously invited to bring awareness to her body in the present moment, allowing her to notice the existence and dissipation of the lump in her throat.

> In our last class, when you had us lay on our back [grounding and connecting to the breath] I realized that I had never felt my lower back. I noticed it touched the ground at that moment. I felt my back!...After class I paid closer attention to how still I hold my body. Now I notice this often and I choose to loosen my body...I can clearly feel that I have a body now. I notice my bones...At nighttime I am often tense when I sleep and wake with a stiff jaw. But now, thank God, I take a few deep breaths in bed and I sleep well. I feel lighter now.

A few days later I bumped into one of the camp psychologists, and once he learned that I was the yoga teacher he shared that one of his clients attended my class: "Thank you for what you do," he said, "I don't know what has happened but she speaks more freely in our session and there's a light in her eyes." I knew that he was talking about Yusra.

When looking back on the footage of my interview with Yusra, you can see the shift in her body language and facial expressions when she describes being able to notice aspects about her body. I was reminded of Marianna Caplan's words from the book, *Yoga and Psyche*. Caplan writes, "It can be a life changing revelation to discover that we experience all emotions as sensation in the body, and subsequently to learn to process emotions through somatic awareness" (Caplan 143). Similar to Javad's experience, the practice of *pratyahara* comes forth, the tuning inward, quieting of the external, and returning to the present sensate experiences remind Yusra that she has a physical body to tend to.

Neda

Neda is a 27-year-old female residing with her husband, 6-year-old son, and sister. Neda and her family were living in a rural village in Afghanistan. They fled due to fear of persecution by the Taliban.

I met Neda towards the end of my time in the camp. She attended one class and the following day she sat down with me in private to share her experience. She began stating that the main reason she showed up for class was because she had just heard that there was a Farsi-speaking yoga teacher. She shared that she had been feeling unmotivated, hopeless, and emotionally drained for over two years. Her sister was highly active working as an interpreter, participating in sports, and working at a factory in the city, Neda was desperately trying to find the energy to be an active participant in her own life again. She wanted to participate in camp activities including English classes, volleyball, swimming lessons, but she struggled to get out of the house.

> "My brother was a policeman" she said. "Two years ago, he was martyred by the Taliban. I had lost all hope, I had lost the desire to live...and yesterday, when you asked us to listen to the sound of our breath, it was the first time

in two years that I felt alive. I heard my breath and realized that I have been living out of my body since his death."

Tears came to my eyes, we hugged. She then shared that she left class and signed up for the English classes. She also expressed her commitment to get out of her house more often. I started seeing her more often while walking through the camp.

Neda was committed to her newfound practice of yoga. Knowing that my time in the camp was coming to an end, she used her mobile phone to record my voice during the guided practices. "Your voice calms me; I will use these to practice at home." During the healing circle she also shared her recent experiences of yoga with the other women. She shared that parts of her body had been forgotten and she is now reconnecting to them. She also described starting her practice of conscious breathing every night before bed because it calms her mind and deepens her sleep.

A few months after my departure I reconnected with Neda to check on her wellbeing during the pandemic lockdown. The topic of yoga arose, and she reminded me of her heartfelt and moving experience of yoga. She shared:

> The Taliban martyred my brother. Nine months later the Taliban attacked our village and overtook everything. We fled, left our homes and emigrated. Ever since my brother's martyrdom I forgot about myself entirely. You and the yoga reminded me that I have a body, that I can breathe and that I'm alive… After I met you, I found myself. When I am feeling uneasy or upset, I go to the breath you taught us [slow, deep diaphragmatic breaths] and it calms me down. I also continue to practice the postures you taught me.
>
> As long as I am alive, I will love yoga.

Deeply immersed in a haze of grief, the yoga space offered an accessible healing environment. For two years, Neda's body was disconnected from the felt experience of her body. Both Yusra and Neda's experiences, and many others, remind me of Rae Johnson's account of feminist theorist Bonnie Burstow and the direct link between oppression and trauma; Johnson explained that the "trauma of oppression often results in some degree of alienation from the body, and there is now some support in the research literature to suggest that systemic oppression and socially constructed imperatives about the body combine in ways that support marginalized subjects to experience their bodies as if they were outside them" (Johnson 2019). Also known as *dissociation*, it is when the body is experienced as unrelated to the self, or there is an inability to feel all or parts of the body (Johnson 2019; van Der Kolk 2015). Like Yusra's experience, the yoga healing space offered Neda an opportunity to be present, to look inward, and practice the invitation of noticing. The sound of her breath became her anchor as it allowed her to reignite awareness back into her felt experience of her body.

Pause. Notice.

Conclusion

Healing from trauma begins in the body, yet demands collective care. I want to be clear that we cannot discuss the experience of trauma in forcibly displaced communities without acknowledging oppressive systems at play and highlighting the importance of collective healing through community care. Our most vulnerable communities are being used as pawns in political warfare and it is imperative that we leverage our privileges. We can donate to refugee support and advocacy groups, we can reach out to our elected officials, and advocate for the hundreds of thousands of refugees at our borders today, and much more. This too is yoga, the call to action and advocacy for basic humanitarian rights and collective healing. With that said, the pathway towards collective healing begins within our body.

When the body (mind, body, and spirit) feels safe, connected, and honored, we have greater opportunity to access our innate and restorative wisdom. When we practice redirecting our attention inward and compassionately communicate with the body, we begin to disrupt old patterns and form new ones. We reignite neural pathways that allow us to explore forgotten terrains and muted experiences that trauma robbed us of. Sounds and sensations reawaken, new breath fills our lungs, and new light enters our spirit. The hope is that we find respite as we begin to honor, exist in, and ultimately embody our present, the liminal state between our past and our future.

Pause. Notice.

In their own words

Finally, below I've included a list of some additional reflections from various participants accumulated over the course of the six months. Their feedback was based on their experience of the *Circle of Hope* and/or the *OMPowerment* yoga leadership training:

> I feel lighter.
> Now, I know that I can find joy in the little things through my day
> My sleep is better, I focus on my breath before bed, slow deep breaths, every night.
> My lungs have expanded, it's easier to breathe.
> I have found calm.
> I am more calm, agreeable…I have more control over my emotions
> I teach my children every night and my 13-year-old son is eager to learn more.
> I practice being more present and more engaged with my children and husband.
> I feel good, that's why I keep coming back.

My body feels lighter.

Thank you for reminding me of the joy in my life.

I love myself more, I give myself time and I ask myself "what do I want and need?"

I let things out and I leave here feeling more at peace.

My breath is deeper.

I am beginning to care more about myself and my needs.

I've noticed a 180° change in how I am with my children, I felt I didn't understand them and I didn't have the energy to connect. I would just nod my head when they would speak, but now I listen to understand, I speak with them, I offer guidance.

I use the power of my breath when I get angry, it has been very powerful and calming. I also understand what it means to "ground" now.

As I was eating breakfast today, I decided I have to like my body.

I listen to my children, before I was so preoccupied with my stress that I pretended to listen. My relationship with them is deepening.

I've learned that the most important person is me.

I want to live more, I don't think about dying.

Despite being a refugee, we can be in the present moment more and worry less.

Thank you for reading and for your practice.

Acknowledgement

I would like to acknowledge appreciation for the Indigenous practices and wisdom of sharing circles and the philosophical teachings and ancient art form of yoga. I also wish to recognize the Malakasa refugee camp community and express my gratitude for all who showed up to the yoga circles, and finally, a heartfelt thanks to those who contributed their stories to this chapter.

Notes

1 Direct quotations from the refugee community are translated and paraphrased from Farsi to English by the author.
2 www.refugym.org.

Work cited

Adele, Deborah. *The Yamas & Niyamas: Exploring Yoga's Ethical Practice*. On-Word Bound Books, 2009.

AIDA The Asylum Information Database. "Country Report: Greece." *European Council on Refugees and Exiles*, 2018, pp. 1–191, www.asylumineurope.org/reports/country/greece.

American Psychiatric Association. *Mental Health Facts on Refugees, Asylum-Seekers, & Survivors of Forced Displacement*, www.psychiatry.org

Amnesty International. "Key Facts about Refugees and Asylum Seekers' Rights." *Refugees, Asylum-Seekers and Migrants | Amnesty International*, www.amnesty.org/en/what-we-do/refugees-asylum-seekers-and-migrants/.

Amnesty International. "Afghanistan's Refugees: Forty Years of Dispossession." *Amnesty International*, 20 June 2019, www.amnesty.org/en/latest/news/2019/06/afghanistan-refugees-forty-years/.

Anagnostopoulos, Dimitris C., et al. "The Synergy of the Refugee Crisis and the Financial Crisis in Greece: Impact on Mental Health." *International Journal of Social Psychiatry*, vol. 63, no. 4, June 2017, pp. 352–358, doi:10.1177/0020764017700444.

Ansa. "Migrant Deaths: 19,000 in Mediterranean in Past 6 Years." *InfoMigrants*, 9 Oct. 2019, www.infomigrants.net/en/post/20055/migrant-deaths-19-000-in-mediterranean-in-past-6-years.

Arian, Farhad. "Iran's Mistreatment of Afghans: Human Rights Violations of Refugees and Asylum Seekers." *Refugee Research Online, University of Melbourne*, refugeeresearchonline.org/irans-mistreatment-of-afghans-human-rights-violations-of-refugees-and-asylum-seekers/.

Associated Press. "A Timeline of Key Events in Afghanistan's 40 Years of Wars." *AP NEWS*, 29 Feb. 2020, apnews.com/7011b5086a21f7f57c3cb218947742b2.

Axworthy, Michael. *Revolutionary Iran*, Kindle Edition. Oxford University Press, 2013.

Caplan, Mariana. *Yoga & Psyche: Integrating the Paths of Yoga and Psychology for Healing, Transformation, and Joy*. Sounds True, 2018.

Christides, Giorgos, and Steffen Lüdke. "Videos and Eyewitness Accounts: Greece Apparently Abandoning Refugees at Sea - DER SPIEGEL - International." *DER SPIEGEL*, 16 June 2020, www.spiegel.de/international/europe/videos-and-eyewitness-accounts-greece-apparently-abandoning-refugees-at-sea-a-84c06c61-7f11-4e83-ae70-3905017b49d5.

Dwyer, Sonya Corbin, and Jennifer L. Buckle. "The Space Between: On Being an Insider-Outsider in Qualitative Research." *International Journal of Qualitative Methods*, vol. 8, no. 1, 2009, pp. 54–63. doi:10.1177/160940690900800105.

FRA. "2020 Update - NGO Ships Involved in Search and Rescue in the Mediterranean and Legal Proceedings against Them." *European Union Agency for Fundamental Rights*, 27 July 2020, fra.europa.eu/en/publication/2020/2020-update-ngos-sar-activities.

Gard, Tim, et al. "Potential Self-Regulatory Mechanisms of Yoga for Psychological Health." *Frontiers in Human Neuroscience*, vol. 8, 2014, doi:10.3389/fnhum.2014.00770.

Haines, Staci. *The Politics of Trauma: Somatics, Healing, and Social Justice*. North Atlantic Books, 2019.

Human Rights Watch. "Greece: Investigate Pushbacks, Collective Expulsions." *Human Rights Watch*, 29 Aug. 2020, www.hrw.org/news/2020/07/16/greece-investigate-pushbacks-collective-expulsions.

International Rescue Committee (IRC). "As Greece Reaches Breaking Point, the International Rescue Committee Urges Europe to Step in." 3 Mar. 2020, www.rescue.org/press-release/greece-reaches-breaking-point-international-rescue-committee-urges-europe-step.

Johnson, Rae. "Oppression Embodied: The Intersecting Dimensions of Trauma, Oppression, and Somatic Psychology." *Embodied Philosophy*, 3 Apr. 2019, www.embodiedphilosophy.com/oppression-embodied-the-intersecting-dimensions-of-trauma-oppression-and-somatic-psychology/.

Kuo, Lily. "This Poem Is Now the Rallying Call for Refugees: 'No One Leaves Home Unless Home Is the Mouth of a Shark.'" *Quartz Africa*, 30 Jan. 2017.

Lavallée, Lynn F. "Practical Application of an Indigenous Research Framework and Two Qualitative Indigenous Research Methods: Sharing Circles and Anishnaabe Symbol-Based Reflection." *International Journal of Qualitative Methods*, vol. 8, no. 1, Mar. 2009, pp. 21–40. doi:10.1177/160940690900800103.

Lighthouse Reports. "The Borders Newsroom." *Lighthouse Reports*, 5 Apr. 2020, www.lighthousereports.nl/ourprojects/2020/4/5/borders-newsroom.

Meierotto, Lisa, and Michail Fragkias. "The Refugee Crisis in Greece: Lessons for the United States." *Essays on America's Future: Refugees, Migration and National Security, Frank Church Institute*, 23 Oct. 2017, www.boisestate.edu/sps-frankchurchinstitute/publications/essays/essays-meierotto-fragkias/.

Menakem, Resmaa. *My Grandmother's Hands: Healing Racial Trauma in Our Minds and Bodies*. Penguin Books, 2019.

Mobasher, Mohsen. "Cultural Trauma and Ethnic Identity Formation Among Iranian Immigrants in the United States." *American Behavioral Scientist*, vol. 50, no. 1, 2006, pp. 100–117. doi:10.1177/0002764206289656.

Sabol, William J., Thaddeus L. Johnson, and Alexander Caccavale. *Trends in Correctional Control by Race and Sex*. Council on Criminal Justice, Washington, DC, December 2019.

Satchidananda, Swami. *The Yoga Sutras of Patanjali: Commentary on the Raja Yoga Sutras by Sri Swami Satchidananda (Kindle Location 3755)*, Kindle Edition. Integral Yoga Publications.

Shire, Warsan. "Home" *Facing History & Ourselves*, www.facinghistory.org/standing-up-hatred-intolerance/warsan-shire-home. Accessed 17 Aug. 2020.

UNHCR: Protracted Refugee Situations. Standing Committee 30th Meeting. EC/54/SC/CRP.14, 2004.

United Nations Office of Drugs and Crime. "Smuggling of Migrants by Sea." *Smuggling of Migrants by Sea, United Nations*, 2011, pp. 1–71.

UN Refugees. *United Nations*. United Nations, www.un.org/en/sections/issues-depth/refugees/.

Van der Kolk, Bessel. *The Body Keeps the Score: Brain, Mind, and Body in the Healing of Trauma*. Penguin Books, 2015.

Part III

Yoga in Educational Spaces

Chapter 13

Yoga, engaged pedagogy, and the process of *becoming*

Explorations of a socially just yoga intervention

Kimberly Nao

Western society is experiencing a yoga revolution. If popular media is any indication, and it clearly is, yoga has found its way into almost every aspect of Western life. References to yoga can be found in advertising, social media memes, and the imagery and lyrics of pop music icons such as Janelle Monáe. Both *Newsweek* (2018) and *Time* (2016) magazines have devoted entire editions to yoga and mindfulness[1], respectively. The appeal is understandable as the demands and pressures of the social, professional, and political landscapes are increasingly daunting and even apocalyptic. Seekers of spiritual comfort and "self-care" practices can find relief in yoga and adopt the physical asanas, breath work, and meditation for this purpose. Despite the spiritual aims of yoga at its roots, its reputation as a means of attaining physical fitness and reducing stress is most prominent in the West. According to *Yoga Journal*'s "Yoga in America Study" (2016), yoga has increased in popularity with a 90% increase in awareness about yoga since 2012 and one in three Americans trying yoga on their own. Seventy-five percent of Americans agree that "yoga is good for you." The same report found that 72% of yoga practitioners are women and 37% of practitioners have children under 18 who have practiced yoga. It would only follow that as adults begin to experience the benefits of yoga, they would want to transfer these benefits to youth in their families and communities. Indeed, yoga practices (primarily meditation and physical postures) are increasingly being implemented in schools. As the West integrates, interprets, and repackages yoga for consumption by American adults, with a practitioner base composed primarily of White, middle class, well-educated, physically fit women, it would only follow that those women with children would eventually seek out these benefits for their own children. Teachers, many of whom are also middle class,[2] White (80.1% of public school teachers), women (77% of public school teachers) (National Center for Education Statistics, 2019), could potentially be inspired to include yoga practices in schools (Taie, Goldring, & Spiegelman 2017). Yoga is, indeed, finding its way into America's schools in various forms. As it does, how will it be implemented? What will be the goals of its implementation? More precisely, to what extent will yoga practices – whether physical or contemplative – serve to discipline and control students' bodies, aim for the narrow goals of physical fitness, or aid in the project of managing student stress through an often alienating system of schooling? Alternatively, to what extent can yoga work toward student self-awareness, engaged teaching practices, and a socially just pedagogy? Rather than serving the interests of state mandated testing, discipline policies that disproportionately "push out" youth of color, and increasingly stringent university entrance expectations, how might yoga practices connect students to school, to their teachers, to each other, and to themselves in nurturing and transformative ways? Furthermore, going beyond the schooling context and in keeping with the true purpose of yoga, to what extent can yoga help students attain the broader goals of yoga itself – calming the "modifications of the mind-stuff" (Satchidananda, 2012), attaining non-attachment to the physical world with the intent of self-knowledge and self-liberation?

My personal experience with yoga demonstrates that it is not a means of discipline, control, and stress reduction with the hope of controlling bodies toward high achievement and good behavior, but is instead a means of self-awareness, self-actualization, and agency. As a researcher and certified yoga teacher, I have piloted or taught in yoga programs as both a separate physical education class in a local high school and as an after-school intervention in a middle school combined with a focus on literacy. Programs outside of the core content have their place in potentially helping students manage stress, change problematic behaviors, and increase focus in studies. However, these are residual effects of the ultimate goals of yoga.

What is the purpose of yoga as stated in yoga philosophy and as initially practiced within its cultural and spiritual context in India? In her introduction to Satchidananda's transliteration and interpretation of Patanjali's Yoga Sutras, Rev. Vidya Vonne writes, "[Yoga's] ultimate aim is to bring about a thorough metamorphosis of the individual who practices it sincerely. Its goal is nothing less than the total transformation of a seemingly limited physical, mental and emotional person into a fully illumined, thoroughly harmonized and perfected being" (Vonne in Satchidananda xiii). Yoga master Sri Aurobindo (1948) emphasized that Rajayoga's aims were not only at "self-rule or subjective empire" but also at controlling one's "outer activities and environment" (37). In other words, yoga is more than a management of student bodies by teachers, yoga allows the practitioner to master the self and shape the outer world. It would be difficult to imagine that schools hold these same goals if their main emphasis is on stress management and the discipline of student bodies in the service of curricular aims. But if schools can become sites of student consciousness raising with social justice aims, then the goal of individual illumination and transformation is fully in line with educational theorists and practitioners who work toward these goals. Indeed, as will be discussed, Freire's text *Pedagogy of the Oppressed*, seminal in its influence on social justice educators, articulates many assertions about the purpose of education that align with yoga philosophy.

Research on school-based yoga programs is relatively new but quickly growing as schools recognize yoga "as a strategy to enhance students' mental and physical health, behavior, and performance" (Butzer, et al. 2015). Studies point to some positive affordances for yoga programs, although there is a need for more quality empirical studies to truly gauge effectiveness. Hence, yoga is a burgeoning and necessary area of rigorous research as programs proliferate and as the benefits are yet to be clarified.

Aside from their use for stress management, yoga and contemplative practices have been popularized in the media as an alternative to traditional discipline procedures such as in-school detention (Bloom, 2016; Denver Post, 2018; Upworthy, 2017). In contrast scholar, educator, and spiritual leader, J. Krishnamurti, who was not a yoga philosopher but a spiritual teacher, infused a holistic approach to teaching and learning in his philosophy of education. Contemplative practices were central to the pedagogical practices at the schools he founded in India and in the U.S. (Valsiner, J. 2000; Moody, D. 2011). For Krishnamurti (1953), "Discipline is an easy way to control a child, but it does not help him to understand the problems involved in living" (32). He adds, "Implicit in right education is the cultivation of freedom and intelligence, which is not possible if there is any form of compulsion, with its fears. After all, the concern of the educator is to help the student to understand the complexities of his whole being" (33). There are benefits to replacing punitive, non-reflective detention with calming techniques and self-reflection that can come from meditation, but schools could look beyond using yoga as a method of control and move toward a contextualized effort toward self-awareness and personal transformation.

My own personal experiences with yoga as a means of attaining self-healing and personal empowerment through a steady practice over several years, inspired me to implement a more contextualized yoga program for adolescents. Best practices in yoga implementation suggest that students undertake a consistent practice within, rather than separate from, core content areas (Childress and Harper, 2015). I wanted to further explore what would happen if such a program included reflective engagement with their personal lives in the service of social justice aims.

Yoga philosophy and the purposes of education

Through the implementation of an action research project at a local high school, I, along with a Spanish and Social Studies teacher, Claudia Bautista Nicholas, sought to answer these questions in an eight-week program of yoga asanas and meditation within the core curriculum of a Freshman Seminar class. The class is a required, introductory ninth grade Social Studies course designed to prepare students for college and career readiness, familiarize students with social issues in the U.S. currently and historically, facilitate individual identity development and community building, and engage students in a service learning project. The course description states that the course encourages students to "make informed choices" related to issues of "academic, career, health and lifestyle goals, now and in the future." In the second semester, the course uses the Facing History and Ourselves[3] resources to encourage students to "confront the complexities of history by analyzing the American Eugenics movement, the Holocaust, and other examples of genocide and atrocity and the moral choices they confront in their own lives." Another course goal is to "engage students of diverse backgrounds in an examination of racism, prejudice, and anti-Semitism in order to promote the development of a more humane and informed citizenry." Finally, the course culminates in a service learning project "that challenges students to become upstanders in their school and community." These goals align with Freire (1993), who critiques traditional schooling as a passive and alienating process of "banking education" – treating students as receptacles for deposits of information by a presumed expert teacher. "The more completely she fills the receptacles, the better a teacher she is. The more meekly the receptacles permit themselves to be filled, the better students they are" (53). He states further that, "[t]he more students work at storing deposits entrusted to them, the less they develop the *critical consciousness* which would result from their intervention in the world as transformers of that world" (54, emphasis mine). Much like Freire, Krishnamurti states that schooling should not simply encourage students to "cling to formulas or repeat the slogans." For him, "Education should awaken the capacity to be self-aware and not merely indulge in gratifying self-expression." Self-awareness and consciousness, or as Freire calls it, conscientization, is crucial since, "[s]ystems, whether educational or political, are not changed mysteriously; they are transformed when there is a fundamental change in ourselves" (15–16). The goals of education for both are personal liberation and meaningful engagement in the social world.

Affordances of social justice pedagogical strategies have clear connections to the aims of yoga (Berilla, 2016). To the extent that the Freshman seminar course lives up to its stated goals of empowering students to both reflect upon and transform themselves and their world, it is an ideal location for an engaged yoga intervention. I use the term "engaged" in much the way bell hooks (1994), who was a former student of Freire and was also influenced by Buddhist monk Thich Nhat Hanh, defines an "engaged pedagogy" – that is, a social justice approach to education that encourages students to become self-aware, while exploring their place in a world and systems that can be oppressive towards the ultimate goal of self-liberation. This engaged form of education also requires teachers to break down the traditional student–teacher relationship of all-knowing and all-powerful expert to instead lead with a loving approach that engages students' body, mind, and spirit in a more holistic approach to education.

The yoga asanas and meditation intervention, then, would incorporate yoga into the curriculum strategically and purposefully engaging with yoga philosophy as an organizing framework for the pedagogical practices within the course. We, therefore, implemented an eight-week yoga (asanas and meditation) session based on the traditional Freshman Seminar curriculum in conjunction with philosophical concepts that encourage education for a larger purpose. Each of these goals is related to the main purposes of yoga – self-awareness, self-actualization, increased focus and calm for optimum decision-making, and service to others.

As the teacher of the Freshman Seminar class, Ms. Bautista had additional goals for her own teaching practice. For her, the study's aims were to help give her and her students tools to manage trauma, stress, and the caretaker empathy that she experienced as their teacher. As a researcher, I had to be careful to state that the intervention might not mitigate stress or trauma (although these may be by-products of the yoga practice) but remained interested in the impact of yoga on resilience and self-awareness. In other words, I did not want to put yoga forth as a cure for mental health issues but wanted to see if there were any impacts on teacher and student self-healing as a complement to a curriculum that emphasized understanding the self and how these traumas might be implicated in the content they were studying.

Furthermore, Ms. Bautista stated that many of the students came with serious personal challenges. She was concerned about opening up these discussions without having the tools to appropriately address the emotional needs of students and their ability to negotiate these topics while potentially being triggered around situations in their own lives. Therefore, Ms. Bautista wanted to collaborate with me to provide tools for self-examination, self-regulation, and resiliency. To this end, some main characteristics of yoga philosophy that are leveraged in the service of how the curriculum is taught are: self-awareness, conscious communication, learning to focus and concentrate, self-compassion and compassion for others, self-realization/empowerment, and service to others.

Ms. Bautista: The empathic caregiver

Claudia Bautista advanced levels of Spanish and Freshman Seminar for Immersion students at Pacific High School[4]. She is a beloved teacher due to the care and nurturing which she joyfully showers onto her students. As an immigrant from El Salvador who experienced the trauma of living in a war-torn country, she is very cognizant of the necessity of supporting students' academic and emotional needs. As students enter her class, she greets them warmly often with hugs as she questions them about how they slept, how their classes are going, and how things are at home. Upon entering the room one day, I found Ms. Bautista dressing a student's wound using the classroom first aid kit, while a second student entered and asked "Ms. Bautista, are you good at math?" The student with the wound expressed fear that the wound wasn't healing fast enough, and Ms. Bautista hugged her while making cooing, nurturing "oh *pobrecita* (poor baby)" sounds. Every student, or even I, might have a chance to be called *mija/mijo, mi amor*, or *corazón* as she employs these terms of endearment regularly throughout the class. She knows all about the challenges of immigrant students and students of color in a school that has historically been predominantly White, and which has a very academically competitive culture. Her students often expressed their stress, anxiety, and trauma to her through their class assignments or personal conversations. She empathized with them, but she wanted tools to address both her students' and her own emotional needs.

For this intervention, I observed and taught yoga in two Freshman Seminar courses in the Immersion program both taught by Ms. Bautista. The Spanish language immersion program starts in kindergarten and continues in select courses throughout middle and high school. It maintains a balance of native and non-native English speakers; hence the classes are diverse ethnically and have an even gender balance. Pacific High has no clear racial majority; the population is 39.2% White, 35.7% Latinx, 8% Black, and 7.9% Asian (including Filipino and Pacific Islander). Students reporting two or more racial identities also make up 7.9% of the student population. Ms. Bautista's classes are a microcosm of that ethnic breakdown with perhaps fewer Black and Asian students represented proportionally (there is one Asian male and one Asian female and one African American male and one biracial female who is mixed African American and White). There are 11 male and 11 female students in one class and 8 male and 13 female students in the second. A visitor to the classroom will witness the behaviors of a room full of 14- and 15-year-olds who have known each other since kindergarten. As soon as they see each other they may either tease each other, celebrate each other, hug each other, or playfully punch each other. Indeed Ms. Bautista feels like they are the family and she is the outsider trying to negotiate a close-knit family over which she is supposed to reign. It takes all of her energy, of which Ms. Bautista has barrels full. It is perhaps for this reason, that when they complete assignments that allow them to draw on personal experience, they go openly and deeply rather quickly.

Ms. Bautista assigned an identity mask activity that alerted her that she would need extra support to attend to the emotional needs of students. On the front of the mask, students were asked to write or creatively depict markers of their identity that people can observe externally, and on the back, they wrote markers of identity that people cannot see – their more internal or truer self. Each student presented their[5] mask to the class. Ms. Bautista gave them the option of only sharing the front of the mask. Many students opted to share the back of the mask, even with me – an outsider and researcher – in observance. The level of sharing was indicative of the community that they had built over the course of their years together and of the sense of safety that students felt in the space that Ms. Bautista created.

Through this activity, students revealed experiences related to psychological issues such as eating disorders, depression, ADHD, and social issues such as stress and/or trauma related to sexual orientation and coming out, gender identity, physical and sexual abuse, and undocumented immigration status. There has been some evidence that yoga can ease symptoms of these mental health concerns (Macy, et al, 2018, Yamada and Victor, 2012). Of course as mandated reporters we would have had to report issues of abuse that came up during class time. Nothing rose to that level, but Ms. Bautista felt that she needed the tools to both integrate and respond to students' needs and to manage her own empathic response as someone who cared deeply for them.

In the push to study the impact of yoga on students, it would be helpful to understand its effect on teachers. One study found that yoga transformed teachers' thinking about their own dilemmas – either eliminating them or shifting their thinking about them. Mindfulness also allows teachers to respond to chaos more thoughtfully. Teachers in the study "gradually began to let go of unhelpful thoughts and beliefs about themselves and their dilemmas and began taking some personal and professional responsibility for how they were affected by them" (Burrows, 2015, p. 135). Ms. Bautista would readily admit that the yoga helped her as much as it did her students. When we meditated and practiced physical postures, she was often right there in a chair or on the floor with the students modeling engagement despite her own physical limitations. At the time of the intervention, Ms. Bautista had health challenges that made her days difficult, required missed classes on occasion, and was a source of stress. Ms. Bautista often shared her experiences of meditation with the class. She was very open, for example, about having been at a doctor's appointment and using breath work to calm her nerves.

Throughout the course of the yoga intervention, I watched as Ms. Bautista rethought her own practice out of a need to accommodate the new style of teaching that was required. She would allow for independent work, discussion, and small group work where students chatted as they completed assignments in her traditional classroom practice, but this led to off-task discussions and delays in proceeding forward with new activities where more focus was required. This environment definitely allowed students to feel comfortable and engaged, but when it was time to transition to teacher-led discussion it proved difficult to redirect students to a more single focused activity. The meditations provided a single focus activity – and one that was not focused on the teacher, but on the self. Students were asked to become still and silent and to close or lower their eyes in meditation. Their focus was on breathing, on the body, and on the workings of the mind. The newness of this type of focus was evident as some students had a hard time settling in without looking at each other to see who was engaged and who wasn't, giggling or trying to inspire each other to giggle, or physically moving their bodies in self-soothing actions. As a result, Ms. Bautista made some classroom adjustments, such as moving students and rethinking seating charts. The problem of excess chatter lessened and there were smoother transitions between activities as classroom shifts in practices allowed for students to experience less chaos and more calm. Furthermore, her participation in the intervention, as a beloved and trusted teacher, encouraged students to take the practice more seriously than if she sat to the side grading papers while students meditated, providing much-needed motivation since these students had their own concerns, misconceptions, and previous experiences with yoga that didn't always lead to full compliance with related activities.

What follows are case studies of students who had markedly different responses to practicing yoga. They challenged their own perceived limitations and shortcomings as the yoga introduced them to practices that urged them to flex new muscles – both metaphorically and literally. I could have chosen any of the 43 students to highlight as each presented compelling personal stories and reactions to the yoga, both positive and negative. I chose these five because each stood out for behaviors that were impacted by the yoga practice. Each presented a story of yoga that went beyond classroom management toward personal transformation.

Thomas: "I'm just going to push through"

Thomas knows how to make an entrance. As soon as he enters a room, you know he's there. He usually announces his arrival with a statement about how he feels or with a warm hello to Ms. Bautista. When he hugs her in greeting, he envelops her small frame and short stature with his large portly body. The curls of his hair and his brown skin give him a soft, warm look. His voice is more high pitched than one would expect given his size. But perhaps it's his size that amplifies it so that when he talks he can be heard throughout the room. Thomas is of Oaxacan origin and strongly identifies as such. Ms. Bautista states that Oaxaca is a Zapotec area of Mexico where cultural pride is identified with indigenous roots. Thomas lives with his father, a waiter, and his mother, who cleans houses. Neither of his parents speaks English fluently and they do not know how to navigate schooling in the U.S., so his older brother serves as a father figure. He is both role model and academic advocate.

Thomas speaks often in class, usually with great humor although it seems he is being absolutely serious. Often humorous, if only because of his almost whiny tone, are his pronouncements about how much his math teacher hates him and how stressed he is about the next test. When he expresses anxiety about his math teacher, other students chime in their agreement. It will often require some coaxing and comforting from Ms. Bautista to get the class to quiet down.

His size is also a source of shame for Thomas. Unlike his table mate who is equally large, Thomas does not leverage his size as a source of cultural capital by joining the football team. During a class discussion about negative self-talk, I gave a few sample statements, and Thomas chimed in with, "I'm too fat." I was impressed with his willingness to name this shame publicly. Despite the fact that Thomas has no filter and tends to narrate his life, this is a very open admission for a freshman in high school to announce in front of his peers.

Thomas's ambivalence about his body didn't impact his willingness to participate in yoga, although it did limit his ability to perform some of the physical exercises. During one of our yoga sessions, Thomas struggled even through the warm ups. He couldn't touch his toes and even had a hard time reaching his shins. He noticed this and said out loud, "I can't do any of these moves!" As the asanas became increasingly difficult and many students were outwardly complaining and groaning through the yoga, Thomas stated loudly, "I'm just going to push through!" In this instance, Thomas expresses both the difficulty of the task but also his strategy for surviving it. Simultaneously, whether he knew it or not, he modeled for his classmates what to do when things become difficult. I would draw on this wisdom with the class later when discussing what to do when things get tough.

Pedro: "I'm just gonna not come to school"

Much like Thomas, Pedro is hard to miss in a room, but unlike Thomas, he has a tall, lanky frame and a wide smile. No matter if he is chatting with friends or being chastised by Ms. Bautista, the same smile remains giving him an endearing quality. His hair is cut close on the sides and back, but the hair on top and upfront is long enough to either be in a bun at the top of his head or individually braided as he often wears it. Like Thomas, Pedro is a bit of a character, but while Thomas is directly engaging with the teacher, Pedro is frequently off task and distracts the class by engaging with peers.

When we meditate, it is impossible for Pedro to find any type of stillness. He moves incessantly. He often talks to his friends and giggles during meditations and even when he tries, he cannot sit still either shaking his leg or playing with his hands. Once when he had a hard time meditating without talking to his table mates, Ms. Bautista asked him to come sit with her at the back of the room. He went willingly and, of course, with the same smile. When he was at the back sitting next to her, he was more focused and able to participate in the meditation.

Ms. Bautista tells me that Pedro comes from a strict Mormon family. His father is White and his mother is Mexican. She states that he identifies more strongly with his religion than with race. Pedro struggles academically. He is the disruptive kid that is always trying to get kicked out of class, or he says he has to go to the bathroom and takes a long time to return. Ms. Bautista feels that he almost "refuses to be engaged in school."

As a result of the meditation, which was requiring him to find silence and stillness and which challenged Ms. Bautista to keep him involved without excluding him by sending him out, Pedro learned his own solution to his lack of focus. After that one time of being called to the back to sit by Ms. Bautista, when we began to meditate, Pedro would ask, "May I sit somewhere else?" and then he would voluntarily and without prompting go sit away from his peers. He did this same thing during our focus group interview. The task was to write before I engaged them in conversation. He had a hard time focusing and asked if he could write outside and then come back in when he was done. I was amazed at both his willingness to regulate his own body and attention through this strategy of voluntarily moving and being on task when he did move. More impressive than the classroom management aspect of this shift in behavior, is the ownership that Pedro took over his own body and over his own learning. Pedro expressed the benefits of yoga in his own words, which was actually surprising to read given the difficulty he had with meditation: "The meditation was a big help for me during the past few weeks. It helped me concentrate in class and do my work and not mess around cause I was melo [sic] and chill and I felt like I didn't need to play around or be distracting."

Meditation in this instance is not to be lauded as a means of ensuring that Pedro behaves, but instead as a means for him to observe his own behaviors and make some choices on his own. If Ms. Bautista had asked him to sit near her when completing an academic task, would Pedro have had the same realization? Clearly, that tactic had not worked for Pedro in the past. Most significantly, it became clear that Pedro was motivated to engage in school during the meditation. As he left the group interview on that last day he asked, "You're not doing it anymore? Why?" When I told him that the intervention had ended and therefore we would no longer practice together, he quipped, "I'm just gonna not come to school," as he bounced out the door.

Nicole: "I don't focus on anyone while we do the meditation and yoga so I can get the most out of it"

Aside from the boys, several girls had experiences with yoga that proved meaningful. One such young woman was Nicole, a brown-skinned, petite Latina whose size should not detract from the fact that she is a very tough and hard-working student. Nicole stood out almost immediately as a star student both academically and socially. She had been out of school due to a sports injury and when she returned Ms. Bautista and the students joyfully greeted her. She is clearly well liked in class. Academically, Nicole shines. She is a straight A student in the advanced math and honors classes, perhaps inspired by an older brother who attends U.C. Berkeley. She also has two younger siblings. Ms. Bautista describes her as extremely bright and diligent. Her challenge is that she is undocumented and lives in constant fear that her mother will be deported. Ms. Bautista reports that she didn't immediately go to the doctor after her injury for fear of deportation.

Each time we practiced meditation, Nicole took the practice very seriously. Eyes closed, breathing as instructed, Nicole could easily appear on a brochure for yoga and mindfulness. Once, when we tried a meditation where other students were giggling and talking, she mentioned publicly that it was hard to meditate because some of her classmates weren't taking it seriously. When it came to the physical asanas, there too she challenged herself to keep up and sustain tough poses and exercises. Nicole's meditation journal was peppered with instances of when Nicole chose to employ the breathing practices at home.

> Entry #1 Today isn't the best day. I hate that it came back. It hadn't happened in so long. I was scared, anxious I wanted to go home. It was the feeling you get when you can't control anything and just stand there hopeing [sic] the feeling will go away. I got in the car and I cried, that helped, it really did. Seeing my mom also made it better, she always knows how to help, always… I cried it all out before practice and I did some breathing that helped me get ready and just enjoy the rest of the night. It was a pretty character building day.

> Entry #3 OMG!! Today is my first game back from my surgery and I'm sooo excited. I've missed it sooo much. To be honest I'm kind of scared. I couldn't help but think of all the things that could possibly go wrong…Before I played I prayed and did some breathing, that helped calm me down and every thing [sic] went well. It felt amazing.

Clearly, she was experiencing stress and anxiety and breathing proved to be one of many tools that she used to mitigate it. Aside from those two instances, Nicole mentioned using breathing when she was scared watching a scary movie and before presentations that made her nervous including the presentation for the service learning project for Freshman Seminar.

After Nicole stated that she couldn't meditate because of the distractions, I mentioned to her that people have different challenges with yoga. Some have a hard time being quiet and still, and her challenge with the meditation would be to focus even with the distractions present. In her last entry Nicole wrote about class: "I don't feel judged when I'm in this room and all the adults are kind and understanding. It also helps that I don't focus on anyone while we do the meditation and yoga so I can get the most out of it." She had managed, over the course of the intervention, to move from being frustrated with others to blocking them out so that she could meditate for whatever benefits that the meditation would give.

Florence: "Without [meditation] I would be sitting in class right now high"

Florence and her best friend Vanessa are the dynamic duo in class and not always in the most productive ways. They feed off each other's very sometimes frenetic energy, often dominating class with their astute commentary on the issues discussed but equally with tales of their weekend exploits. Florence is a thin, blonde girl who identifies very strongly with her Irish background. She often brings Irish history up in discussions around race, ethnicity, and oppression. She seems to use this framework as a lens through which to empathize with other oppressed groups. But behind this happy-go-lucky façade lies other facets of her personality that she readily shares when she presents her mask to the class. She publicly shares mental health challenges for which she is receiving help and the details of how they make life challenging for her. Vanessa does the same when she presents her mask, and they call out support to each other as each presents her mask. But Vanessa and Florence have very different reactions to yoga. Vanessa is distracted during the yoga. The stillness is very hard for her. She often looks to Florence to see if she is meditating or not but finds no partner in crime to distract her, so she sometimes resorts to asking to go to the restroom. In the focus group Vanessa reveals that the meditation and stillness bring up thoughts that she doesn't want to address. This is common. Despite the view that meditation is calm and peaceful, it can actually bring our most difficult problems to the surface. This is why many practitioners refer to meditation as "peace and calm" but also as "practice and work." Vanessa did not find calm in meditation. She wrote, "Since the only thing I had to focus on when I was meditating was my breathing, I felt the negative thoughts become louder & louder." Vanessa chose not to do the work of meditation, to practice calming the thoughts. It does take much practice when thoughts may be particularly troubling. While another student in our focus group mentioned that meditation helped the thoughts come up so she could deal with them, Vanessa felt the thoughts come up and had to run, both metaphorically and physically. As a facilitator, I let her take the time and space she needed away from class during meditation. When students face trauma, forcing yogic practices is not productive.

Florence, on the other hand, dove wholeheartedly into the meditations. She was in her own world eyes fully closed remaining seated, back straight, eyes closed well past the time the meditation had ended. If breathing or a mudra (hand gesture) were involved, she would sometimes forego those exercises for sitting in complete stillness. Florence, when asked how the meditation went, once responded, "The hardest part about doing this is that I never want it to end." Florence also writes prolifically in her meditation journal. In her first entry she writes that she likes that she can go deep in meditation because it makes her feel "completely free, in control, and content." In another entry, she writes,

> The other night I was having a manic episode and I felt like I was going crazy. After laying awake for 3 hours trying to go to sleep, and it wasn't until I did the meditation for a calm heart [taught in class] that I was able to fall asleep. I'm so tempted to smoke, I've been clean for months, but all I want is something to help me escape the constand [sic] tugging and pulling of my heart. The meditation helps me escape, and without it I would be sitting in class right now high.

While Vanessa wants to escape the meditation because of the thoughts it unearths, Florence finds meditation to be the escape, because it helps calm her mind and give her what she often lacks – a sense of control over her thoughts and healthy responses to them.

Lauren: "If it might work, I want to give it my best shot"

Lauren is perhaps the student who wanted the yoga the most. She knew she needed it. Lauren identifies as Chicana, but she can easily pass for White. Her parents are divorced so she lives between their two households. When presenting her mask to the class, she cried as she recounted her parents' divorce and abuse she had suffered. It is perhaps for this reason that, as Ms. Bautista notes, she has a very protective mother. Ms. Bautista says that she is a lovely, outgoing, and empathic young woman who had in the past seen herself as a victim but now sees herself as a survivor. Ms. Bautista also says that she has straight As and is a positive and natural leader. I noticed that students in class made off-hand comments that she is new, since she came in the seventh grade. But the community embraced her, and she felt that embrace. As she tearfully shared her mask and her story, students cried with her and she stated that their support helped get her through those tough times.

When it came to yoga, Lauren decided that she was going to take it seriously because she thought, "If it might work, I want to give it my best shot." She was very optimistic about the role yoga would play in achieving her dreams. In an early journal entry, she wrote:

> So much homework! I am stressing about college. I hope that I get accepted into an ivy league or possibly Berkeley. I want to strive to do the best I can. I want good grades, be in a club, and stick with lacrosse. I will use breathing and yoga along the way to accomplish my goals. I will get into a college. I can do it. I am a powerful young lady.

Interestingly, many students had this perception that yoga was going "to work" for them – it was going to accomplish something. One student thought it wasn't working because it wasn't helping her sleep better. Other students didn't even try to make it work. Still others did see results. Lauren is one of those students. But yoga "didn't work" for Lauren. Lauren worked the yoga. What came through in her journal was that the consistency of the meditations and even the practice itself was often hard for Lauren. But she kept up the practice. In one entry she wrote:

> Today was a great/good day…Breathing today was hard though. Our mantra made my hands feel uncomfortable and tingly. I did like repeating a positive affirmation in my head. I picked f.l.y. first love yourself. I feel like I have felt ugly and bad about my body. I am blowing out all those thoughts and just flying.

When you look at her exterior, it's hard to imagine that Lauren has been through so much. She sits in class wearing a Berkeley sweatshirt with bright eyes fixed on whoever has the floor. When she speaks, she often has a wide smile that lights up her face and is contagious. After one meditation session, Lauren opened her eyes and was the first to speak. She said "Can I say something? I just think it's *so* beautiful that out of all the billions of people in the world, we're just 30 people in a room taking time to breathe together."

Embodied self-reflection and the praxis of becoming

As students simultaneously engaged in what Freire refers to as a "problem-posing education" that exposed them to social issues in the world while simultaneously allowing them to reflect on their own individual places within it and an embodied practice that allowed students to work through their own emotional and physical strengths and challenges, these students made moves toward self-awareness and transformation. Most significantly these embodied practices revealed mind patterns and behaviors that shifted or became noticeable as a result of asanas and meditation. Thomas outwardly named his frustrations with his body, with the way it looks, with what it can and cannot do. He also began to address this "problem" by expressing standpoints of resilience and determination. Pedro realized his own habits and patterns and of his own accord began to shift them. He went from being a distraction to himself and others to knowing when he needed to move himself to a different location in order to focus. Out of a need to hold space for meditation rather than out of a need to discipline Pedro, Ms. Bautista initiated a suggestion to move near her, but henceforth, he began to move himself without shame or as an exclusionary practice, but as a result of his own self-awareness and willingness to contribute to the meditative environment. This new strategy translated to academic activities as well. Lauren decided to give the asanas and meditation her wholehearted effort out of her desire to heal herself. She heard it "worked" and if she had a chance at improving her mental health, she was going to give it a shot. During meditation she found peace and, despite being a very ambitious student, was not concerned with her grade, her school work, or being "good" but with healing the extreme abuse she had been experiencing. Nicole, too, could manage the pressure of the need to "perform" both on the field and academically by breathing and calming her mind and body. She learned that she could focus less on the behaviors of others so that she could focus on finding her own sense of peace. This focus on herself allowed her to use yoga to perform on the soccer field at optimum levels despite the physical and emotional limitations due to injuries. While Vanessa became aware that meditation brought up disturbing thoughts that immediately highlighted both her need to run from the thoughts and her need to run from the room during meditation, Florence allowed herself to find relief each day and never wanted the meditations to end. She used them at home and at school as a means of calming herself and even as an alternative to drugs. She learned that she had another choice. Another way to *be*. We cannot expect but we can hope that these students will continue to transfer this learning to other areas of their life. We did not measure the extent to which the practice led to increased academic achievement, but clearly it did give students a new way of experiencing and "doing" life. Freire describes a problem-posing education as a "process of becoming" that affirms humans as "unfinished, uncompleted beings in and with a likewise unfinished reality." As such it is characterized by constant change as students engage in the process of becoming themselves and transforming their world. Referring to passive, objectifying pedagogies, which, he states, "emphasizes permanence and becomes reactionary", a problem-posing education, by contrast, "accepts neither a 'well-behaved' present nor a predetermined future [but] roots itself in the dynamic present and becomes revolutionary" (65). What can be more yogic than rooting in the now with a clear and open consciousness and self-awareness in order to experience liberation? As Patanjali states in the first sutra, "Now the study of yoga begins" which, given the structure and syntax of Sanskrit, can also be interpreted as "Yoga is the study of the now." Through meditation and a focus on some object in the present, one detaches from the mind-stuff – the false perceptions, the limited reality, the false identities – that consume us all and disturb our minds. Once we see clearly, we can see ourselves in our true nature. Giving us the power to liberate ourselves and transform our outer world.

Notes

1 In the West, yoga is often defined by the physical postures as yoga in its totality. In the context of this paper, yoga refers to the practice and philosophy of yogic living as out-

lined in Patanjali's Yoga Sutras, which includes meditation, breath work, the physical postures, and as a guide to living as a conscious human being. Mindfulness is a specific practice derived from Buddhist form of meditation. Thus in the West yoga is bifurcated in two strands yoga as physical postures and mindfulness as meditation whereas in its roots yoga is a holistic practice with meditation and physical practices forming only two aspects of a whole way of living.

2 According to the National Center for Education statistics, the average base income for teachers at the time of the Yoga Journal Study was $57,950. The extent to which this income would provide a middle class lifestyle would depend largely on where they lived and if they were part of a one or two income household.

3 Facing History and Ourselves is an organization that provides curricula, professional development training, and pedagogical modeling to help teachers and schools teach students about the historical implications of bigotry and hatred and to encourage students to stand up to these forces in their communities. https://www.facinghistory.org/.

4 The name of the school has been changed to protect the anonymity of the students.

5 The use of their here is meant to present a gender inclusive singular pronoun rather than the plural pronoun.

Works cited

Asmar, Melanie. "Denver Elementary School Replaces Detention with Yoga." *Denver Post*. February 27, 2017. https://www.denverpost.com/2018/02/27/denver-school-detention-yoga-class/

Berilla, Beth. *Integrating Mindfulness into Anti-Oppression Pedagogy: Social Justice in Higher Education*. New York: Routledge, 2016.

Bloom, Debora. "Instead of Detention, These Students Get Meditation." *CNN*, Updated 12:16 PM ET. November 8, 2016. https://www.cnn.com/2016/11/04/health/meditation-in-schools-baltimore/index.html

Burrows, Leigh. "Inner Alchemy: Transforming Dilemmas in Education Through Mindfulness." *Journal of Transformative Education* 13, no. 2 (February 2015): 127–139.

Butzer, Bethany, Marina Ebert, Shirly Telles, and Sat Bir Khalsa. "School-based Yoga Programs in the United States: A Survey." *Advances* 29, no. 4 (Fall 2015): 18–26.

Childress, Traci, and Jennifer Harper. *Best Practices for Yoga in Schools*. Atlanta: Yoga Service Council, YSC-Omega Publications, 2015.

Freire, Paolo. *Pedagogy of the Oppressed*. London: Penguin Books, 1993.

hooks, bell. *Teaching to Transgress: Education as the Practice of Freedom*. London: Routledge, 1994.

Macy, Rebecca J., Elizabeth Jones, Laurie M. Graham, and Leslie Roach. "Yoga for Trauma and Related Mental Health Problems: A Meta-Review with Clinical and Service Recommendations." *Trauma, Violence, & Abuse* 19, no. 1 (January, 2018): 35–57.

Moody, David. *The Unconditioned Mind: J. Krishnamurti and the Oak Grove School*. Wheaton: Quest Books, 2011.

National Center for Education Statistics. *Digest of Education Statistics*. December, 2019. https://nces.ed.gov/programs/digest/d19/tables/dt19_211.10.asp

Newsweek. Special Edition "Yoga", 2018.

Satchidanda, Sri Swami. *The Yoga Sutras of Patanjali*. Buckingham: Integral Yoga Publications, 2012.

Taie, Soheyla, Rebecca Goldring, and Maura Speigelman. "Characteristics of Public Elementary and Secondary School Teachers in the United States: Results From the 2015–16 National Teacher and Principal Survey." *National Center for Education Statistics, US Department of Education*, August, 2017. https://nces.ed.gov/pubs2017/2017070.pdf

"The 2016 Yoga in America Study Conducted by Yoga Journal and Yoga Alliance." *IPSOS Public Affairs*. January 2016. https://www.yogaalliance.org/2016YogaInAmericaStudy

"This School Sends Kids to Meditation Instead of Detention and the Results Are Incredible." Upworthy. January 4, 2017.

Time Magazine. Special Edition "Mindfulness: The New Science of Health and Happiness." September 2016.

Valsiner, Jaan. *Culture and Human Development*. London: SAGE, 2000.

Yamada, Kiyomi, and Tara Victor. "The Impact of Mindful Awareness Practices on College Student Health, Well-being, and Capacity for Learning: A Pilot Study." *Psychology Learning and Teaching* 11, no 2 (2012): 139–145.

Chapter 14

White teachers, Brown yoga
Teacher candidates learning yoga

Erin Adams, Sohyun An, Jillian Ford, and Sanjuana Rodriguez

Introduction

Each year, our university's Division of Global Affairs themes its programming around a particular country in a program called "Year of." The year 2017–2018 was the "Year of India" with the various Colleges preparing associated programming. This chapter is about how the four of us conceptualized, prepared, and executed a series of events called "Global Learning and Mindfulness Through the Study of India" that specifically focused on mindfulness and yoga as a form of civic engagement.

Context

The four of us are professors at a regional university in the southeastern U.S. The project was a university-wide project hosted in the College of Education. Like much of the teaching population in the United States, the teacher candidate population in the College of Education is majority middle class, female, and White. Our goal was to help these teacher candidates, our students, engage in mindful practices and also to expose students to a more global perspective through the activities focused around the "Year of India" program in 2017–2018.

According to our university's Division of Global Affairs website, the "Year of" program; "helps students break down stereotypes, build connections across cultures, and develop the intercultural competencies needed to act responsibly in today's complex interdependent world" (https://dga.kennesaw.edu/yearof/). Programming typically consisted of an invited lecture from a noted scholar in the field. These scholars were invited by a group of select faculty. In the previous year, "Year of Russia," lectures were held at the same time and place every Thursday and primarily planned by the Division of Global Engagement. While this method provided consistency, it meant that the speakers were not very diverse in terms of their subject areas. It also largely excluded students from places like the College of Education who, due to demanding course schedules that allow for few electives, rarely venture to other parts of campus. Participants sat in auditorium-style seats and were mainly talked at instead of actively engaged. In 2017, financial awards were given to individual colleges within the university, not departments or groups. Thus, the four of us had to come together and merge our interest in the "Year Of" program.

In order to depart from the previous year's format, we planned four events that included a keynote speaker, yoga practice, and a series of workshops designed to help teacher candidates (our students) make sense of the themes discussed in the keynote as well as to increase their understanding of India, Asia, and global engagement and citizenship in general. The program and its components were open to everyone in our university community. We hoped that the mindfulness component would help preservice teachers to develop skills to reduce stress and increase focus, two elements with which early-career teachers struggle. Through yoga and meditation, we hoped that our students would gain knowledge, skills, and dispositional assets that increase their retention in the teaching profession. We saw mind/body development as a necessary component of civic and global mindedness among students, faculty, staff, and community. The workshops and speakers were designed to foster more globally-minded teachers in Georgia and, by extension, more globally-minded K–12 youth who are prepared for 21st-century life. Thus, we wanted to help preservice teachers grow as practitioners by engaging in practices that nourished their minds, bodies, and souls. We hoped that students would see the connections between their mind and bodies and learn to appreciate, not denigrate, that connection.

In this chapter, we share our experiences and the themes from these workshops, as well as findings from our research into how our students made sense of two keynote addresses and workshops. Through students' written responses, we found a few success stories as well as entrenchments in thought that signal ways in which we might help White preservice teachers think differently, and better, about the role of mindfulness and yoga practice in schools and the world.

Our yoga stories

Before moving forward, we feel that it is important to position ourselves in relation to yoga and mindfulness, as this shapes our attitudes and approaches to the project.

Erin is an Assistant Professor of elementary social studies education. She teaches courses in social studies methods, teacher leadership, and classroom management. Her academic background includes doctoral coursework in geography, social studies, teacher education pedagogy, and poststructural theories. Erin's main area of scholarship is an investigation into the power structures, namely capitalism, that frame K–12 economics curriculum in her state as well as the United States. Erin is a White woman who does not consider herself an active practitioner of yoga (i.e. postural yoga) or specific and intentional mindfulness practices. Some of her disinclination towards yoga is due to some bad past experiences and associated with cost and inconvenience. In past years, she occasionally practiced the types of whitened yoga this chapter, and volume, problematizes, most of which consisted of a few classes taught at the university fitness center and one ill-fated visit to "hot yoga" with friends in 2015. In graduate school, mind/body classes at the university fitness center ranged from $65 to $135 per semester. This was in addition to fitness center membership fees, lockers and a dollar to borrow a towel (which was mandatory) if a patron forgot to bring their own. The classes were held in rooms farthest away from the fitness center's entrance, and were strictly regulated by staff who checked IDs and did not admit latecomers. Erin is an Assistant Professor of elementary education. She teaches courses in social studies methods, teacher leadership, and classroom management. Her academic background includes doctoral coursework in geography, social studies, teacher education pedagogy, and poststructural theories. Erin's main area of scholarship is an investigation into the power structures, namely capitalism, that frame K–12 economics curriculum in her state as well as the United States. Erin is a White woman who does not consider herself an active practitioner of yoga (i.e. postural yoga) or specific and intentional mindfulness practices. Some of her disinclination towards yoga is due to some bad past experiences associated with cost and inconvenience. In past years, she occasionally practiced the types of whitened yoga this chapter, and volume, problematizes, most of which consisted of a few classes taught at the university fitness center and one ill-fated visit to "hot yoga" with friends in 2015. In graduate school, mind/body classes at the university fitness center ranged from $65 to $135 per semester. This was in addition to fitness center membership fees, lockers and a dollar to borrow a towel (which was mandatory) if a patron forgot to bring their own. The classes were held in rooms farthest away from the fitness center's entrance, and were strictly regulated by staff who checked IDs and did not admit latecomers. There was also no parking on weekdays. Needless to say, she did not attend many classes and eventually dropped the gym membership altogether.

Erin decided to give yoga one more shot by attending a hot yoga class with friends. Hot yoga was the latest fitness trend. The class was held in the evening in a bourgeois neighborhood in her college town. During the hourlong ordeal, she was only mindful of: surviving the stifling heat, not slipping on her sweat, that she was not wearing the "right" wicking, slipproof clothing (which was for sale at the studio for $88) and the fact that her water was hot and undrinkable because, unlike her friends, she had not paid $40 for a special insulated water bottle. All of this was in addition to $25 for a single class session! A specialist in economics education, she wondered about the capitalistic gimmick of this sort of commodified yoga. At the end of the day, who, or what really benefited from all that heat? Who was this sweat for? It certainly wasn't for her; she suffered from dehydration and heat-related headaches for three days afterward. That really was her last yoga class. As a result of these experiences, for a long time Erin mainly associated yoga with cost and aspirational lifestyles although she now knows there is much more to yoga than what she has experienced. She was open to, and excited about, learning about yoga and mindfulness from decolonized viewpoints and perspectives.

Sohyun is an Associate Professor of elementary social studies education. She is a mother-scholar and teacher educator of critical race theory, AsianCrit, and critical pedagogies (An, 2020). She teaches courses in social studies methods, educational equity, and action research in undergraduate and graduate programs. She seeks to "get it right" in critical race parenting of her two daughters who are Korean/Asian American. Sohyun began to take yoga classes in 2014 when she gave birth to a second child. She felt physically and emotionally weak and overwhelmed with parenting and working as an Asian immigrant mother/scholar/teacher educator. She had zero knowledge of yoga when she started taking yoga practice sessions at a local gym, and slowly she fell in love with yoga and its mindful practices. For her, yoga is a place and time where she can fully focus on herself and take gentle care of her mind and body.

Sanjuana is an Assistant Professor of literacy education. She teaches undergraduate and graduate literacy courses. She began her career as a kindergarten teacher and later became a literacy coach for a school district.

Sanjuana does not consider herself to be an active practitioner of yoga. She does attend beginners yoga on a weekly basis since learning more about the practice in the activities that will be described in this paper. Her interests in participating in this project stemmed from her interests in diverse children's literature. Through the project, she was able to introduce literature to teacher candidates that included the topics of mindfulness and yoga.

Jillian is an Associate Professor of social studies education in the Secondary and Middle Grades department. She is a Black/White biracial cisgender woman who uses womanist theory to research civic participation, contemplative practice in education, and queer identities in schools. She teaches undergraduate and graduate courses on social studies methods, social justice pedagogies, and qualitative research methods. Jillian began practicing yoga about five years ago, and has since explored other contemplative engagement with meditation, altar building, pilgrimages, and sound healing. Yoga has played an integral role in her healing journeys.

Planning the Year of India events and how we thought of mindfulness and yoga

Global Learning and Mindfulness through the Study of India was intended to bring the "Year Of" program to the College of Education. Despite the critically important role they play in society, our students, preservice teachers' schedules are arranged so that they have few opportunities for electives or time to attend other campus events. As they advance further into their junior and senior years, their schedules become more and more dictated by the demands of their majors which are increasingly confined to courses in the College of Education and in local K–12 schools. Moreover, if students do not see a direct connection to their chosen profession and the topic in a lecture or campus event, they might be understandably reluctant to attend.

We were each attracted to Year of India (YoI) for what it could offer. As professors of social studies education, Erin, Sohyun, and Jillian were interested in helping students grow in their global understanding and competency. Jillian contributed an interest in yoga and contemplative practices. Erin and Sohyun sought to find ways to help preservice teachers reconceptualize what social studies is and why and how it is taught. For Sohyun, who is an Asian immigrant, the Year of India was a good chance to counter curricular/instructional silence on teaching about Asia and the U.S.'s current and historical involvement with/in Asia. Although similarly concerned about an additive model of global content, Jillian saw the YOI opportunity as a way to address topics such as coloniality, spirituality, and energy. Sanjuana specialises in language arts education and was interested in bringing diverse books to the College of Education (see https://diversebooks.org). Through the Spotlight grant and funding from our Dean, Sanjuana was able to build a small collection of children's books about India for the College's Literacy Center.

We specifically wanted to help the preservice teachers that we teach increase their global understanding, engage in mindfulness practice(s), and develop more nuanced understandings of how to use (or not use) yoga and mindfulness practices in their future work in K–12 public schools. Collectively, we are concerned about the increasingly technocratic nature of teacher education, and saw this institutionally-funded grant as an opportunity to help our students imagine a more holistic approach to planning and instruction.

Global understandings are essential for teachers to develop as a means to help support the well-being of all humans. Pointing to the reality of immigration, forced migration, multinational organizations, and international trade, 17Zong asserts the necessity of global education to promote students' critical thinking and decision-making skills. Recognizing the largely skills-based undergraduate curricula (Kinchloe), we sought to provide time for students to experience both scholarly and community-based lectures about India, elements of the Indian Diaspora, and yoga in the West. Having introduced her class to a series of contemplative practices the previous semester, Jillian was struck by how positively her students responded to attention to breath and intentional silence. By providing the asana element of hatha yoga practice in our series, our aim was to allow students the time and space to experience embodied lessons along with the more common cognitive information delivered in the lectures. In Teaching for Tenderness, Thompson explains the contemporary imperative "to nurture a yin environment (an opening up, making space for thought and feeling, making room for listening, breath, air)," in our classrooms. The yin is important, given the accelerated pace of life and information production that "fuel a yang culture (condensed, compact, concentrate)" (56). Although a few of our student participants had practiced yoga prior to this experience, it was the first time for the majority of our students. We were intentional about inviting only People of Color to deliver the lectures and to facilitate the yoga practices; all but one with ancestral roots in south Asia. We facilitated a total of four events, two in the fall semester and two in the spring (although the fourth event was abbreviated). We themed the series of events around the social studies disciplines of history, geography, and civics. These are the four most common disciplines taught in K-12 schools in the U.S. Fall events related to history and civics while Spring events engaged with geography and economics, although elements of each discipline could be found in each event.

Fall events

The first event featured Roopa Singh, an attorney, academic, and founder of the Yoga Standards Review Project[1]. Singh delivered a keynote address entitled "What is this place- Mapping Yoga as American Property." Singh spoke about the whitening of yoga via the patenting of yoga in the United States using theories of whiteness as currency and critical race theory. For example, Singh discussed the history of yoga practice in the United States and the ways in which yoga has become simultaneously Americanized and whitewashed. That is, it has become the commodified, trendy, and private practice many of us, and our students, know it as today. Consequently, yoga has been separated from its Indian-subcontinental roots and "whitened." Yoga, which was a public practice, now often (but not always) is practiced behind a paywall. It thus became a personal, individualized good rather than a public good. Singh discussed the various ways the U.S. copyright and patenting process and the protection of "privat(iz)e(d)" property has led to this commodification. One of the major takeaways from Singh's presentation was the idea of yoga as a form of cultural appropriation. Singh taught that cultural appropriation is not just about dress, but also about practices. In the case of yoga, this appropriation does harm in a variety of ways, including separating yoga from its people.

For the second event, "yoga as civic engagement," Sonali Sadequee, founder of Sustainable Wellness and specialist in trauma-informed yoga[2] discussed mindfulness and yoga as restorative justice practices as well as yoga as a philosophy and way of life rather than the programmed arm and leg movements of the whitened Americanized version. In short, "doing yoga" is not limited to a mat. Yoga is a way of life. This realization complements Singh's work and the violence of co-opting, commodifying, and whitening of yoga. Sadequee led the audience, consisting of faculty and college students, in exercises in listening and engaging with others. Students commented that this activity was one of the most meaningful to them, because we often do not take time to listen to others. It was also a good teaching example. As future teachers, the students we teach will inevitably ask their K–5 students to "listen" but what that is and how to do it might not be clear and teachers might not be modelling engaged listening. Democratic societies require people to listen to one another. In addition to listening to one another speak, Sadique discussed listening to our bodies and to see the body as a site of knowledge. Sadequee spoke about her work using yoga for healing, particularly the generational trauma that is carried in the body. Healing the body and the mind is a way to heal society from the horrors of the past including slavery.

Critical examination of the commodification of yoga was a common theme between the two keynote addresses. Both of these speakers radically flipped the narratives of civic engagement, yoga, and race familiar to the predominantly White, suburban, middle class students that we teach. These speakers expanded what it means to be civically engaged and showed a way forward from the traumas we have both experienced and inflicted as actors in current manifestations of coloniality. As people with Asian, Indigenous, African, and European ancestry, our histories are marked with genocide, enslavement, land theft, state imposition, and other mechanics of colonialism (Blu Wakpa, 2018; Linklater, 2014). The keynote speakers reminded us that we are all connected, a difficult reality to hold given our varied ancestral lineages. Healing ourselves, one another, and the Earth can be forms of embodied civic engagement.

Spring Events

The third event happened in the spring of 2017 and was on the social studies topics of economics and geography. Sarasij Majumder, a professor of anthropology at our university, spoke about issues of land and identity in India-Bharat. The talk engaged with diaspora, development, land and capitalism, and culture[3].

The fourth event was a chance for faculty to engage in yoga practice during one of our college's monthly faculty and staff research/writing days. Occuring on the final Friday of each month, these days are used for faculty to present their research, give and receive editorial feedback and peer review, and dedicated writing time. Though undoubtedly helpful for faculty, these sessions are also in service of fulfilling the goals of the neoliberal university and its compulsions to produce "to fit the template of managerial best practices" within "narrowly defined measures of value and success" (p. Petersen & Davies, 2010, p. 103). This time, however, Sadequee conducted faculty through restorative practices to heal us from the pain and posture accrued by academia, writing, and days and nights lived at laptops.

After each keynote speaker, a local yoga instructor creator, organizer, life enthusiast and joy seeker zahra alabanza led students, staff, and faculty in yoga practice. Then, we led small workshops on topics such as Asian immigration, religion (and who gets to determine what "counts"), yoga in the classroom, civic engagement, and the importance of picture books in classrooms that can act as both windows and mirrors for children (Tschida, Ryan and Tiknor, 2014).

Mind-ful teachers and the neoliberal teaching machine

One of our goals was to create more mindful and contemplative teachers. By this, we mean teachers who engage in mindfulness practices themselves and who can be mindful of the practices they employ in their classrooms. It would seem natural that schools and classrooms would be natural sites of mindfulness and contemplation, that is, places to think, to dream, to consider multiple possibilities, to be in touch with one's body and soul and the Earth, to heighten our awareness of ourselves and others in a space of productive silence. However, our experience tells us this is not the case. Instead, schools and classrooms are busy. They are excessively noisy and repressively silent.

Much has been written about neoliberalism as it relates to the U.S. economy and to schools and education. Neoliberal "reforms" include charter schools, standardized testing, and "accountability" measures "overall, the nature of educational reform over the last 30 years has been characterized by increased accountability, standardization and testing, the professionalization of schooling at all levels, increased federal administrative authority and corporate influence, a nod toward privatization and the infusion of technology into the classroom" (Heertum, Torres and Olmos, 4). Time is the greatest commodity in schools that are constantly under pressure to produce standardized test scores. To do this teachers are instructed to teach "bell to bell," to control their bodies and their students', to minimize recess and time outside, to constantly make work for themselves and their students. Teachers are inundated with tasks and expectations that often feel impossible. It is no wonder that the teaching profession is plagued by high turnover and toxic stress.

Issues in teacher education

Collectively, we are concerned about the increasingly technocratic nature of teacher education, and saw this institutionally-funded grant as an opportunity to help our students imagine a more holistic approach to planning and instruction. Global understandings are essential for teachers to develop as a means to help support the well-being of all humans. Pointing to the reality of immigration, forced migration, multinational organizations, and international trade, Zong (2009) asserts the necessity of global education to promote students' critical thinking and decision-making skills. Recognizing the largely skills-based undergraduate curricula (Kinchloe, 2011), we sought to provide time for students to experience both scholarly and community-based lectures about India, elements of the Indian Diaspora, and yoga in the West.

Having introduced her class to a series of contemplative practices the previous semester, Jillian was struck by how positively her students responded to attention to breath and intentional silence. By providing the asana element of hatha yoga practice in our series, our aim was to allow students the time and space to experience embodied lessons along with the more common cognitive information delivered in the lectures. In *Teaching for Tenderness*, Thompson explains the contemporary imperative "to nurture a yin environment (an opening up, making space for thought and feeling, making room for listening, breath, air)," in our classrooms. The yin is important, given the accelerated pace of life and information production that "fuel a yang culture (condensed, compact, concentrate)" (p. 56). Although a few of our student participants had practiced yoga prior to this experience, it was the first time for the majority of our students. We were intentional about inviting only People of Color to deliver the lectures and to facilitate the yoga practices; all but one with ancestral roots in south Asia.

Yoga in schools

Jain (2015) writes that postural yoga "often betrays a desire to repair what is perceived as an imbalance of 'body–mind–soul'" (172). That is, Americanized yoga is supposed to fix something that is out of place, and in this case, children are assumed to be in need of fixing or correction.

Yoga is selectively applied and accessed in schools and other institutions. Yoga can be one more form of enrichment for children from more affluent homes and a trendier and seemingly more benign, and even benevolent version of gaining compliance from and control over children from less affluent families. Moreover, Norman points out that community resistance to yoga for marginalized populations can stem from a "principle of less eligibility" (5). That is, the belief that incarcerated people or poor children, for example, are undeserving of a commodity (yoga classes and instruction) that the general public cannot afford.

Shopping at organic, health-oriented grocery stores like Whole Foods, attending postural yoga classes, enrolling children in enrichment activities and hockey are practices of the "aspirational class"-a class that relies on knowledge acquisition and cultural signfiers, rather than material possessions like expensive cars or flashy clothes and jewelry (Currid-Halkett). In this class, Currid-Halkett observes, people are not defined by how much money they spends, per se, but by their "informed" choices. "Inconspicuous consumption" creates a new class divide because those who participate do so in a way that is "nonvisible except to those in the know and it is difficult to emulate without tactic information or a significant amount of money." Status-signalling activities can contribute to inequality when practitioners shore up informational, sociocultural privilege and pass it on to their children. Yoga, for example, allows this group to "experience the idea of another culture while focusing on the self" (Gandhi & Wolff). While none of these activities are harmful on their own, collectively, the aspirational class aims to own, control and access the means of cultural and knowledge production that functions as a kind of social currency (Klein). This mindset may add to the drive to commodify, copyright and privatize yoga in order to make it an exclusive social signifier.

Yoga is particularly salient to us, as our university and our preservice teachers are located in a community (White and affluent) that recently made national news when it was embroiled in a controversy over yoga in schools. An elementary school assistant principal was transferred after introducing yoga and mindfulness practices into her elementary school (3French). One of the primary complaints was that yoga was "anti-Christian." This seeemd to be a classic case of "Christian yogaphobia." Jain describes yogaphobia as;

A social anxiety characterized by suspicion and fear of modern yoga... expressed by certain religious institutions and individuals [it] emphasizes the incompatibility between yoga and certain doctrines or moral codes. [This] perpetuates essentialist and Orientalist stereotypes, which are often buttressed by social and political ideologies and agendas and relies on a sense of shared otherness (133).

Christian yogaphobia appears to intensify "in direct proportion to the industry's growth" (Jain, 2017, 47). The district's parents seemed to be under the impression that students were engaging in a religious practice that included the use of healing crystals. Despite being whitened and Americanized, the kind of posturing yoga practiced in schools was somehow viewed as promoting the Hindu religion.

A parent told the local news that the school was "pushing ideology" on children (Wolfe and Hoff). As a result, yoga was allowed to continue but teachers were directed not to have students color pictures of mandalas, say "namaste" or put their hands near their hearts. This shows the complexity of doing something like yoga in schools. The use of "namaste" is a problem for reasons including "somatic Orientalism," and the word's appropriation as white speech" (Putcha, 7). However, parents had a problem with the word, allegedly, due to its perceived religious connotations rather than its use in the popularizing and commodification of yoga in America.

In these suburban "secular" schools in the south, yoga is only viewed as acceptable when it is fully appropriated and commodified "without respect for or knowledge of its cultural roots" (Bharadway, 2016) and when people from India are made invisible. As yoga instructor Lakshmi Nair (2019) expressed it "your superpower of invisibility is on point when a billion of you go unnoticed" (Nair 34). Similarly, "the yoga industrial complex profits from romanticizing the culture of India while excluding real people...of South Asian heritage from taking up space or positions of leadership" (Ansari, 21). Eliminating any seemingly religious or spiritual practices from yoga further Americanizes, whitening it away from its multicultural spiritual roots on the subcontinent and from the same texts and traditions from which Hinduism, Buddhism, and Jainism formed (Kremer).

Selected findings/implications for yoga and mindfulness in (teacher) education

We analyzed preservice teachers' written responses to the two "Year of India" lectures. Preservice teachers were required to attend one of the "Year of India" events as part of Erin's elementary social studies methods course. Then, they were asked to write about their experiences and how they might frame their future teaching. Preservice teachers were asked to frame their responses in terms of Harshman's (2015) six questions for teachers to reflect on their global citizenship. The six questions are:

1.) Whose perspective is missing?
2.) What influences my global perspective and how does my perspective inform my decision making as an educator/student?
3.) In what ways are the people we intend to help involved in deciding what we intend to do?
4.) How do we guard against perpetuating inequity and social injustice while promoting responsible and active global citizenship education?
5.) What role does privilege play in my ability to be a global citizen?
6.) To what extent do the actions I consider to be positive examples of global citizenship adversely affect people and places I do and do not know?

Harshman's goal was to help students develop more critical global dispositions through investigating their own biases and perspectives. Although teachers might normally be positioned as question-posers, Harshman encourages teachers to question their own understandings so that they can be global citizens who do no harm even when attempting to help; "by acknowledging that how we think about the world is only one of many valid perspectives, we begin the important work of reflecting on the deeper influences that consciously or subconsciously influence our worldviews" (Harshman, 2015, para. 3).

Brain Breaks

We found that Erin's students overwhelmingly conceptualized "using" yoga and mindfulness practices as a brain break. "Brain break" is a popular term in K-5 education to signify a break from formalized academic instruction. Teachers can find a host of brain break activities, including yoga, on the Internet. One site notes brain breaks are good to use "anytime your students are feeling restless and are struggling to pay attention." Afterwards, "you can get back to the lesson with your students ready to focus on the lesson at hand" (Lynette & Noack).

Here are two representative examples the preservice teachers' responses: "The teacher could use yoga as a transition in the classroom or for a brain break for the students. This allows the students to take a break and relax from the curriculum giving the students an opportunity to optimize their learning when they are done. It is giving the students a chance to relax and take a break from learning and regain their focus back." Another preservice teacher expressed a similar sentiment about yoga as a "brain break:" "I believe that yoga is a great 'brain break' to incorporate into the classroom. When young children practice yoga, they are helping their bodies physically by stretching and they are also learning focus and concentration. If yoga is practiced as a 'brain break' students will be receiving a mental break from their schoolwork, and will receive a feeling of accomplishment, and when they return to their school work they will be more relaxed and able to focus on what they are working to accomplish."

The examples contains language and signifies preservice teacher beliefs that are concerning to us for several reasons.

Yoga as mind-lessness

First is the idea of a "brain break" from the curriculum. That is, the teacher candidates saw yoga practice as separate from "the curriculum" which we presume means the "official curriculum" such as math, language arts, science, and social studies. Here, yoga is viewed as as disconnected from schoolwork, as absence of learning. It is as if yoga is not in itself a teacher, but is subservient to teachers and to the official curriculum who use it as a means for an end. This totally misses what yoga is all about. Yoga, by definition is about the union between body, spirt and mind (Johnson). This "absence" is part of a larger Western tradition of mind/body separation, a "mutually reinforcing dichotomy" (Ruth, 1) wherein the mind is privileged and the body is viewed as distracting.

Rehabilitation

Second, the teachers' statements suggests that learning and yoga practice are separate, as indicated by the statements "optimize their learning when they are done" and "take a break from learning." Our biggest worry here is the preservice teacher's appropriation of yoga and mindfulness practices for the sake of supporting a neoliberal educational agenda. Yoga is viewed as a way to correct the body for the sake of the mind. It is not only about correcting, or controlling the body, but punishing it. Jain (2015) argues that "in postural yoga contexts, yoga's aim is to surmount some types of suffering, but other types of suffering, which involve the disciplining of desire for the sake of body enhancement and healing, is worth pursuing" (108). This is a kind of repentance through denial and pain that has become popular in American exercise culture and a "no pain, no gain" workout ethos (e.g. Crossfit). In the case of schools, it is not so much that yoga is meant to be physically strenuous, but that when applied with certain ends in mind, repressive; to keep desire in check.

We are not saying yoga should not be in schools, far from it. We believe it has tremendous revolutionary and healing potential, which the authors in this volume have illustrated. However, we worry about how postural, Americanized yoga could be used and for what (and whose) ends. Practicing yoga itself is not necessarily an issue. The issue lies with "how yoga is commonly practiced and commercialized" in culturally appropriative ways that "takes a traditional practice from a marginalized group and turns it into something that benefits the dominant group-ultimately erasing its origins and meaning" (Johnson). In schools, yoga and mindfulness practices are being viewed as an alternative to detention and more punitive practices (e.g. Jones). We question some of the motives for using (or appropriating) yoga and mindfulness in schools. 11Norman wrote of a similar phenomenon in prison yoga, whereby the practice is thought to "contribute to incarcerated people's rehabilitation and well-being through encouraging behavior and psychological changes" (4).

There, yoga is approached from a "what works" standpoint that "attempts to pinpoint precise behavioral outcomes for participants" (4). Programs like these are forms of social control that "contribute to a neoliberal agenda that individualizes criminal behavior" (Norman 4). Used in this way, yoga becomes both social control and good public relations for the prison. Norman sheds light on one of the many ways yoga is appropriated in carceral institutions like schools and prisons, and yoga in schools ought to be interrogated as resisting, not contributing to, the school to prison pipeline. We also acknowledge that the teacher candidates' sentiments are part of this larger cultural discourse which needs to be interrogated and interrupted.

Focus

Finally, it seems that the preservice teacher sees yoga as a means to "focus." "Focus" is education-speak for both children's bodily compliance in the classroom and their "learning" which, in turn, means students' performance on standardized test scores. The preservice teacher presumes that yoga has a start and endpoint, indicated by "when they are done." Again, this stems from the belief that yoga is merely a series of physical movements divorced from social and spiritual response-abilities instead of as "preparation for meditation…[for] mental quiet and rigor" (Bharadway). The ultimate goal of yoga practice in the classroom, as the second preservice teacher conceptualized it, is "accomplishment" of some sort. We take "accomplish" to mean class assignments, tests, and success in the neoliberal economy. However, "a breath isn't always benign" when "yoga and meditation are seen as a way to gain a 'competitive edge'" (Strauss). In short, the teacher misunderstood what yoga is meant to prepare practitioners for.

Understanding and appropriation

Despite these problematic statements about her future "use" of yoga, first teacher candidate wrote a thorough and thoughtful summary of Roopa's talk, writing: "The more that yoga becomes profitable the narrower, and narrower the term yoga becomes, which brought to sharing the modern day term of yoga. Today people see yoga as going to a class, making sure you have the right outfit, the right mat, and making sure you feel good about yourself. However, yoga is something that we are supposed to be doing at all times. It does not end, nor begin at a certain time; it is about how we hold our physical mortal shell in alignment with our energy." The teacher candidate provided a succinct and thoughtful critical analysis of yoga practice in America. Nevertheless, the student later reinforced the very discourses she critiqued. Thus, there is a disconnect between what the preservice teacher has learned to be true of problematic practices in the appropriation of yoga for capitalistic ends and her intentions to use it as a method of intervention, of "fixing" her future K-5 students. By "fixing" we mean the teacher's impetus to do things such as "refocus" children for the purpose of achieving better test scores.

Like the previous student, this second preservice teacher was able to summarize Roopa's main points; the whitening of yoga and whiteness as property, the history of copyrighting in the United States and the problematic practices of copyrighting of yoga. However, the student had trouble connecting these ideas with her own life, writing: "Before her speech, I did not know that yoga was a practice that transformed from India and was known as a free meditation. I have always had a bias of yoga until just last year when my [relative] opened her own yoga studio in my home town. I now have a love for yoga because of the sense of relaxation it gives. It is interesting to reflect and think about how if it were not for the first person who introduced yoga to individuals in the United States and copyrighted yoga, we may not have this wonderful type of relaxation that we practice and now make a part of everyday lives as Americans."

The preservice teacher wrote, uncritically, about the very thing Roopa problematized; White women copyrighting/commodifying/privatizing yoga practice. Moreover, the student adopted a problematic, America-centric, "celebratory" approach to yoga and its Indian roots. In the preservice teacher's narrative, yoga was freely practiced, and freely given, by people from India to Americans who can now enjoy "this wonderful type of relaxation" for themselves. This echoes an eerily similar, and just as problematic, settler-colonialist narrative of Native Americans freely giving over their resources to white European settler/invaders (i.e. Americans) "to enjoy." Blu Wakpa hypothesizes yoga's popularity among European Americans as due, in part, to a "case of misplaced 'imperialist nostalgia' since the practice foregrounds the interconnections among body, mind and spirit, which European Americans have attempted to destroy through the assimilation of Native practices, but simultaneously long for" (ii). Settler colonialism and yoga intersect in several ways, including problematic histories of cultural commodification and erasure. The teacher's statement is indicative of a particular feeling of entitlement to yoga and other knowledge and practices as if they were created for them. Such a "pursuit of happiness" and subsequent commodification through copyrighting comes at the expense of Brown bodies.

Theory/practice divide

Although these students, and others, missed the mark, their responses are not surprising. Not only are they part of the very (colonial, White, copyrighted, neoliberal) systems Roopa and Sonali critiqued, their responses are part of a larger theory-into-practice problem that is pervasive in teacher education. By understanding the preservice teachers' misconceptions and disconnects, we (teacher educators) can see ways to improve our practice. We can see what needs to be made intentional. In this case, we know that preservice teachers have trouble translating theory into practice. As Leonardo (2009) stated, we believe that the theory is not generated for theory's sake but, rather, for "the production and application of theory as a part of the overall search for transformative knowledge" (p. 13). Theories are then not "something separate from practice" (13), but rather "ways of knowing with habits of knowing" (hooks, 43). Practice and theory are, therefore, married entities, incomprehensible in isolation. However, we see preservice teachers have a hard time translating theories to practice. We teach educational theories and theorists *so that* preservice teachers will take them into their classrooms, yet they do not seem to use theory to inform their practice. We often hear them say "I didn't learn anything" or "Why do we have to read this?" In fact, many teacher education scholars have noted the theory/research divide. According to Segall, "For theory to become more than that [a body of someone else's knowledge that students are required to learn] it must be practiced, explored as a form of cultural production, examined for what it yields and for what it conceals" (157). Thus, we realize that although we want students to apply theory or identify how theory informs practice, not just summarize/memorize a theorist's ideas, we maybe are not providing appropriate outlets in which to put theory to work. In our own work with students, we have found it both challenging and helpful to invite our students' "whole selves" into the classroom by drawing our collective attention.

We also know they are, largely, products of No Child Left Behind (NCLB) and neoliberal educational "reforms" that largely quantify "success" for both students and teachers as grades on standardized tests. Due to what Lortie (1975) called the "apprenticeship of observation" wherein teachers reproduce their own 13 years of schooling, they may have trouble conceptualizing different kinds of classroom life, purposes for schooling, and relationships to learning. Moreover, these preservice teachers' middle class whiteness positions them in the very process of whitening the curriculum, and yoga, that the keynote speakers discussed.

For example, Michael Apple (2000) writes about the contradictions between the rhetoric of individuality and autonomy and the reality of standardization and centralisation.

"Rather than moving in the direction of increased autonomy, in all too many instances the daily lives of teachers in classrooms in many nations are becoming ever more controlled, ever more subject to administrative logics that seek to tighten the reins on the processes of teaching and curriculum. Teacher development, cooperation, and 'empowerment' may be the talk, but centralization, standardization, and rationalization may be the strongest tendencies, even with the increasing media focus on privatization, marketization and decentralization" (p.114).

These are the conditions for teachers that are then passed on to students. Substitute "students" or "children" for "teachers" in Apple's paragraph. Personal empowerment and personal sovereignty might be the rhetoric but in reality these discourses are used as a persuasive leveraging tool when conformity and standardization is what is really meant.

For example, Michael 1Apple writes about the contradictions between the rhetoric of individuality and autonomy and the reality of standardization and centralisation; Rather than moving in the direction of increased autonomy, in all too many instances the daily lives of teachers in classrooms in many nations are becoming ever more controlled, ever more subject to administrative logics that seek to tighten the reins on the processes of teaching and curriculum. Teacher development, cooperation, and 'empowerment' may be the talk, but centralization, standardization, and rationalization may be the strongest tendencies, even with the increasing media focus on privatization, marketization and decentralization (114). These are the conditions for teachers that are then passed on to students. Substitute "students" or "children" for "teachers" in Apple's paragraph. Personal empowerment and personal sovereignty might be the rhetoric but in reality these discourses are used as a persuasive leveraging tool when conformity and standardization is what is really meant. When used a certain way, yoga in schools and classrooms can support an illusion of empowerment while at the same time reinforcing discipline, docility and compliance. Americanized, postural, commodified yoga which markets itself as redemptive, harmless and enriching is well positioned for misapplication.

On the other hand, imagine the revolutionary possibilities if yoga, not just posturing, was actually practiced in schools. What if yoga in schools was "about sustaining ourselves in ways that have nothing to do with money or material possessions"? (Johnson). What if yoga was used not simply as an additive, but as an attitude that frames and reconceptualizes the entire school expereince. As Ansari expresses it;

When I invite someone to raise an arm or breathe into their belly, I am thinking about how to stay in connection to the humanity of this person, to consider this individual's experience moving and being moved in this world. I stay curious about what personal memories, difficulties, or hidden potentials there are for this person. I understand that the power of racism and patriarchy lies in how it dissociates the personal from the political, building a private interiority away from sociocultural context. Therefore, I aim to promote an intimate process for people to slow down, to be in touch with the truth of their emotions and their experiences" (22).

Sophia Ansari's description of yoga, especially the notion of slowing down and processing difficulties, seems wholly at odds with the kind of hyper-competitive, fast and outcomes-based culture in American schools.

Takeaways

We noted several important takeaways from this project. First, critical approaches to addressing mindfulness and yoga for teachers and schools take systematic program-level incorporation. That is, a one-time discussion is not enough and might provide students with just enough interest in mindfulness and yoga to be "dangerous" in the sense of Roopa's work on the whitening, colonizing, and copyrighting of yoga. The preservice teachers' responses are indicative of larger neoliberal forces at work in K–12 schools and teacher education. Where we see mindfulness and yoga as a tool to dismantle and resist neoliberalism, our teacher candidates may see it a tool to reify the status-quo. It is also important to remember that "what is healing/liberating for one group may cause suffering/violence for another" (Blu Wakpa). Although we have recounted examples of problematic responses from preservice teachers who "missed the mark" the program was not all bad. Weeks later, in class, one student remarked that she could not get Roopa's speech out of her mind. She connected Roopa's talk with her job at an organic grocery store, remarking about the store's role in the commodification and branding of health as trendy and aspirational. She noted that the store seemed to make customers feel healthy and therefore gave them license to buy cookies and cakes and other snack food. Without realizing it, the student connected her work at the grocery store with the aspirational lifestyle theory (Currid-Halkett). This is an example of the "lived experience of critical thinking, of reflection and analysis" that is theory and theorizing and that we would like our teachers to recognize and practice (hooks, 61).

Moreover, just because students' written responses are not what we would have liked them to be does not indicate failure. The preservice teachers had the opportunity to observe masterful teaching and were exposed to concepts and ideas that were very new to them. Thus, we never know when, where, or how this learning will materialize. We hope that we can continue to help our preservice teachers view yoga and mindfulness as mind-full rather than mind-less and seek out these practices for the sake of healing and not the neoliberal regime, as a respite from the world not an offering to it.

Notes

1 https://yastandards.com/roopa-singh/.
2 https://www.sustainable-wellness.com/.
3 Dr. Majumder's talk can be accessed here; https://ksutv.kennesaw.edu/play.php?v=00130012.

References

An, S. (2020). Disrupting curriculum of violence on Asian Americans. *Review of Education, Pedagogy, and Cultural Studies*, 42(2), 141–156.

Ansari, S. (2020). Decolonizing yoga: Restoring my seat of consciousness. *Race and Yoga*, 5(1), 18–23. https://escholarship.org/uc/item/3v8504zx

Apple, M. (2000). *Official Knowledge*. New York: Routledge.
Bharadway, A. (2016). *Why Understanding the Roots of Yoga Is So Important*. https://fitbottomedgirls.com/2016/09/appropriation-the-roots-of-yoga-is-so-important/
Blu Wakpa, T. (2018). Decolonizing yoga? And (un)settling social justice. *Race and Yoga*, 3(1), x–xix. https://escholarship.org/uc/item/8nz498zt
Currid-Halkett, E. (2017). *The Sum of Small Things: A Theory of the Aspirational Class*. Princeton University Press. [Kindle Edition].
French, R. (2016, March 21). Classroom yoga exercises prompt parent concerns in Cobb. *Atlanta Journal-Constitution*. https://www.ajc.com/news/local-education/classroom-yoga-exercises-prompt-parent-concerns-cobb/fJOGtzRYXr8UP56OsM5DFJ/
Gandhi, S. & Wolff, L. (2017, December 19). *Yoga and the Roots of Cultural Appropriation*. Praxis Center. https://www.kzoo.edu/praxis/yoga/
Harshman, J. (2015). Reflection, action, and variation within global citizenship education. Education Week. https://blogs.edweek.org/edweek/global_learning/2015/11/reflection_action_and_variation_within_global_citizenship_education.html
Heertum, R.V., Torres, C.A., & Olmos, L. (2011). *Educating the Global Citizen in the Shadow of Neoliberalism : Thirty Years of Educational Reform in North America*. Oak Park, IL: Bentham Science Publishers.
hooks, b. (1994). *Teaching to Transgress: Education as the Practice of Freedom*. Routledge.
Jain, A.R. (2017). Yoga, Christians practicing yoga and God: On theological compatibility, or is there a better question? *Journal of Hindu-Christian Studies*, 30, 46–52. https://doi.org/10.7825/2164-6279.1658
Jain, R.R. (2015). *Selling Yoga: From Counterculture to Pop Culture*. Oxford University Press.
Johnson, M.Z. (2016, May 25). 8 signs your yoga practice is culturally appropriated-and why it matters. Everyday Feminism. https://everydayfeminism.com/2016/05/yoga-cultural-appropriation/
Jones, S. (2019, May 23). Ditching detention for yoga: Schools embrace mindfulness to curb discipline problems. Education Week. https://www.edweek.org/leadership/ditching-detention-for-yoga-schools-embrace-mindfulness-to-curb-discipline-problems/2019/05
Kincheloe, J.L. (2011). Meet Me Behind the Curtain. In *Key Works in Critical Pedagogy* (pp. 85–99). Sense Publishers.
Klein, E. (2019, November 14). How Whole Foods, yoga and NPR became the hallmarks of the modern elite. Vox. https://www.vox.com/podcasts/2019/11/14/20964420/whole-foods-yoga-npr-elite-ezra-klein-elizabeth-currid-halkett-inequality
Kremer, W. (2013, November 21). Does doing yoga make you a Hindu? BBC. https://www.bbc.com/news/magazine-25006926
Leonardo, Z. (2009). *Race, Whiteness, and Education*. New York: Routledge.
Linklater, R. (2014). *Decolonizing Trauma Work: Indigenous Stories and Strategies*. Halifax: Fernwood Publishing.
Lortie, D.C. (1975). *Schoolteacher*. The University of Chicago Press.
Lynette, R. & Noack, C. (2021). Brain braks: 20 awesome ways to energize your students fast. Minds in Bloom. https://minds-in-bloom.com/20-three-minute-brain-breaks/
Nair, I. (2019). Even spirit has no place to call home: Cultural appropriation, microaggressions, and structural racism in the yoga workplace. *Race and Yoga*, 4(1), 33–38.

Norman, M. (2019). Transforming space? Spatial implications of yoga in prisons and other carceral sites. *Race and Yoga*, 4(1), 1–16.

Petersen, E. & Davies, B. (2010). In/difference in the neoliberalised university. *Learning and Teaching*, 3(2), 92–109.

Putcha, R.S. (2020). Yoga and white public space. *Religions*, 11(12), 669–683. doi:10.3390/rel11120669

Ruth, D. (2012). White minds, black bodies; The dichotomies of labour at the edges of empire. *Bi-Annual Journal of the Asian School of Business Management*, 5(1), 1–7.

Segall, A. (2002). *Disturbing Practice: Reading Teacher Education as Text*. New York: Peter Lang Publishing.

Strauss, E. (2016, March 2). Being mindful about mindfulness: Is the push to teach meditation in schools just a way to mold shiny corporate humanoids? Slate. https://slate.com/human-interest/2016/03/teaching-mindfulness-meditation-in-schools-a-skeptics-investigation.html

Tschida, C.M., Ryan, C.L., & Ticknor, A.S. (2014). Building on windows and mirrors: Encouraging the disruption of "single stories" through children's literature. *Journal of Children's Literature*, 40(1), 28–39.

Wolfe, J. & Hoff, V. (2016, March 22). School apologizes for "mindfulness" yoga after complainst. 11Alive. https://www.11alive.com/article/news/education/school-apologizes-for-mindfulness-yoga-after-complaints/96838332

Zong, G. (2009). Developing preservice teachers' global understanding through computer-mediated communication technology. *Teaching and Teacher Education*, 25(5), 617–625.

Chapter 15

Trials and transformations
Ruminations of a community college yoga teacher

Shyamala Moorty

Fall 2010: "I don't have anything to be grateful for"

It is the third week of school and the room is packed with students still trying to do late adds at West LA College, where I have been teaching yoga for the past two years. I glance around and count 45 students in the room, over three-quarters are Latinx and African American, with a smattering of White and Asian students. Squeezed into a large circle, each person takes a turn sharing something they are grateful for while I simultaneously take roll. "I am grateful for my Mom, she helps me take care of my daughter while I'm in school" says a young Latinx woman. A Black woman in her 40s shares, "I am so grateful that I am going to graduate this year!" Everyone applauds, then she adds "I dropped out of school 10 years ago, but I came back last year and have a whole different perspective on learning. I'm here to tell you all, don't give up." There are many vocalizations of approval. The students continue with a variety of sweet and inspiring answers. Toward the end of the sharing, a petite young Black woman walks in and sits apart from the circle in the area where we keep shoes and personal belongings. After a few more students share their grateful thoughts, I welcome her and ask her to share one thing she is grateful for. She responds "Nothing," in a mad voice. I pause a moment, surprised at her tone and then gently encourage her to see if there's something even very small that she might appreciate. Her anger escalates and she growls, "I don't have *anything* to be grateful for. I just want to be left alone. I'm only here because I have to be." I tell her, "I'm so sorry you feel that way and I'm grateful that you made it to class today." I awkwardly wrap up the gratitude practice and direct the class into a restorative heart-opening posture to start off our physical practice of yoga. After I make sure everyone is comfortable and has some breathing instructions, I quietly ease over to the latecomer, who has stayed on the side-lines, and inquire in a whisper if everything is ok. She tells me her brother was killed, she doesn't want to do yoga, she only came to class so it wouldn't hurt her grade. I express how terrible this must be for her, and excuse her from class, promising that she'll get credit for showing up today, even in such challenging circumstances.

She leaves. She never returns. I am left with questions.

I felt terrible for her loss and pain. I wondered about her brother and what may have happened to him. I worried about how I had handled the situation, hoping I hadn't made things worse. It is always hard for me to lose a student, and I can only hope and trust that this young woman found her own way to cope with this terrible situation. In retrospect, I take solace in Sheena Sood's words:

> I do not expect to heal and liberate people. I do not have all the knowledge about healing; in fact, communities that have experienced suffering due to systemic oppression are more equipped than me to define their healing path. Humbling myself to build deep, honest relationships and to not be seen as the healing savior when I hold space for collective healing is an ongoing reflective part of my practice. (Sood, 2018)

In my experience, I have found that integrating the physical practice of yoga, *pranayama* (breathwork), and some of its tenants or philosophical practices can offer a powerful toolkit of life skills for college students. However, as seen in the example above, the structure of our school system, as well as the systemic injustices students face, can undermine the possibilities of some being able to access and use these tools. What follows are memories of various students, some of whom faced obstacles and injustices that blocked them from utilizing the tools of yoga, and others that have found the yoga philosophies transformative. In doing this, I hope to open the door for further conversations on how to support, include, and use yoga as a tool of liberation for all who wish to utilize it.

These reflections are based in my memories of ten years of teaching yoga in a large classroom, converted into a yoga space at West LA College[1]. The students at West LA College are typically 44.5% Latinx, 27.7% Black, 13% White and 8% Asian (Wlac.edu, 2016). They come in all shapes, sizes, and abilities. While most are young adults, a few are high school students getting their P.E. credits, some are older adults returning to college later in life, and a few are retired folk from the community doing recreation classes for fun. Although I appear young enough and Brown enough to often be mistaken as a student on the first few days of class, I am a middle class, mixed South Asian and American, able-bodied, cis-woman trained in a commercialized yoga chain in Costa Mesa. Costa Mesa is 70% White and is fairly affluent (https://www.census.gov/quickfacts/costamesacitycalifornia, 2019), while West LA College is populated by bordering communities such as Inglewood, Baldwin Hills, and Crenshaw that are primarily Latinx, Black, and mixed, with poverty levels higher than the national average, and high rates of single-parent households (maps.latimes.com, 2020). Clearly there are great differences between the student population, my own life experiences, and the place at which I had chosen to do my teacher training that color my perspective in writing these memories.

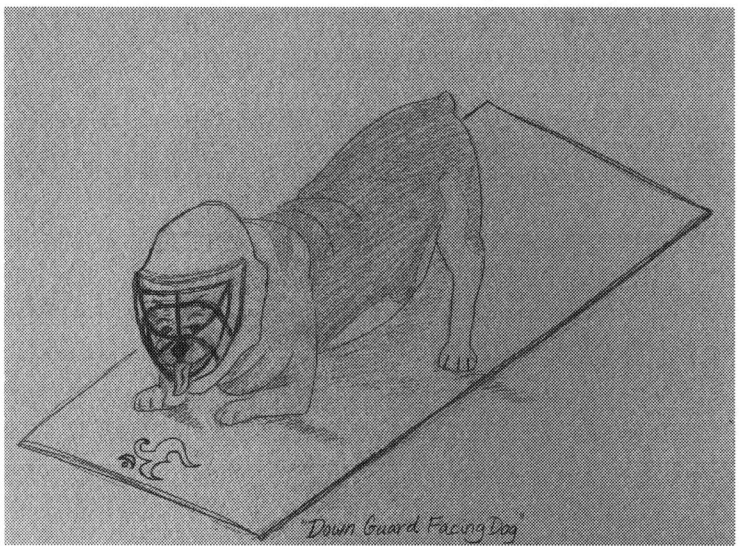

Figure 15.1 "I did Down-guard facing dog." (Student Journal, 2012)

I have chosen to write my memories in present tense, like a journal; however, they are put in order by theme instead of time frame, which I have roughly indicated by semester and year. I have changed the names of the students involved to protect their identities and, where it is pertinent to the content of a story, I note a person's ethnicity and their gender based on my own assumptions (I started asking the yogis in my class their gender pronouns in the spring of 2016, but some of these stories occurred before that). Following the memories are a few reflections, made in retrospect. I also have illustrated a few funny and pertinent quotes from students that I have collected over time as they relate to the stories. For example, I found the quote in the illustration above, a funny mis-writing of "down-ward facing dog" by one of my students, but also find it a way to recognize the need for some of us to be "guarded" in a world where many don't feel safe, even on the yoga mat (Figure 15.1).

Spring 2017: *"a moment of peace to someone somewhere"*

This semester, I assigned a daily gratitude journal to give students practice with Yoga Sutra 33, *Pratipaksha Bhavanam* – a yogic tool of changing negative thoughts to opposite (neutral or positive) thoughts[2]. Reading the journals is uplifting as expected, but this time one stands out. A middle-aged woman, Darya[3], writes her daily grateful thoughts in great detail, they are mundane but I can tell they are truly heartfelt. At the end, she explains that as an Iranian refugee, she had lost everything. She describes how her home was bombed and destroyed, and both her parents were killed. Ever since that traumatic time, even though she had escaped, she was stuck in the mentality that life was terribly hard, and that she was a "martyr"[4] – always doing everything for others with nothing in return. Now, in taking the time to be grateful every day, Darya realizes how much is actually good and positive in her life. She also discovers that she can control how she thinks about things, so that she can choose to be appreciative of the present moment instead of perseverating about the past.

Reading it, I too am affected by witnessing her journey, for I see that even through the most challenging life experiences, it is still possible to find joy and positivity. All week, I can't stop thinking about her writing, and so the next class, I ask Darya if we can share it with the rest of the class. She is pleased and readily agrees. As others hear her experiences, they are moved as well. Several other Iranian refugees come forth with their own stories of challenges and growth as well. One older woman describes the challenge of losing her husband, and migrating to the United States with two kids. She started life all over again, didn't know how to do anything in a new country, and had never worked before. However, through these trials, she discovered her own strength and abilities as a single working mother and grew tremendously because of the experience. She is so proud of herself, explaining that she never knew what she was capable of until she had to rise to such a challenge.

In response, one student says that hearing these stories makes her feel even more grateful for her own life. Another beautifully articulates that each of our attitudes affects one another and that we can collectively practice positive thoughts. Yet another adds that utilizing tools of yoga, not just as individuals, but as a community, can be far more powerful than isolating ourselves and our experiences. Together as a class we feel how the practice of *Pratipaksha Bhavanam*, changing negative thoughts to the opposite, is profoundly transformative, not just to one person, but also to those around her.

Many of us have experienced the power of practicing yoga asana in group classes – as each individual sets aside other distractions for a set period of time and the group keeps us accountable – our experience is often deeper than if we try to focus by ourselves. At West LA College, I enjoyed the benefit of long two and a half hour yoga classes, which left plenty of time for a full physical practice, as well as explorations of meditation, pranayama, and yoga philosophy. To facilitate the possibility of evolving collectively, I utilized the practice of putting our mats in a circle, like spokes of a wheel, that I had learned from another college yoga teacher, Carol McDowell. She articulated it as a non-hierarchical way of organizing a yoga room, and I also used it as a way to foster a sense of community, dialogue, and inclusiveness.

In Spring 2017 I had the unusual situation of having four students who were refugees from Iran, and so our discussions of yoga philosophy became a way to process the collective trauma of the 1978–1979 revolution in Iran and the consequent challenges of being a refugee in the U.S. The willingness of these students to engage in self-study, or *svadhyaya*, helped the entire class feel our inter-relatedness to them and each other. As B.K.S. Iyengar wrote:

> When people meet for svādhyāya, the speaker and listener are of one mind and have mutual love and respect. There is no sermonizing and one heart speaks to another. The ennobling thoughts that arise from svādhyāya are, so to speak, taken into one's bloodstream so that they become a part of one's life and being. The person practicing svādhyāya reads his own book of life, at the same time that he writes and revises it. There is a change in his outlook on life. (Iyengar, 1979)

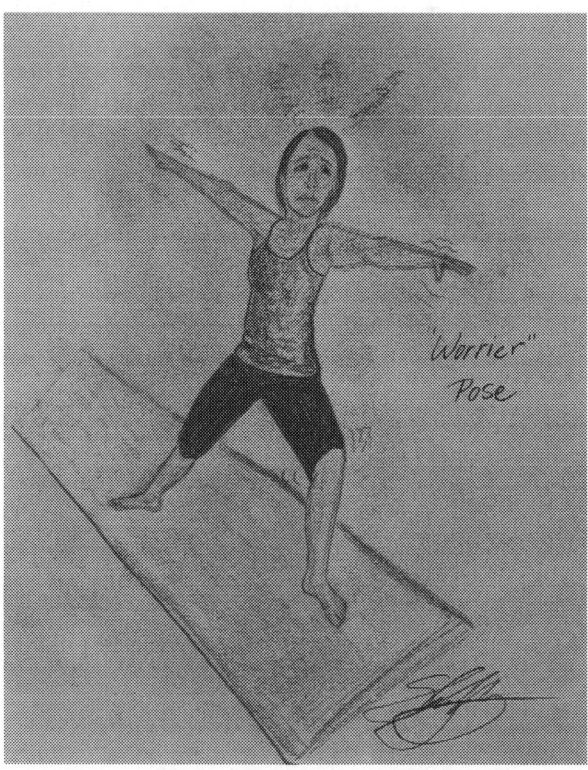

Figure 15.2 "I practiced Worrier Pose." (Student Journal, 2012)

Even though this specific trauma was experienced by only a few in the room, we all could relate to the universal experience of working through past experiences and controlling our current mindset with our attitude. For a moment, the veil of difference and separation from one another was lifted and we felt our deep connection. The feeling of interconnectedness and the awareness of how we all affect each other naturally re-occurred throughout the term, as exemplified by one Latinx student's introduction to her final project. The assignment was to create a personalized sequence for herself[5], but still she thought of others as she wrote, "I don't expect to be able to give someone such a gift but maybe the sequence will give a moment of peace to someone somewhere" (Student Journal, 2017).

The illustration on page 237 was inspired by a funny mis-spelling of Warrior, and yet an apt description of many who are living life as worriers instead of spiritual warriors (Figure 15.2).

Spring 2012: Savasana in sunglasses

Chris and Blake[6] are the jokers of the class this semester. These two young Black men are always together cracking jokes and testing boundaries with their humor. Chris is always complaining about *virabhadrasana* (warrior pose), and Blake likes to wear his sunglasses during the final deep relaxation, *savasana*. The first time he wore them, I laughed at this cool dude version of *savasana* and mused out loud "Why not, it's kind of like using an eye pillow to block out the outside world and rest inward more deeply." He grinned and seemed able to relax a bit more deeply when I validated that all of him was accepted and invited into the yoga space, even his sunglasses.

This past week I have been worried about them, because they didn't show up for the midterm project, which is often an indicator that someone will not complete the class. But today, just before the end of class, they arrive looking disheveled. I guide the class into *savasana*, and take Chris and Blake off to one side to ask how they are doing. Chris complains that they had just spent two nights in jail and didn't get any sleep. Blake adds that they just got out and came straight to class. Shocked, I inquire about what happened. They explain how a police officer had searched their car and found a gun in the dashboard. I stiffen at the thought of a gun, and a million thoughts rush through my mind, but I sense no aggression in them. I feel they pose no threat to myself or to the other students in the classroom; the young men simply seem tired and a bit flustered. So, I follow my gut and welcome them to join the class for *savasana*. Out come the sunglasses and they settle in for a well needed rest.

By the end of class they have fallen asleep and remain sleeping, even as the other students get up, pack up their belongings, and chat amongst themselves. I leave them be, knowing they are exhausted and turn to ask a long time yogi, who attends my class, for advice. Vitaly is not a college student but a community participant in the class, and runs a nearby, one-room continuation school for teens who have been pushed out and/or kicked out of traditional high school. I have come to respect him deeply and his unique ways of treating students as equals, co-creating curriculum with them, and guiding them to take a lead in transforming their own lives. Surely he can suggest a way to support Chris and Blake, and perhaps dissuade them from guns.

But Vitaly doesn't talk about the gun as I expect, and instead he asks me what kind of help they might need: lawyers for protection against police, or maybe information about groups who are challenging the laws on gang injunctions[7]? He also questions my assumptions of the situation by asking if the car actually belongs to either young person? Was there actually a gun in the car before the police searched it? And if so, did it belong to either of the two young people? Did they even know it was there? He briefly educates me on the world of police injustice towards youth of color in the area, the curfews for perceived gang members, and the negative effects of these on Black and Brown youth. It is my first time hearing about these sorts of prejudices in the police system. Unsure and overwhelmed, I tell him that any resources he's able to give will surely help. He leaves me with the name and number of a non-profit that can help the students with their rights and to get legal representation if needed.

While they continue in their much-needed *savasana*, I ponder the sad irony of the meaning of the word *savasana:* corpse pose. I contemplate the violence I associate with guns and I wonder how yoga might help Chris and Blake? Clearly they have come to yoga in need of refuge. Is there anything more that I can do? Chris and Blake stir from their slumber and jar me from my thoughts. I give them the information from Vitaly as they stumble out the door, groggy in the bright afternoon light. They never return.

At the time of this incident, the number of mass shootings in schools was not at the heightened level that it is today. I am not sure how I might react now after the many lockdown drills on college and elementary school campuses where I have taught. Would my own fears overcome my compassion and instincts around the harmlessness of these two students? This was also just before the Black Lives Matter movement helped to widely disseminate knowledge of the systemic police violence toward Black people into mainstream media and helped to disentangle my own misinformed notions of the community that I worked in.

So what use is yoga to young people who are facing normalized systemic violence like economic ghettoization, racial violence, and police profiling? If they even have access to yoga, can it give them the mental space and clarity to "liberate" themselves from the injustices they were born into, or is it instead a tool to appease their spirits while keeping them in their place? As much as I value yoga philosophies as tools toward our individual and sometimes collective spiritual liberation, I believe that they can also be utilized for societal discrimination and protection of the status quo. In India, yoga has been inter-tangled in the inequities of the caste system since its inception: Dalits (underprivileged castes, who were often dark skinned as well) were traditionally not allowed to even read the Vedas, an important Hindu scripture that is considered to contain the knowledge of yoga (Jeremiah, 2013); and Karma yoga, as it is taught in the spiritual verses of the Bhagavad Gita, blatantly justifies the caste system.

This is relevant to us in the U.S. as well, as the Bhagavad Gita is often quoted from and taught here. In it, Arjuna is a legendary archer who is riding into battle with his charioteer, who is also the God Krishna. Arjuna pauses on the way, distraught at the moral dilemma of fighting against his own cousins and teachers on the battlefield. In their seminal conversation, Krishna encourages Arjuna to continue into battle by teaching him that Karma yoga or the act of fulfilling one's "natural" duty or Dharma, will lead eventually to samadhi/enlightenment. One's duty, in all the different English translations of the Sanskrit text that I've seen so far, is determined by the caste that one is born into, rather than by choice, talents, or interests. Thus, the message is to find liberation within your predetermined life path, rather than seek to change it. To me, it is an obvious justification to uphold the status quo of discrimination[8].

While there are many other sources of yoga, the oft quoted Gita contains the sort of philosophy that has been ingrained in the psyches of Hindu Fundamentalists across the globe and that is currently upheld by the Indian Government as a symbol of Hindu superiority[9]. As NPR reported in 2017:

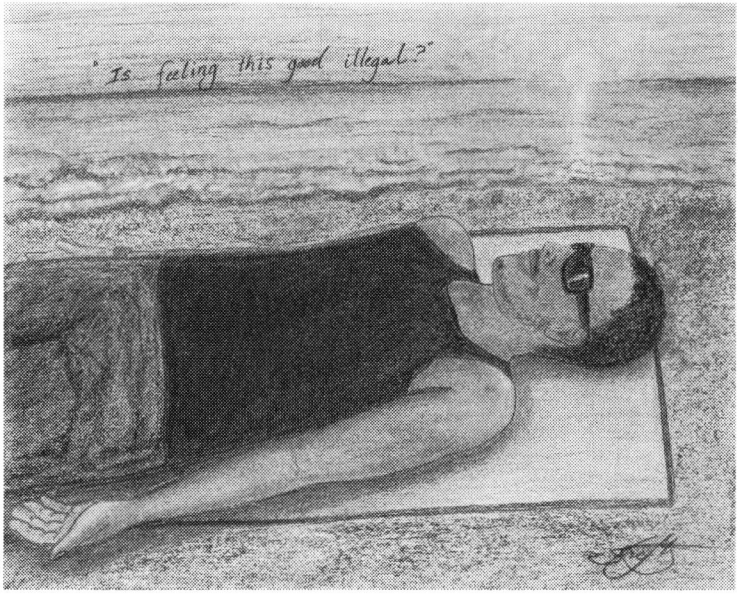

Figure 15.3 "Is feeling this good illegal?" (Student journal, Fall 2015)

a lot of Muslims in India feel like yoga is being weaponized. And the Western adoption of yoga as exercise has provided the perfect mask for a really insidious agenda. Prime Minister Modi came into office with a lot of support from the Hindu nationalist movement. That is a movement that wants to create a Hindu religious state. There's been a lot of anti-Muslim violence in India. (Morning Edition, 2017)

Three years since that report. Prime Minister Modi's Hindu Nationalist legacy has culminated in new discriminatory citizenship laws, violent backlashes against protestors, and a pogrom against Muslims (*New York Times*, 2020).

While we are far from this use of yoga in the U.S., it is still important to note the existence of these inequities within the ever evolving history and writings on yoga. As Susanna Barkataki invites us, *"Let's ask ourselves 'For whom is yoga accessible today and how might that be a legacy of past injustices that we have the opportunity to address through our teaching practice and our lives?'"* (Barkataki, 2015).

One of my students wrote the quote in the illustration of page 240 after taking a day off from school and doing yoga on the beach (Figure 15.3). Meant in jest, it is still a terrifying reality for Black folk, especially for those identifying as queer or transgender.

Fall 2017: "the only kind words I had heard all week"

The students and I are going over the syllabus on the first day of class when I begin to sense some mild discomfort in the room. An older Black man who appears to be in his 50s occasionally rolls his eyes and groans whenever a younger student asks questions a bit slowly due to a disability. I do my best to take my time and clarify everything, explaining to everyone that if one person has these questions, it is likely that others do too. Suddenly someone jumps up, surprised by a spider on their mat. Another student runs to get a shoe and is ready to squash it. I stop them, telling them that I'll take care of it. I get a couple pieces of paper, scoop the spider up, and explain that one of the tenets of yoga is non-violence, or *Ahimsa*, and so rather than kill the spider we can choose to remove it and put it outdoors.

We finish the syllabus and then take a break, during which, I invite students to get permission numbers to enroll in the already full class. The man who had been groaning approaches for a number to enroll and while signing the paperwork, he introduces himself as Jackson[10]. He shakes my hand and tells me that he appreciates how I saved the spider, and that he'd never seen someone do something like that before. Then he gestures toward the student with the disability and half-whispers, "you know he's *different*, right?" I am surprised at this and tell him that I do my best to make yoga accessible to everyone. He mutters that he just wanted to make sure that I knew and walks away.

At the end of class one of my returning students, Henry[11], asks to speak with me privately. I oblige and we step outside into a little courtyard. Henry, a slight framed young Latinx, proceeds to tell me that an incident happened between himself and Jackson that I should know about. He describes how during the class break, he had smiled at Jackson in a friendly sort of way, but Jackson had retorted, "Don't look at me. Look at me again and I'll sock you!" Henry backed off and avoided eye contact for the rest of the time. Henry worries that somehow he is bothering Jackson. I remember that Henry identifies as gay (information he shared when he took my class in a previous semester) and note to myself that Jackson may have negative associations with that. I express how shocked and sorry I am that this happened to him, while internally regretting that I gave Jackson permission to add the class.

Henry and I discuss what to do. I tell him that we can report it to campus police, but suggest that if Henry is ok with not taking that more extreme action right away, that I can try to talk to Jackson before or after class next week. I can see if he's willing to talk to me about things or people that might be bothering him in yoga class and help him find better strategies for dealing with those problems. I am thinking that maybe if Jackson has a supportive outlet to talk and express himself, then he will not feel the need to be violent physically or emotionally toward Henry and others in the class. Henry agrees that I should talk to Jackson first and we both decide to not voice that there was a complaint about Jackson just yet, since Jackson may guess who that was and maybe retaliate.

I am relieved and hopeful, as I have been learning a lot about restorative justice, a non-punitive way of holding individuals accountable for their wrong-doings. Through restorative justice, I have been learning how important it is to listen to both sides in order for the participants to feel supported enough to be able to see the harm they have created and hopefully make choices to rectify and heal that harm. I am also terribly nervous because I haven't had much experience in dealing with violent threats. I send an email to the chair of our department to let him know that a violent threat has been made in my class, but that the student did not want to report the situation just yet. I ask for resources for student conflicts, other than campus police. He thanks me for writing, asks me to keep him informed how things go, and does not offer any further resources.

I ask other colleagues for help as I consider my next steps. Cynthia Ling Lee, who had gained much experience with race-related issues while working at a university in the South, warned against bringing in campus police unless I really needed to, considering the climate of police violence against Black males in America, even on college campuses. I agreed, remembering how a student of Iranian heritage was tased by campus police at UCLA in 2006[12]. As I continue to weigh the situation, I begin to see the parallels between restorative justice and the tenet of *Ahimsa* in yoga.

I decide to make the theme of the next class about the yogic principle of *Ahimsa*. However, neither Jackson nor Henry show up to school that day. The following class, Jackson arrives late, so I do not have a chance to talk to him before-hand. Since the class has already talked about Ahimsa in a general way, I spontaneously decide to carry the theme farther and explore how we can be non-violent toward ourselves for Jackson's benefit. We discuss how self-judgment or lack of self-care are forms of violence towards oneself. Interestingly, Jackson gets excited about the topic and reveals to the class that he has been feeling a lot of anger lately. He realizes aloud that this is because he is over extended and exhausted: everyone he knows needs something from him and he is trying to help them all, but in the process he's not taking care of himself and consequently feeling miserable and lashing out. He articulates that learning to say no would help him be less violent to himself, have less anger, and ultimately be less violent to others. I feel amazed and hopeful by his deep self-inquiry. After class he tells me that he is working on reacting differently to folk, like I did with the spider. I am impressed that he still is thinking about the spider from the first week of class.

Meanwhile I begin to worry that Henry has not been coming to class since the first day and that he may not feel comfortable returning. I sense that I need to be proactive to get him back to class. I email him and stress how I am dedicated to supporting him to feel safe and that Jackson has been responding favorably to the idea of *Ahimsa*. He writes back that he'll be there, and expresses that it means so much to him that I wrote. It turns out he has been in and out of the hospital with ongoing anxiety issues. I worry about how the situation with Jackson may be adding to his anxiety and I emphasize that I am there to help. When Henry returns, he and I are able to have a more in depth conversation and he seems open to seeing how things go again with Jackson.

As the weeks roll by, no more groaning or eye rolling from Jackson, no more threats, and both he and Henry add insightful contributions to the conversations when they are present (attendance is a bit spotty for both). Feeling a need to continue the class conversations on non-violence, one week I focus on the stories of famous people such as Mahatma Gandhi and Dr. Martin Luther King, Jr. who have used Ahimsa as a method of resistance to create great political and social changes. Another week, we chat about how to incorporate Ahimsa in everyday life.

On the final day, I see the payoff when Jackson expresses how he is now approaching his work, relationships in life, and care for himself in an entirely new way. He says he feels calmer, happier, and kinder. Indeed there have been no more incidents in class that I am aware of, though I have done my best to keep him separated from Henry when assigning small work groups. While reading the end of the semester reflections, I discover that all this in-depth focus on ahimsa has had effects on other students as well. The following is written by a young Latinx woman:

> This semester has challenged me in every respect; morally/mentally, emotionally, physically. There were times I wanted to stay in bed, but somehow I managed to get up and keep going. I remember coming to yoga class and hearing the only kind words I had heard all week. In those moments

I let the tears stream down my face. It made me grateful to still be alive.
Yoga brought healing into my life and allowed me to practice non-violence.
(Student Journal, 2017)

Sadly Henry never had the benefit of getting an apology or even a recognition of the situation from Jackson. As far as I know there are no Restorative Justice circles at West LA College. Rather, Restorative Justice was an inspiration for my actions to find alternative ways to help ease the conflict instead of escalate it. My exposure to Restorative Justice came through volunteering with the Restorative Community Conferencing program run by the California Conference for Equality and Justice (CCEJ)[13].

As I realized at the time, Restorative Justice is strongly related to the principle of *Ahimsa*, or non-violence, in yoga. In Patanjali's Yoga Sutras, *Ahimsa* is one of the Yamas or principles of morality that are meant to guide us in our social interactions and behaviors in order to help us toward the ultimate goal of yoga: peace and liberation (Satchidananda, 2007). Restorative Justice, as I understand it, is a non-punitive way of approaching justice that will ultimately help to restore harmony in a community. It is a structure to hold those who have done harm accountable in a way that helps them listen, communicate, and offer reparations to those that have been harmed. One of the fundamental principles of Restorative Justice according to Howard Zehr is: "Fairness is assured, not by uniformity of outcomes, but through provision of necessary support and opportunities to all parties and avoidance of discrimination based on ethnicity, class, and sex" (Zehr, 2002). A contract of actions to make amends is ultimately agreed upon by both parties, rather than a punishment imposed from the outside. This method was created by the Maori people in New Zealand and current practices of Restorative Justice around the world have been influenced by the circle practices of various other indigenous populations.

The language that I was trained in around Restorative Justice at CCEJ, included naming the participants as "one who has done harm" and "one who has been harmed" (rather than "perpetrator" and "victim"). This language mirrors master yogi B.K.S. Iyengars' explanations on *Ahimsa*:

> The yogi opposes the evil in the wrong-doer, but not the wrong-doer... Opposition to evil and love for the wrong-doer can live side by side... Opposition without love leads to violence; loving the wrong-doer without opposing the evil in him is folly and leads to misery. (Iyengar, 1979)

As in Iyengar's words above, Restorative Justice does not create further ripples of harm by causing violence to the one who has done the harm with punitive judgments inflicted upon them from the outside. Instead, as in yoga, they are encouraged through this process into self-inquiry to work with the one harmed to find an agreeable solution to "repair" the situation and thus to transform their relationship to the one they have caused harm to, to themselves, and to the community. This approach has the possibility of being truly transformative.

Iyengar's writing about violence further gives me insight into Jackson, as a mirror to all of us, and his actions:

> Violence arises out of fear, weakness, ignorance or restlessness. To curb it what is most needed is freedom from fear. To gain this freedom, what is required is a change of outlook on life and reorientation of the mind. Violence is bound to decline when men learn to base their faith upon reality and investigation rather than upon ignorance and supposition. (Iyengar, 1979)

It is my hope and belief that Jackson truly did undergo such a "reorientation of the mind," though as a parent and human, I understand that reorientation as a constant practice. I see myself in him, as I too struggle with drawing boundaries as a form of *Ahimsa* for myself so that I don't lash out my frustrations on my child when exhausted and overwhelmed.

I often use Darth Vadar as an example of how to imagine the sound of Ujjayi Pranayama (Victorious breath) for students. In the illustration below, a student not only mis-remembered the name of the breath control but even of Vader himself (Figure 15.4). Still it is an apt example of someone considered "evil" doing the inner work to transform.

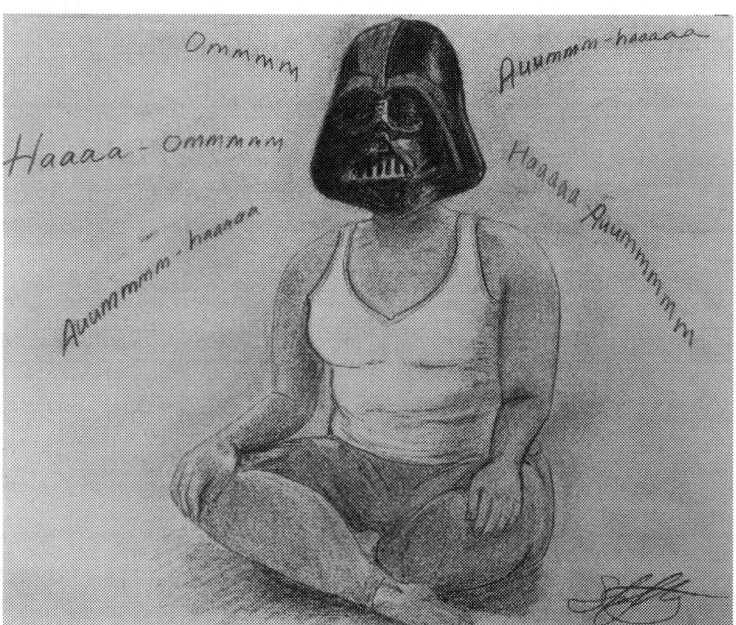

Figure 15.4 "When I do Dark Vader I feel more calm and end my day great." (Student Journal, Spring 2013)

Spring 2018: WE are yoga

My keys jangle as I walk to class on the last day of the semester. Several students are waiting, anticipating sharing their final projects. We exchange greetings as I unlock the hallway where the yoga mats are usually kept in a tall cage. We peer in only to discover that there are no mats there. I make a series of calls to track them down while more students arrive. After multiple calls and an inquiry to the friendly pod of custodians who are taking a break in the next room, it becomes clear that the yoga mats have been taken on purpose by someone in my department. Why they took them and how to get them back in time for the final projects remains a mystery. As the students organize themselves into a circle, I see that a few have brought their own mats, but most have not. I am reminded of the conflict I am always having about attaching a grade to yoga, and so I decide to be flexible. I check-in with the students, we discuss the situation, and together we decide to shift the plan: instead of sharing their personalized sequences with each other, we will take some group pictures to share on social media to show the diverse faces of yoga for the International Day of Yoga. All are excited to be in the photos, except for one who volunteers to be the photographer.

I first explain that I had received an invitation from Susanna Barkataki, a prominent yogi in the movement for diversifying yoga in the U.S., to participate in a disruption through education of the otherwise commercialized International Day of Yoga[14]. In her invitation she states three main goals:

1. Disruption through education
2. Educate to Diversify (honor the history and the roots, the history of yoga has ALWAYS been DIVERSE: Yoga emerged as syncretic and fringe, pre-Hindu, influenced and interrelated with by Islam, Sufism, Buddhism, Jainism, etc). Let's harness and expand on this Diversity
3. Yoga as relationship; non-commercial/non-transactional (Barkataki, 2018).

The students share what kind of images they have seen of yoga in the world so far and discuss what they would like to see more of. We all agree that we need to see more diverse bodies, that mirror those in the room. Then we playfully and joyfully document our complex space of inquiry, growth, questioning, and support.

When we join together, interconnecting our bodies of various shapes, ethnicities, and life experiences, I feel we are also metaphorically exploring the possibility of universal connectedness through yoga. We are *yuj* – the "yoke" that the root of the word yoga comes from – that joins body, mind, spirit, and community. We are *Ahimsa* as we continually practice to minimize harm to each other and ourselves. We are filled with gratitude as our practice deepens inward and simultaneously ripples outward.

In tree pose we rooted our trees together, like redwood trees whose roots are interconnected with each other to create a strong enough base to allow their great height (Figure 15.5). In this chapter, I brought out some heavier situations in order to spark the dialogue and increase the network of support so that we all might rise together. In the spirit of *Pratipaksha bhavanam* (changing negative thoughts to the opposite) I wish to end by celebrating some of the blossoms of the practice that came out of the network of support at West LA College in a few short examples.

There was a young Latinx woman who came to class for over a year, even when she couldn't get credit anymore, because it helped her through her depression. She ultimately claimed the practice as her own and would do yoga on the beach as her own practice in creating joy and healing for herself. An older Black man liked to brag that he had shocked the doctors that he was able to lower his blood pressure with the *Ujjayi Pranayama*, breathing technique that we had practiced in class. A young White woman quit her nightly glass of wine and found greater clarity of mind, focus, and lost a considerable amount of weight. And there was Santa Monica Sam, a Black man who had already gone through his own inspirational journey from addiction to spiritual awareness, who shared his amazingness through his music, which we played during our practice[15].

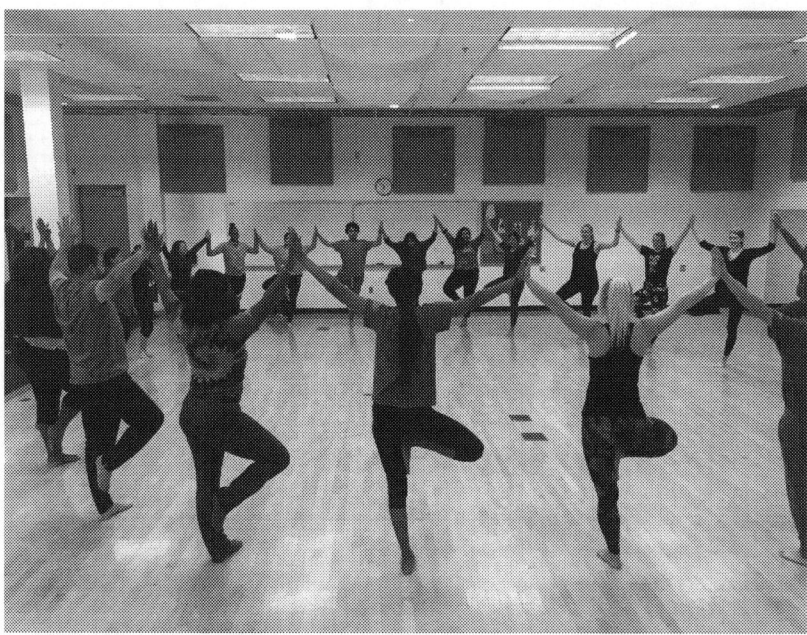

Figure 15.5 A forest of Tree Poses, photo taken with permission of West LA Yoga students.

Recently, I ran into a former West LA yogi, Christina S. Wherry, and she told me she had gone on to get trained as a yoga teacher and had since started her own yoga business "Thick Girl Yoga Full Embodied Expression." As she wrote on social media, "Sharing yoga and meditation wasn't the initial goal, my emotional healing journey was I wanted to quiet my mind and embrace my body. Through my practice the awareness that these are tools that can empower us all came to light" (Wherry, 2019).

As always humans are resilient and find our ways for healing and resolution in many ways. As yoga can be one of those ways, I hope that we as a community of practitioners can do the deep work of self-inquiry to see who we are including, develop our networks to make it more accessible, and be conscientious how we utilize it, so we do not blindly teach parts of the practice that may inherently carry harm embedded within them.

Notes

1 I also taught yoga at Cerritos College in Cerritos and Rio Hondo College in Whittier, with variations in the populations but overlapping issues.
2 Sutra 33: Vitarka badhane pratipaksa bhavanam, translates as "When disturbed by negative thoughts, opposite [positive] ones should be thought of" (Satchidananda, 2007).
3 The name of this individual has been changed to protect their identity.
4 While I did not keep a copy of her paper, I distinctly remember her using the word martyr.
5 Our final project in class is often for students to create their own sequence to reflect their own interests and needs. The hope is that they will be able to use it on their own after the semester is over. This is a practice that was inspired by Jamie Hammond, another college yoga teacher.
6 The names of these individuals have been changed to protect their identity.
7 Gang injunctions were court orders that placed curfews and restricted individuals from meeting friends or family in certain neighborhoods if they were identified by the police as potentially being a gang member. Injunctions had been in place since the 1980s were finally barred in court in March 2018 (LA Times, 2018)
8 Gita Verses 18.41.39–18.41.48. Some translations or explanations that I have cross-referenced in English are by Eknath, Mitchell, and Rutt. Full citations are in the works cited section.
9 For other examples see Sheena Sood's "Cultivating a Yogic Theology of Collective Healing: A Yogini's Journey Disrupting White Supremacy, Hindu Fundamentalism, and Casteism" (Sood, 2018).
10 The name of this individual has been changed to protect their identity.
11 The name of this individual has been changed to protect their identity.
12 For more information on this incident, see "UCLA student stunned by Taser plans suit" (LA Times, 2006)
13 This program is now called "Healing Harms" https://www.cacej.org/cause/healing harms/.
14 I found out only recently about India's Prime Minister, Narendra Modi's, involvement as one of the primary proponents of International Yoga day, which aligns it with a more Hindu Fundamentalist agenda than I knew at the time.
15 Music by Santa Monica Sam can be found on his YouTube channel: https://youtu.be/o2Z3yULW6gU.

Works cited

Barkataki, S. (2018). *Potentially Disrupting/ Educating on IYD- June 21st Together*. [email].
Barkataki, S. (2019). *How To Decolonize Your Yoga Practice*. Decolonizing Yoga. Available at: http://www.decolonizingyoga.com/decolonize-yoga-practice/ [Accessed 3 Jan. 2019].
Eknath, E. (2019). *The Bhagavad Gita*. 2nd ed. Tomales, CA: Nilgiri Press, pp. 261–262.
Iyengar, B. (1979). *Light on Yoga*. New York: Schocken Books Inc, pp. 31–32, 38.
Jeremiah, A. (2013). *Community and Worldview among Paraiyars of South India: 'Lived' Religion*. 1st ed. New York: Bloomsbury Academic, p. 7.
Los Angeles Times (2006). *UCLA Student Stunned by Taser Plans Suit*. Available at: https://www.latimes.com/archives/la-xpm-2006-nov-17-me-ucla17-story.html [Accessed 12 Apr. 2020].
Los Angeles Times (2018). *Los Angeles Barred from Enforcing Nearly All Gang Injunctions, Federal Judge Rules*. Available at: https://www.latimes.com/local/lanow/la-me-ln-gang-injunction-court-order-20180315-story.html [Accessed 25 Mar. 2019].
Los Angeles Times (2020). *Mapping L.A. Neighborhoods*. Available at: http://maps.latimes.com/neighborhoods/ [Accessed 6 Mar. 2020].
Mitchell, S. (2000). *The Bhagavad Gita*. 1st ed. New York: Harmony, pp. 190–191.
Morning Edition. (2017). *Rough Translation: Why Many Muslims In India Feel Yoga Has Been Weaponized*. [podcast] Available at: https://www.npr.org/2017/09/18/551726470/rough-translation-why-many-muslims-in-india-feel-yoga-has-been-weaponized [Accessed 25 Mar. 2019].
New York Times (2020). *Why Delhi Police Did Nothing to Stop Attacks on Muslims*. Available at: https://www.nytimes.com/2020/03/03/opinion/delhi-pogrom.html [Accessed 17 Apr. 2020].
Rutt, S. (2006). *An Ordinary Life Transformed*. New Hampshire: Hobblebush Books, pp. 217–218.
Santa Monica Sam. (2013). *I Am*. Available at: https://youtu.be/o2Z3yULW6gU [Accessed 16 May 2020].
Satchidananda, S. (2007). *The Yoga Sutras of Patanjali*. Yogaville: Integral Yoga Publications, pp. 125–130, 127.
Sood, S. (2018). Cultivating a Yogic Theology of Collective Healing: A Yogini's Journey Disrupting White Supremacy, Hindu Fundamentalism, and Casteism. *Race and Yoga*, 3(1), p. 18. Available at: https://escholarship.org/uc/item/0wn4p090.
Tagore, R. (1955). *Fireflies*. New York: Macmillan Publishing Company, p. 67.
The United States Census Bureau. (2020). *QuickFacts Costa Mesa City, California*. Available at: https://www.census.gov/quickfacts/costamesacitycalifornia [Accessed 11 Apr. 2020].
Wherry, C. (2019). Christina S. Wherry. *Facebook.com*. Available at: https://www.facebook.com/ChristinaSWherry [Accessed 10 Oct. 2018].
Wlac.edu. (2016). *Fall 2016 Student Profile*. Available at: http://www.wlac.edu/WLAC/media/documents/research/planning/Student_Profile_Fall_2016.pdf [Accessed 11 Oct. 2018].
Zehr, H. (2002). *The Little Book of Restorative Justice*. Intercourse, PA: Good Books, p. 69.

Chapter 16

Situating girls of color in K–12 yoga research

Reflections and results from studying an after school yoga program for at-risk youth

Michele Tracy Berger

Introduction

In the last decade, there has been an explosion of public interest and research about the effects of yoga and meditation practices on children and adolescents[1]. Yoga is considered a mind-body intervention by the National Center for Complementary and Integrative Health (2011) that often incorporates physical postures, relaxation, meditation, and breathing exercises. The presence of yoga and meditation programs in educational settings has quietly but steadily increased over the last five years, making its way from the periphery (e.g. after school programs and yoga clubs) to a central part of school culture and curriculum through innovative programs all across the country (Serwacki and Cook-Cottone 101; Butzer et al. 18). Research suggests that providing yoga practices within the school curriculum may be an effective way to help students develop self-regulation, mind-body awareness, and physical fitness, which may, in turn, foster additional and positive student outcomes such as improved classroom behavior, mental state, health, and academic performance (Butzer 19; Khalsa, et al. 80).

This trajectory of research is indeed promising, but it typically does not acknowledge or explore the impact of racial and gender disparities in school settings that increasingly structure many adolescent experiences. Nor does it take into account how different communities of students may experience stressors that are related to identity, including but not limited to race and gender. Finally, many of these studies compare groups across single categories of analysis (either comparing across gender, or race, or socioeconomic status). These three features that characterize much of this literature should give us pause when thinking about the gains of yoga interventions. Researchers may inadvertently overstate the gains for girls of color. Monocausal analyses have been theorized and shown empirically to create gaps in addressing women of color and girls of color's life experiences (Bowleg 313–314, Cole and Sabik 175, Harnois 159–160, May 21–28).

Since 2014 I have been co-investigator on a series of collaborative projects that seek to measure and assess the health, emotional, and physiological effects of yoga and meditation interventions on children enrolled in middle and elementary public schools. We have created and evaluated yoga interventions in several afterschool programs that serve academically and behaviorally marginalized middle school students[2]. Girls of color (i.e. Latina, African American, Chinese, and Laotian) made up the majority of the research participants. Given that experiences of girls of color in public school settings are under-theorized in much of the emerging research on yoga and meditation in K–12 settings, this chapter focuses on the girls of color in our 2016–2017 study. It offers some preliminary findings about the impact of yoga and meditation on their stress levels and ability to self-regulate before and after the intervention.

In this chapter, I also situate myself as a woman of color scholar and yogini, reflecting on the tensions, challenges, and opportunities while working in the emerging area of K–12 yoga research. In the conclusion, I also raise the possibility that yoga research in K–12 schools may replicate ways that girls of color experiences are ignored, minimized, or made invisible due to the lack of attention to how overlapping systems of oppression impact girls of color differently than their White female and/or male counterparts. I argue that it would behoove researchers to acknowledge the prevalence of racial and gender disparities in schools, and engage with critical theories about race and gender.

Situating myself: Yogini and researcher

There are several pathways that led me to this current research. Since 2000, I have been interested in the field of what was once called complementary and alternative health and is now referred to as "integrative medicine" or "integrative health." While a postdoctoral fellow through the Robert Johnson Foundation in the early 2000s, I interviewed breast cancer survivors about their use of herbs, acupuncture, and other healing modalities. I also spent time working on a pilot project trying to understand the professionalization practices of yoga teachers. After completing several other projects, I returned to yoga. I was interested in continuing my research on yoga and studying its impact on underserved communities.

I have also been a yoga student for many years, since 1995. For most of that time, my sense of what it meant to have a yoga practice was highly individualized and focused on personal growth and health. After a decade of practicing yoga, I made the decision, in 2005, to become a certified yoga teacher. This decision was precipitated by a powerful experience I had attending the 2004 International Association of Black Yoga Teachers conference in Washington, D.C. (IABYT). It was the first time that I was in a yoga space with primarily Black and POC yogis and yoginis and where the focus of conversations centered around the intersection of yoga and social justice. I met many people who were teaching outside of the conventional yoga studio system and teaching yoga to communities of color, both in the United States and abroad. This catalyzing and full-bodied consciousness-raising experience convinced me to become a yoga teacher and to offer yoga as a resource, primarily to communities of color.

Around this same time, I met my future colleague, Keval Kaur Khalsa, and began taking yoga classes with her. Eventually our friendship spilled out from the confines of the yoga studio. Given her social justice interests and history of anti-racist activism, we found ourselves having long conversations about racial health disparities and yoga's possible usefulness as a tool to support individual and collective health. For many years, we worked together on creating community health fairs and offering yoga to diverse communities. In 2013, we received seed money from Duke University that led us on the long journey of researching yoga interventions in K–12 settings. In our early formulation of the importance of the project, we held a long-range vision about the possibilities of successful interventions as a scalable resource for schools that would support empowering young people.

There are various degrees of insiderness and outsiderness that I bring to our research. My colleague is White and I am African American. We are friends as well as collaborators. For many years I took yoga classes from her. She is a dance professor at Duke University and I am in the Department of Women's and Gender Studies at the University of North Carolina-Chapel Hill. I have been aware of my own uniqueness as an African American yogini and scholar at many conferences on yoga research. Given the racialized and gendered stratification in the academy where less than three percent of all full time faculty in degree-granting postsecondary institutions are Black women[3], it should not be surprising that in the emerging field of yoga research there are few women of color, particularly African American female researchers conducting empirically based research.

Girls of color in K–12 yoga research

Despite the scholarly interest in children and adolescents in K–12 yoga research, there has been little theoretical or empirical attention specific to the experiences of girls of color and indigenous girls (i.e. Asian/Pacific Islander, Native American, Asian American, Latina, African American) and the ways that school experiences (and yoga interventions) may impact them differently than their counterparts. This kind of unidimensional framing, as Crenshaw has argued, can erase the lived experiences of race and gender as systems of oppression that mutually reinforce each other (Crenshaw 140).

Why should we pay special attention to girls of color in K–12 in yoga research? Given the well-documented, complex, and often challenging issues that girls of color face in K–12 public institutions, this group warrants heightened consideration. Girls of color in K–12 face numerous educational disparities as compared to their White peers including experiencing a higher risk of suspensions, being more likely to be tracked into special education and remedial classes, increased risk of punishment from school authorities, and high rates of sexual harassment (Cammarota 54; Crenshaw, Ocen and Nanda 1). Suspensions for girls of color are particularly alarming and begin as early as kindergarten. In California, the suspension rate for Native American girls is almost four percent higher than their peer group. According to the most recent data from the U.S. Department of Education, nationally, Black girls were suspended *six times* more than White girls, while Black boys were suspended three times as often as White boys (Crenshaw, Ocen and Nanda 16). Kimberlé Crenshaw, gender and racial equity pioneer, co-authored a report titled, "Black Girls Matter: Pushed Out, Overpoliced and Underprotected" that highlights the ways that schools reinforce sexism and racism and thus blunt Black girls' educational opportunities. The report highlights how schools curtail their "educational opportunities, and marginalize their needs, while pushing them into low-wage work, unemployment, and incarceration" (Crenshaw, Ocen, and Nanda 7).

Although scholars have begun to note the institutional and discriminatory issues involved as girls of color navigate K–12, there is little attention in yoga in school intervention research that thinks about how perceived concepts like stress, anxiety, and depression may manifest differently across different communities and may be triggered by a variety of factors within school settings and at home.

Description of the project and methods

For the purposes of this chapter, using descriptive statistics, I compare the social and emotional outcomes of girls of color in an afterschool program with a yoga intervention to a control group of girls of color and their White female counterparts. The primary aim of the overall study is to compare the effects of the yoga program to the control condition on self-reported emotion dysregulation, depression, anxiety, stress, and mindfulness.

Demographics

One hundred and nineteen adolescents in sixth (53%; 11–12 years old), seventh (25.6%, 12–13 years old), and eighth (21.4%, 13–14 years old) grade classes from four middle schools in North Carolina enrolled in the study through a passive consent, opt-out procedure. Twenty-one students participated from School A, 44 from School B, 28 from School C, and 26 from School D. In our total sample, 50.4.% were female, 15% were White, 42.9% were African American, 24.4% were Latinx, 10.1% were Asian, and 5.93% did not identify with these categories. This chapter reports on 21 African American girls, 6 Asian girls, 18 Latinx girls, and 12 White girls[4].

All students and parents or guardians were informed that the students would be participating in a yoga study and could choose either the Y.O.G.A. for Youth after-school program or an alternate activity, our control condition. Participants in the control group (depending on the school) participated in a range of activities including completing homework, free time, music class, or outdoor play. There were no exclusion criteria. There were no measurable systematic differences between students who opted-in to the study. The research protocol was approved by the Institutional Review Board of Duke University.

Students participating in the research study were enrolled in after school programs at public schools in the Chapel Hill-Carrboro, NC school system.

Intervention: The Y.O.G.A for Youth Program

The non-profit Your Own Greatness Affirmed dba Y.O.G.A. for Youth (Y4Y) organization provided a series of two weekly yoga classes for six weeks, offered as one of the after-school programs. Y4Y classes teach Kundalini Yoga as taught by Yogi Bhajan© (Bhajan, 2007), adapted for educational settings. The Y4Y program utilizes Kundalini yoga because of its accessibility to people of different ages, as it requires no special equipment or particular physical flexibility. In addition, previous evidence has demonstrated its benefits on psychological functioning. For example, Kundalini yoga emphasizes cultivating self-awareness and has demonstrated effectiveness in treating depression (Devi, Chansauria, and Udupa 115), stress (Granath, Ingvarsson, von Thiele, and Lundberg 7), and several other types of psychiatric disorders (Shannahoff-Khalsa 92). The Y4Y program prioritizes serving youth who are at risk for behavioral and emotional problems (Sarkissian et al. 210). One study found that this program significantly improved students' self-reported stress, affect, and resilience (Sarkissian et al. 216).

Each class consists of chanting an opening mantra, breath practice, physical warm-ups, a kriya (specific sequence of physical postures that may incorporate specific breath patterns, eye focus, and hand positions), meditation, relaxation, and a closing song. Additionally, a Y4Y class includes social-emotional learning based on eight Y4Y principles derived from the Eight-Fold Buddhist path. These principles are incorporated through games and group discussion. In this program, specific breath practices are utilized and each posture or movement in Kundalini Yoga is intended as physical exercise, meditation, and a method of increasing self-awareness (Bhajan 100). Postures are used to isolate specific muscles and put pressure on specific points or areas of the body. Meditation in Kundalini Yoga utilizes specific hand positions, specific eye foci, as well as a specific breath pattern or sound/mantra.

Y4Y teachers are Yoga Alliance-certified 200-hour teachers who have also undergone Y4Y's 40-hour specialty training and have been mentored as Teaching Assistants by a Lead Teacher before becoming Lead Teachers themselves. Each yoga class was taught by a Y.O.G.A. for Youth Lead Teacher, assisted by a Y4Y teacher assistant. At each of the four school locations, classes were divided by students' gender identification (there was a girls' class and a boys' class at each school) and were offered simultaneously. A total of five Lead Teachers and five teacher assistants taught at the four sites. Three of the five Lead Teachers and three of the five Teacher Assistants taught at more than one school in different pairings. The Y4Y training targets the teaching of underserved youth and covers the Y4Y curriculum structure and content, trauma-informed yoga practices, and classroom management. Included in the curriculum content are the eight Y4Y principles: Right Understanding, Right Intention, Right Speech, Right Action, Right Livelihood, Right Attitude, Right Mindfulness, Right Concentration. The same class curriculum was applied in each of the four schools.

Study procedures

The after-school programs (including the Y4Y program and the alternate programs) took place in four public middle schools in North Carolina over six weeks, with two 40-minute classes per week (Monday/Wednesday or Tuesday/Thursday). Two schools held the after-school programs in the fall semester of 2016 and the other two in the spring of 2017.

Participants were recruited for the study from the after-school programs through a passive, opt-out consent procedure. Y4Y North Carolina teachers and one of the study's principal investigators visited each school at the start of the semester to provide orientation sessions for students and staff. These sessions were held to explain the purpose and benefits of a yoga practice, the elements of a Y4Y class, expectations for behavior during yoga classes, and to answer any questions. All students that enrolled in the after-school programs, as well as their parents/guardians, were informed by a parental notification letter that they could participate in a study on the psychological effects of the Y4Y program. Students who provided assent to our study and chose the Y4Y program for the after-school program were included in our yoga condition and students who provided assent to our study and chose an alternate activity for the after-school program (i.e. activities could include completing homework, outdoor play, music class, and free time depending on the school) were included in our control condition.

For all data collection procedures, the research team administered the measures to all participants in paper format during scheduled data collection sessions at the schools. In these sessions, students participating in the study gathered in a large classroom, where members of the research team distributed the questionnaire packets and gave detailed instructions for answering questionnaires with examples. Extra instructions were given for reverse-scored measures, such as the Mindful Attention and Awareness Scale for Adolescents (see below). The research team answered any questions from the students while they filled out the questionnaires (i.e. if they had difficulty understanding the language of the items). The main questionnaires (the Difficulties in Emotion Regulation Scale-Short Form, the Depression, Anxiety and Stress scale, and the Mindful Attention and Awareness Scale for Adolescents) were administered to all student participants at two time points: once during the week before the programs started (time 1) and once during the week after the program finished (time 2). Students were given snacks at the conclusion of each session of data collection to compensate for their participation.

Measures

Mindful Attention Awareness Scale-Adolescent (MAAS-A). The MAAS-A is a 14-item scale designed to assess dispositional mindfulness, defined as a tendency to be in a receptive state of mind of present-moment awareness. Items are rated on a Likert scale from one (*almost always*) to six (*almost never*) and the measure is calculated as the average score across all items. The MAAS-A has been validated for use with community and clinical adolescent populations from ages 14 to 18 years old. Exploratory and confirmatory factor analyses with community sampled adolescents aged 14 to 18 years have confirmed a single factor scale structure. The MAAS has demonstrated high internal consistency (above 0.80), test–retest reliability, and both concurrent and incremental validity. In the present study, the Cronbach's alpha was 0.89 at time 1 and 0.91 at time 2, which indicate high internal consistency.

Depression Anxiety Stress Scale-21 (DASS-21). The DASS-21 is an abbreviated version of the full self-report measure of depression, anxiety, and stress. In this measure, participants rate 21 items on a Likert Scale of zero (*did not apply to me at all*) to three (*applied to me very much, or most of the time*) scale and yields a total score and three subscale scores for (1) anxiety, (2) depression, and (3) stress. This measure has shown strong psychometric properties, as internal consistencies range from 0.82 to 0.93 in large, non-clinical samples. In the present study, the Chronbach's alpha for the entire scale was 0.92 at time 1 and 0.90 at time 2, which indicate high internal consistency.

Difficulties in Emotion Regulation Scale-Short Form (DERS-SF). The DERS-SF, our primary outcome measure, is an 18-item self-report measure of difficulties to regulate emotions effectively. Items are rated on a Likert scale ranging from one (*almost never*) to five (*almost always*). This measure yields a total score that captures general emotion dysregulation and six subscales that capture different facets of emotion dysregulation, including (1) non-acceptance of negative emotions, (2) difficulty in emotional situations with pursuing goal-directed behaviors, and (3) controlling impulses, (4) lack of regulation strategies, and (5) problems with emotional awareness, and (6) problems with emotional clarity. The DERS-SF has high internal consistency within adolescent samples, ranging from 0.79 to 0.91. (Kaufman et al., 2016).[5]

Discussion

Across the majority of the indicators, the treatment group overall fared better than the control group in becoming more mindful, decreasing their anxiety, and being able to self-regulate from pre-test to post-test (Tables 16.1–16.4).

Table 16.1 shows the MAAS scale, from before the program (pre) to after (post).

On the MAAS scale, African American, Latina, and White girls in the treatment group had higher average scores after taking yoga (improved mindfulness).

Table 16.1 Mindful Attention Awareness Scale (1)

MAAS Mean Scores

Row Labels	Average of MAAS_Mean_pre	Average of MAAS_Mean_post
Asian	**4.357142857**	**4.523809524**
Control	3.821428571	4.285714286
Treatment	5.428571429	5
White	**4.357142857**	**4.530612245**
Control	4.232142857	4.196428571
Treatment	4.523809524	4.976190476
African American	**4.185714286**	**4.45**
Control	4.273809524	4.488095238
Treatment	4.053571429	4.392857143
Latina	**4.1**	**4.228571429**
Control	4.523809524	3.880952381
Treatment	3.464285714	4.75
Grand Total	**4.237142857**	**4.437142857**

Table 16.2 Mindful Attention Awareness Scale (2)

MAAS Mean Scores (2 Groups: Group 1-African American or Latina, Group 2-White or Asian)

Row Labels	Average of MAAS_Mean_pre	Average of MAAS_Mean_post
Group 1	**4.157142857**	**4.376190476**
Control	4.357142857	4.285714286
Treatment	3.857142857	4.511904762
Group 2	**4.357142857**	**4.528571429**
Control	4.095238095	4.226190476
Treatment	4.75	4.982142857
Grand Total	**4.237142857**	**4.437142857**

Table 16.3 Mindful Attention Awareness Scale (3)

MAAS Mean Scores (Group 1-Black & Latina, Group 2- White)

Row Labels	Average of MAAS_Mean_pre	Average of MAAS_Mean_post
Group 1	**4.157142857**	**4.376190476**
Control	4.357142857	4.285714286
Treatment	3.857142857	4.511904762
Group 2	**4.357142857**	**4.530612245**
Control	4.232142857	4.196428571
Treatment	4.523809524	4.976190476
Grand Total	**4.220779221**	**4.425324675**

Table 16.4 Mindful Attention Awareness Scale (4)

MAAS Mean Scores pre (Multiple Items) MAAS Mean Scores post (Multiple Items)

Row Labels	Average of MAAS_Mean_pre	Average of MAAS_Mean_post
Asian	**4.357142857**	**4.523809524**
Control	3.821428571	4.285714286
Yoga	3.821428571	4.285714286
Treatment	5.428571429	5
Yoga	5.428571429	5
White	**4.357142857**	**4.530612245**
Control	4.232142857	4.196428571
Yoga	4.232142857	4.196428571
Treatment	4.523809524	4.976190476
No Yoga	4.928571429	5.535714286
Yoga	3.714285714	3.857142857
African American	**4.185714286**	**4.45**
Control	4.273809524	4.488095238
No Yoga	5.095238095	5.404761905
Yoga	3.452380952	3.571428571
Treatment	4.053571429	4.392857143
No Yoga	5.428571429	5
Yoga	3.595238095	4.19047619
Latina	**4.1**	**4.228571429**
Control	4.523809524	3.880952381
No Yoga	5.285714286	4
Yoga	4.142857143	3.821428571
Treatment	3.464285714	4.75
No Yoga	3.071428571	4.214285714
Yoga	3.857142857	5.285714286
Grand Total	**4.237142857**	**4.437142857**

Latina students in particular had a marked increase in average MAAS score after taking yoga. African American students' scores were similar between the control and treatment group both before and after taking yoga.

Tables 16.2–16.3 take into account differences that girls of color may experience across race and ethnicity. Table 16.2 groups together African American girls and Latina girls and compares them to White and Asian girls. Table 16.3 compares all girls of color to White girls. In stratifying out these groupings, we see larger gains for Asian and White girls in improved mindfulness.

When including a measure for yoga history, African American students in the treatment group increased average MAAS scores after taking yoga if they had previous experience with yoga[6], whereas African American students in the treatment group with no prior yoga experience had a slight average decrease in MAAS score. Latina students with prior yoga experience showed greater average improvements in MAAS than those with no prior yoga experience in the treatment group.

The DERS assesses difficulties in regulating emotion, and higher scores indicate greater difficulties. Lower scales correspond to better emotional regulation. On the DERS scales (Tables 16.4–16.8), African American, Latina, and White girls had lower mean scores in the treatment group after taking yoga. African American girls showed greatest improvements in the treatment group, followed by Latina girls, and White girls had slightly lowered mean scores. Asian students in the treatment group had higher average scores in difficulties regulating emotion after taking yoga, which may be due to external factors. When considering whether girls had previous experience with yoga, African American, Latina, and White girls with previous yoga experience in the treatment group showed the greatest improvements (score decrease) in average DERS score. The difference between changes in average score post-treatment for girls who had prior yoga experience versus those who did not is notable for African American and Latina girls.

The DASS assesses self-reported depression, anxiety, and stress. Higher scores correspond to higher levels of depression, anxiety, and stress. On the DASS scale

Table 16.5 Difficulties in Emotional Regulation Scale (1)

DERS Mean Scores

Row Labels	Average of TotalDERS_Pre	Average of TotalDERS_Post
African American	**37.63636364**	**34.81818182**
Control	36.85714286	37.85714286
Treatment	39	29.5
Asian	**34.66666667**	**36.66666667**
Control	34.5	35
Treatment	35	40
Latina	**38.22222222**	**33.88888889**
Control	38	36.25
Treatment	38.4	32
White	**36**	**33.57142857**
Control	44.66666667	44
Treatment	29.5	25.75
Grand Total	**37.13333333**	**34.43333333**

Table 16.6 Difficulties in Emotional Regulation Scale (2)

DERS Mean Scores (Group 1-African American or Latina, Group 2-White or Asian)

Row Labels	Average of TotalDERS_Pre	Average of TotalDERS_Post
Group 1	**37.9**	**34.4**
Control	37.27272727	37.27272727
Treatment	38.66666667	30.88888889
Group 2	**35.6**	**34.5**
Control	40.6	40.4
Treatment	30.6	28.6
Grand Total	**37.13333333**	**34.43333333**

Table 16.7 Difficulties in Emotional Regulation Scale (3)

DERS Mean Scores Multiple Items (Group 1-Black and Latina, Group 2- White)

Row Labels	Average of TotalDERS_Pre	Average of TotalDERS_Post
Group 1	**37.9**	**34.4**
Control	37.27272727	37.27272727
Treatment	38.66666667	30.88888889
Group 2	**36**	**33.57142857**
Control	44.66666667	44
Treatment	29.5	25.75
Grand Total	**37.40740741**	**34.18518519**

Table 16.8 Difficulties in Emotional Regulation Scale (4)

DERS Mean Scores pre (Multiple Items) DERS Mean Scores post (Multiple Items)

Row Labels	Average of TotalDERS_Pre	Average of TotalDERS_Post
African American	**37.63636364**	**34.81818182**
Control	36.85714286	37.85714286
No Yoga	35.75	38.75
Yoga	38.33333333	36.66666667
Treatment	39	29.5
No Yoga	32	28
Yoga	41.33333333	30
Asian	**34.66666667**	**36.66666667**
Control	34.5	35
Yoga	34.5	35
Treatment	35	40
Yoga	35	40
Latina	**38.22222222**	**33.88888889**
Control	38	36.25
No Yoga	35	30.5
Yoga	41	42
Treatment	38.4	32
No Yoga	33	32
Yoga	39.75	32
White	**36**	**33.57142857**
Control	44.66666667	44
Yoga	44.66666667	44
Treatment	29.5	25.75
No Yoga	28	26
Yoga	31	25.5
Grand Total	**37.13333333**	**34.43333333**

(Tables 16.9–16.12), African American students in the treatment group had little change in average score after taking yoga. Latina and White girls had slight decreases in average measure of depression, anxiety, and stress, but there was a similar decrease in both the control and treatment group pre- and post- taking yoga. However, when introducing yoga history as an additional variable, African

Table 16.9 Depression Anxiety Stress Scale (1)

DASS Mean Scores

Row Labels	Average of TotalDASS_Pre	Average of TotalDASS_post
African American	**11.6**	**8.4**
Control	11.42857143	6.714285714
Treatment	12	12.33333333
Asian	**18.66666667**	**19.66666667**
Control	44	35
Treatment	6	12
Latina	**14.11111111**	**9.333333333**
Control	17.5	11.5
Treatment	11.4	7.6
White	**12.33333333**	**10**
Control	11.33333333	8
Treatment	13.33333333	12
Grand Total	**13.32142857**	**10.25**

Table 16.10 Depression Anxiety Stress Scale (2)

DASS Mean Scores (Group 1-African American or Latina, Group 2-White or Asian))

Row Labels	Average of TotalDASS_Pre	Average of TotalDASS_post
Group 1	**12.78947368**	**8.842105263**
Control	13.63636364	8.454545455
Treatment	11.625	9.375
Group 2	**14.44444444**	**13.22222222**
Control	19.5	14.75
Treatment	10.4	12
Grand Total	**13.32142857**	**10.25**

Table 16.11 Depression Anxiety Stress Scale (3)

DASS Mean Scores (Group 1-Black and Latina, Group 2- White)

Row Labels	Average of TotalDASS_Pre	Average of TotalDASS_post
Group 1	**12.78947368**	**8.842105263**
Control	13.63636364	8.454545455
Treatment	11.625	9.375
Group 2	**12.33333333**	**10**
Control	11.33333333	8
Treatment	13.33333333	12
Grand Total	**12.68**	**9.12**

Table 16.12 Depression Anxiety Stress Scale (4)

DAAS Mean Scores pre (Multiple Items) Total DAAS Mean Scores post (Multiple Items)

Row Labels	Average of TotalDASS_Pre	Average of TotalDASS_post
African American	**11.6**	**8.4**
Control	11.42857143	6.714285714
No Yoga	10.33333333	1.333333333
Yoga	12.25	10.75
Treatment	12	12.33333333
No Yoga	9	21
Yoga	13.5	8
Asian	**18.66666667**	**19.66666667**
Control	44	35
Yoga	44	35
Treatment	6	12
Yoga	6	12
Latina	**14.11111111**	**9.333333333**
Control	17.5	11.5
No Yoga	4	9
Yoga	22	12.33333333
Treatment	11.4	7.6
No Yoga	10.5	5.5
Yoga	12	9
White	**12.33333333**	**10**
Control	11.33333333	8
Yoga	11.33333333	8
Treatment	13.33333333	12
No Yoga	7.5	5.5
Yoga	25	25
Grand Total	**13.32142857**	**10.25**

American girls with yoga experience in the treatment group showed an average lower score for depression, anxiety, and stress, compared to African American girls in the treatment group with no previous yoga experience. In contrast, White girls in the treatment group with previous yoga experience had relatively high average DASS scores both before and after the study.

Looking at these three scales, we find a complex set of results. Overall, the treatment groups fared better than the control groups across all the scales. Overall, all the girls of color in the treatment group also had stronger outcomes than those in the control group. Those results conservatively suggest that girls of color can be positively impacted by yoga programming.

Comparing across specific communities of girls, we see varying results. Latina girls in the treatment groups showed strong gains in improving mindfulness and were able to better regulate their emotions while showing small gains in decreasing their bouts of depression, anxiety, and stress. African American girls showed the strongest gain in their ability to regulate themselves. Asian girls had the strongest gains in mindfulness. White girls in the treatment group experienced gains across mindfulness and the ability to self-regulate.

The importance of prior yoga experience is also a part of this picture in that gains for African American girls and Latinas in the treatment group who had prior experience with yoga had noted gains for the MAAS and DERS scales[7].

In looking at this picture, we can ask broader questions about the results including: What experiences might be contributing to girls of color (and White girls) in the control group that lead to less self-regulation during a six-week period? Why did mindfulness show a better outcome for some girls and not others? What are the differences in lived experiences between Black, Latina, and White girls that help to explain the results regarding emotional regulation?

Conclusion

Yoga and meditation programing and research in K–12 schools may offer policymakers, schools, and educators tangible low cost, scalable solutions in reducing some individual obstacles that many adolescents may face. Given ongoing visibility and acceptance of yoga programming in K–12, it is important to consider the ways that girls of color may gain through such programming. From these preliminary results, girls of color in the treatment group tended to fare better than girls of color in the control group.

There are limitations to the study. One is the small sample size. Another is the lack of standardization of the after-school activities in the control group. Students in the control group engaged in a wide range of activities, such as completing homework, having free time, attending a music class, or engaging outdoor play, which makes it difficult to identify what aspects of the yoga program were most effective. Furthermore, students were not randomized to the conditions in the study, which introduces the potential effects of selection bias. Given these limitations, the design of this study balanced empirical rigor with ecological validity, as students would most likely have a choice between yoga programs or a number of other potential activity programs in real school settings. Despite these limitations, these findings suggest that it is important to consider the complexities that girls of color face in schools and how yoga interventions may impact their well-being. The complexities that girls of color face in educational settings can be addressed through careful design and implementation of yoga programming, and should be considered in the analysis of any complementary research.

In this chapter, I have also positioned myself as someone who brings insider and outsider perspectives to this work. Earlier I raised some potential challenges and blind spots that I argue are shaping yoga and meditation research in K–12 settings. In considering these, I want to pose the question: What might help center girls of color in ongoing yoga and mindfulness research in school settings? Overall, it may be useful to investigate intersectional approaches that encourage researchers to think analytically about the interconnected experiences of race and gender. This may lead to new research protocols, different questions, and different methods (May 34). An intersectional analysis yields a lens to evaluate policies, practices, and outcomes that on the surface seem neutral, natural, or inevitable. It allows scholars, as Michelle Fine notes, "to theorize with complexity" (Guidroz and Berger 72), drawing attention to systems of oppression and the inter-connectedness of social identities. This approach may be helpful in asking complex questions about racial and gender educational disparities in public schools and yoga research's integration into schools. It also may require engaging with ongoing critical theories about yoga, embodiment, and race (see Berila, Klein and Roberts, Introduction).

How do we wrestle with understanding how racial and gender disparities impact students' experiences in school? Taking an intersectional approach might allow researchers to consider the ways girls of color are seen and represented in public schools and then review the measures being used in their particular study. As psychologists Elizabeth Cole and Natalie Sabik argue, many psychology measures that seem neutral and universal on their face can be critiqued as biased toward dominant groups (see Cole and Sabik 176). In the framing of the project that is reported on here, my colleague and I looked for scales that would be accessible to a broad group of students with diverse reading abilities. We also thought about the experience of students using scales where language is not their first language. At that time we were new to evaluation based research and we often defaulted toward scales that had been widely used and validated. We did not think about whether the scales themselves had been validated across different communities of students. We, as researchers, however can evaluate scales with an intersectional lens, thinking holistically about the communities of students that are our research participants. For example, does the way a validated scale that measures stress in adolescents account for how stress may manifest for African American girls who are often viewed as less innocent and more adult than their White female counterparts (Epstein, Blake and Gonzalez 4)? In racially diverse classrooms, how are some girls of color, compared to White girls and subtly compared to each other based on biased tropes and gender socialization? And, how might such experiences manifest as depression or challenges with managing one's emotions that may not model how White girls express these same psychosocial states?

Such directions provide opportunities to recognize and support girls of color through the design of yoga programming that is affirming and relatable. There is a need for both yoga researchers and yoga educators to educate themselves about racial and gender disparities and how taking an intersectional approach may affect their researcher stance. We also need to examine measurement tools used in yoga research. And, finally, there is a need for more women of color as yoga educators and researchers.

Acknowledgement

The author would like to thank readers of the 2019–2020 Bass Connections team for their helpful comments on early drafts of this chapter. Thanks also go to colleagues Karolyn Tyson and Lisa Pearce and research assistants Brennan Lewis, Sloan Godbey, and Emma Heasley.

Notes

1 See Galantino, Galbavy and Quinn 66–68 and Land Greenberg and Harris, 16–166 for an insightful analysis of this trend.
2 The data discussed in this chapter is also analyzed in a forthcoming paper. See McMahon, et al.
3 The National Center for Education Statistics in 2017 released "Fast Facts" about information collected on the race and ethnicity of college faculty. Across the categories used of Hispanic females, Black females, Asian/Pacific Islander females the number is approximately less than 12% of all full-time faculty. They did not provide a breakdown of gender for American Indian/Alaska Native faculty. American Indian/Alaska Native faculty make up less than 1% of all full-time faculty.
4 Three girls identified as multi-racial were excluded from this analysis.
5 In the present study, the Cronbach's alpha was 0.91 at time 1 and 0.87 at time 2. Because high values of Cronbach's alpha (about 0.65 or above) indicate high internal consistency of a measure and its ability to capture a particular construct with its individual items, these values suggest that the DERS is a consistent measure of emotion dysregulation.
6 All participants in the treatment group were asked to fill out a "yoga history" form that asked if they had ever taken a yoga class or practiced at home by themselves or with their parents.
7 We also looked at whether there were differences between schools A, B, C, D or between the fall or spring semesters and found that neither category affected the results.

Works cited

Berger, Michele Tracy, and Kathleen Guidroz. *The Intersectional Approach: Transforming the Academy Through Race, Class and Gender*. University of North Carolina Press, 2009.

Berila, Beth, Melanie Klein, and Chelsea Jackson Roberts. "Introduction: What's the Link Between Feminism and Yoga." *Yoga, The Body, and Embodied Social Change: An Intersectional Feminist Analysis*, edited by Beth Berila, Melanie Klein, and Chelsea Jackson Roberts, Lexington Books, 2016, pp. 1–12.

Bhajan, Yogi. *The Aquarian Teacher: KRI International Teacher Training in Kundalini Yoga*. Kundalini Research Institute, 2007.

Bowleg, Lisa. "When Black+ Lesbian+ Woman≠ Black Lesbian Woman: The Methodological Challenges of Qualitative and Quantitative Intersectionality Research." *Sex Roles*, vol. 59, no. 5–6, 2008, pp. 312–325.

Butzer, Bethany, et al. "School-Based Yoga Programs in the United States: A Survey." *Advances in Mind-Body Medicine*, vol. 4, no. 29, Fall, 2015, pp. 18–26.

Cammarota, Julio. "The Gendered and Racialized Pathways of Latina and Latino Youth: Different Struggles, Different Resistances in the Urban Context." *Anthropology & Education Quarterly*, vol. 35, no. 1, 2004, pp. 53–74.

Carlson, Linda E., and Kirk Warren Brown. "Validation of the Mindful Attention Awareness Scale in a Cancer Population." *Journal of Psychosomatic Research*, vol. 58, no. 1, 2005, pp. 29–33.

Cole, Elizabeth, and Natalie Sabik. "Repairing a Broken Mirror? Intersectional Approaches to Diverse Women's Perceptions of Beauty and Bodies." *The Intersectional Approach: Transforming the Academy Through Race, Class and Gender*, edited by Michele Tracy Berger, and Kathleen Guidroz, University of North Carolina Press, 2009, pp. 173–192.

Crenshaw, Kimberlé. "Demarginalizing the Intersection of Race and Sex: A Black Feminist Critique of Antidiscrimination Doctrine, Feminist Theory and Antiracist Politics." *University of Chicago Legal Forum*, vol. 1, 1989, pp. 139–167.
Crenshaw, Kimberlé, Priscilla Ocen, and Jyoti Nanda. "Black Girls Matter: Pushed Out, Overpoliced and Underprotected." *Center for Intersectionality and Social Policy Studies and African American Policy Forum*, 2015, pp. 1–44.
Devi, Sanjenbam Kunjeshwori, J.P.N. Chansauria, and K.N. Udupa. "Mental Depression and Kundalini Yoga." *Ancient Science of Life*, vol. 6, no. 2, 1986, pp. 112–118.
Epstein, Rebecca, Jamilia J. Blake, and Thalia González. "Girlhood Interrupted: The Erasure of Black Girls' Childhood." *Center on Poverty and Inequality, Georgetown Law*, 2019, pp. 1–19.
Galantino, Mary LouRobyn Galbavy, and Lauren Quinn. "Therapeutic Effects of Yoga for Children: A Systematic Review of the Literature." *Pediatric Physical Therapy*, vol. 20, no.1, 2008, pp. 66–80.
Granath, Jens, Sara Ingvarsson, Ulrica von Thiele, and Ulf Lundberg. "Stress Management: A Randomized Study of Cognitive Behavioural Therapy and Yoga." *Cognitive Behaviour Therapy*, vol. 35, no. 1, 2006, pp. 3–10.
Greenberg, Mark T., and Alexis R. Harris. "Nurturing Mindfulness in Children and Youth: Current State of Research." *Child Development Perspectives*, vol. 6, no. 2, 2012, pp. 161–166.
Guidroz, Kathleen, and Michele Tracy Berger. "A Conversation with Founding Scholars of Intersectionality: Kimberle Crenshaw, Nira Yuval Davis and Michelle Fine." *The Intersectional Approach: Transforming the Academy Through Race, Class and Gender*, edited by Michele Tracy Berger and Kathleen Guidroz, The University of North Carolina-Chapel Press, 2009, pp. 61–80.
Harnois, Catherine E. "Different Paths to Different Feminisms? Bridging Multiracial Feminist Theory and Quantitative Sociological Gender Research." *Gender and Society*, vol. 19, no. 6, 2005, pp. 809–828.
Harnois, Catherine E. "Imagining a 'Feminist Revolution': Can Multiracial Feminism Revolutionize Quantitative Social Science Research?" *The Intersectional Approach: Transforming the Academy Through Race, Class and Gender*, edited by Michele Tracy Berger and Kathleen Guidroz, The University of North Carolina-Chapel Press, 2009, pp. 157–172.
Kaufman, Erin A., et al. "The Difficulties in Emotion Regulation Scale Short Form (DERS-SF): Validation and Replication in Adolescent and Adult Samples." *Journal of Psychopathology and Behavioral Assessment*, vol. 38, no. 3, 2016, pp. 443–455.
Khalsa, Sat Bir S., et al. "Evaluation of the Mental Health Benefits of Yoga in a Secondary School: A Preliminary Randomized Controlled Trial." *Journal of Behavioral Health Services & Research*, vol. 39, no. 1, 2012, pp. 80–90.
Lovibond, Peter F., and Sydney H. Lovibond. "The Structure of Negative Emotional States: Comparison of the Depression Anxiety Stress Scales (DASS) with the Beck Depression and Anxiety Inventories." *Behaviour Research and Therapy*, vol. 33, no. 3, 1995, pp. 335–343.
May, Vivian. *Pursuing Intersectionality, Unsettling Dominant Imaginaries*. Routledge, 2015.
McMahon, Kibby, Michele Tracy Berger, Keval Khalsa, Liz Harden and Sat Bir Singh Khalsa. "A Controlled Trial Evaluating the Effects of an After-School Kundalini Yoga

Program on Psychological and Emotional Outcomes in At-Risk Adolescents." *Journal of Child and Family Studies*, forthcoming.

National Center for Education Statistics. *Fast Facts: Race/Ethnicity of College Faculty*. Washington, DC, 2017.

Sarkissian, Meliné, et al. "Effects of a Kundalini Yoga Program on Elementary and Middle School Students' Stress, Affect, and Resilience." *Journal of Developmental & Behavioral Pediatrics*, vol. 39, no. 3, 2018, pp. 210–216.

Serwacki, Michelle L., and Catherine Cook-Cottone. "Yoga in Schools: A Systematic Review of the Literature." *International Journal of Yoga Therapy*, vol. 22, no. 1, 2012, pp. 101–110.

Shannahoff-Khalsa, David S. "An Introduction to Kundalini Yoga Meditation Techniques That Are Specific for the Treatment of Psychiatric Disorders." *Journal of Alternative & Complementary Medicine*, vol. 10, no. 1, 2004, pp. 91–101.

Chapter 17

Yoga and arts
Positive disruptors in the school to prison pipeline

Suzana Plaisant McCalley

Introduction

The school to prison pipeline (STPP) is a devastating national trend in the United States where students of color are interacting with police officers called School Resource Officers (SRO) at increasingly young ages on their school campuses. Increased levels of contact with law enforcement leads youth to engage with the judicial system; creating disastrous "personal, educational and economic consequences" for students (Huguley, "Just Discipline"). As those students enter adulthood interacting with a biased judicial system, they acquire a criminal record which authorizes "legal discrimination against you in employment, housing, access to education, public benefits" (qtd. in "Mutually Reinforcing"). Finally, incarcerated and formerly incarcerated individuals suffer irreversible harm, including trauma, disease, and even premature death (Brown and Patterson).

In this chapter we will explore the ways that yoga and the arts can play a positive role in the disruption of the school to prison pipeline through an organization called "Breathing Access". As part of this exploration, I share the story of how I came to the work I do; increasing access to yoga, arts, and contemplative education in underserved communities across Winston Salem, North Carolina. By sharing research in trauma informed yoga, along with my experiences with both the school and prison systems we work with, I offer a model for building equity in our communities.

Part 1: The school to prison pipeline

It is helpful to begin our journey with an understanding of how the school to prison pipeline works. The school to prison pipeline disproportionately affects students of color who are far more likely to be suspended and arrested for the same disciplinary infractions as their White peers, states the U.S. Department of Education Office for Civil Rights in its report "Data Snapshot: School Discipline." One of the causes of these racial discrepancies is the implicit bias which causes White teachers to misinterpret behavior by students of color and "rate African American students as having worse behavior than they do White students" (qtd. in. Blake and Marchbanks 7). Increases in student suspensions leads to heightened risk of "criminal activity in the future...And since Black kids are disproportionately affected, this pipeline reflects the broader racial disparities in the criminal justice system as a whole" (Andrade 19).

"Zero-tolerance" disciplinary practices is a primary contributor to the STPP. The philosophy of "zero-tolerance" in schools was developed in response to school shootings in the 1990s. The goal of these stringent policies, which often include suspension, expulsion, or engagement with an SRO, are designed to keep students safe and schools gun free. When in fact, students are receiving harsh punitive consequences that criminalize behavior such as "talking back to school personnel, bringing over the counter or prescription drugs on school grounds without a doctor's note, and coming to school out of uniform" ("Zero Tolerance"). This practice contributes to increasing numbers of students interacting with SROs and consequently the judicial system; with Black girls being the "fastest growing population" ("Youth Involved").

Some county judges agree that many of these minor infractions should be addressed at school. In the fall of 2020, I attended a regularly held meeting in our home county of Forsyth, led by County Judge Denise Hartsfield with school administrators to discuss their school justice partnership – a local effort that utilizes alternative methods to address disciplinary issues outside of the courts. The objective of these meetings is to see how the courts can better work with and support the schools to keep students in classrooms and out of the judicial system. The judge advocated for addressing disciplinary issues within the schools to avoid student suspensions. She also discussed her goal of raising the age at which minors are charged as adults. Other judges, like one in Clayton County, Georgia, strongly oppose the presence of Police Officers in schools. This juvenile court chief judge stated to Congress in a 2012 hearing that because of soaring rates of juvenile arrests, prosecutors' attention is diverted from serious crimes in the community to "prosecuting kids [that] made an adult mad" (Nelson and Lind).

The Obama administration worked to address the pipeline and its inherent racial injustice by promoting disciplinary guidelines to reduce racially discriminatory practices. Many large school districts adopted these policies and consequently experienced a decline in suspensions overall. Although there was some progress, "black students [were] still twice as likely as whites to be suspended nationwide. So are students in special education." Yet despite improvements due to the Obama-era guidelines that address "racial disparities in suspensions and expulsions,", the Trump administration recommended rescinding these guidelines ("Devos to Rescind").

What we are left with is a strong trajectory from the school system to the judicial system, especially for students of color who, in many cases, live in poverty and have learning disabilities (some of which is related to the psychological strain of having their own parents incarcerated (Najowski and Noel)). These students would benefit not from harsher discipline but from additional learning and social emotional support. Instead, "they are isolated, punished, and pushed out" (ACLU).

Part 2: My connection to this work

I inherited a passion for social justice and service from my parents who were both missionaries, musicians, and educators in Brazil, where I was born. As a child, I helped deliver food, supplies, and shared music performances with orphanages that we worked with. Witnessing the social and economic inequity in these children's lives made me want to continue to address injustice as an adult.

This passion led me to work with social justice organizations that provide, at no charge, basic necessities such as food, clothing, and medical care. While these services were and continue to be essential, I believed in order to affect meaningful change in people's lives, we also needed to offer resources to support the heart, mind, and spirit. Though I had been singing, writing songs and plays, acting, and playing musical instruments my entire life, it wasn't until my freshman year in college in Texas that I discovered yoga and meditation.

For the first time, in that class, I experienced relief from the anxiety and depression that plagued me as a teenager which I now recognize as symptoms of trauma. Years later, I took a trauma-based yoga training in Asheville, North Carolina in December 2019 as part of my 500 hour yoga instructor certification. Janelle Railey, one of the presenters and a Licensed Professional Counselor, illuminated my experience when she defined trauma as "the body-mind's record of any external or internal experience that overwhelms our normal capacities to process and cope." She explained that "How an event is recorded in one's nervous system is more significant than the actual event."

I had experienced traumatic childhood events including abuse, poverty, and the cultural alienation of immigrating to the United States. Because I had limited resources to cope with these experiences, they were recorded for me as long-lasting trauma. So, in spite of excelling academically, this unaddressed trauma led to my acting out which landed me in In School Suspensions and encounters with law enforcement and the judicial system. Persian Poet Rumi says, "the wound is where the light enters you." I had plenty of wounds, which fortunately led me to my path of healing that includes meditation, reiki and energy work, and yoga.

Part 3: Community building

Because of the role that yoga and healing arts played in my own recovery, I became passionate about sharing this work with others. I became certified as a 200 hour yoga teacher and implemented yoga and multicultural arts education into the non-profit organizations I worked with. Through this work of supporting folks from the inside out, we deepened relationships, provided resources for healing, fostered personal growth, and built community.

Eventually, I opened my own business. In 2012, the Breathing Room was established near downtown Winston Salem, NC in the historic West End Millworks – a former flour mill that brings diverse creative entrepreneurs together. Our mission was and continues to be to build community through yoga, arts, and healing arts. One of my goals with this business is to interrupt the notion that yoga is exclusively for "skinny White women."

To this end, we consciously curate our classes and work with a diverse team of instructors, appealing to people of all sizes, races, genders, and cultural backgrounds. The Breathing Room also serves as an entrepreneurial incubator/platform for women of color to run their dance, music, massage, and healing therapies businesses. Our clients continuously comment on how comfortable and welcomed they feel in our beautiful space.

In addition to our in-house programming, we offer satellite programs at a local behavioral and mental health center, Old Vineyard Behavioral Health. We also teach classes for women inmates at the Forsyth County Sheriff's Office Law Enforcement Detention Center in downtown Winston Salem – a maximum security detention facility which is unfortunately where inmate John Neville lost his life on December 4, 2019 while being restrained by detention officers (Paybarah "Sheriff Apologizes"). Working in the prison provides us with a unique point of view from "the end" of the pipeline because we also serve the cradle of this disastrous trajectory: our schools.

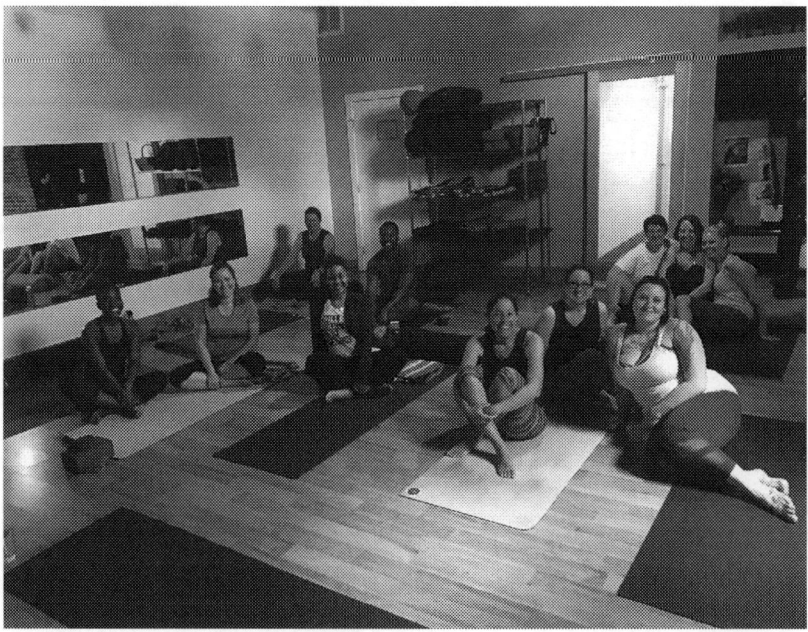

Figure 17.1 Photo by Suzy McCalley

Yoga in schools

After about a year of operating the Breathing Room full time, I realized there was still a big need in our community to bring yoga and mindfulness tools to under-served individuals and communities that wouldn't necessarily seek out, have the resources to attend, or feel comfortable in a yoga studio. I also noticed that my son, who attended a charter school at the time, received yoga and mindfulness education in his classroom, as did many other students throughout the city. However, many of the title one (low income) public schools did not have this programming available.

Winston Salem, where I have lived for the past 12 years, is located near the center of North Carolina. It was founded by the Germanic Moravians of Salem known for their crafts and arts, who joined with the more economically focused Winston. Much of Winston Salem's wealth was acquired by the thriving tobacco and textile industries that were recently replaced by the biotech and medical industries. It also boasts the first Arts Council in the country and strives to live up to its moniker as the "City of Arts and Innovation." Tragically, the city is a segregated one, racially and economically separated by a highway designed for that purpose (Cruise). The city continues to suffer from low upward mobility rates and has some of the lowest performing schools in the state.

The opportunity to work within the schools arose in 2013 when the Winston Salem Mayor, Allen Joines, who is now my husband, invited us to partner with him on an anti-obesity initiative. Although he is not responsible for the schools, as they are run by Forsyth County, he had an existing relationship with a local title one (i.e. low income) school, where the large majority of students live in economic poverty. The racial makeup of the students is mostly Black and Latinx. Families are non-traditional, somewhat transient, and young people have direct exposure to gang activity. The Mayor had already developed a working vegetable garden and brought in nutritional services, as well as health education. Breathing Access 501c3 offered yoga as a program enhancement.

Most of our students are victims of trauma or adverse childhood experiences, including the effects of intergenerational poverty and institutional racism. Yoga supports students who have experienced trauma in regaining inner strength and resilience through the body. Leaders in the area of trauma informed yoga state that "yoga is at the frontier of trauma treatment in promoting mind/body healing." The social and emotional learning that yoga provides, enables our students to better self-regulate which can be a challenge for trauma survivors (Emerson and Hopper 15, 18).

Encouraged by our success with this school, as well as the community's support for Breathing Access, we achieved non-profit status and formed a diverse board of educators and community leaders. While our team and work continue to grow, our mission remains to provide yoga and healing arts for children and communities in need. We work with students, teachers, and staff at elementary, middle, and high schools; delivering trauma-informed yoga and creative instruction and tools to more effectively manage stress, trauma, and difficult emotions. Our vision is to create a physically and emotionally healthy community for all by providing access to yoga and healing arts. With the support of grants, local corporations, individuals, and sometimes the school's budget, we have added five more K-12 schools since 2013 and our roster continues to grow.

Our programs help students relieve stress and manage emotions, which leads to decreases in negative behavioral incidents. The classes also help students increase their ability to focus which improves learning outcomes and academic performance (Kauts and Sharma). However, even though funders and school administrators love this quantitative data, yoga is not and should not be used as another tool to further control students' behavior.

While strong academic performance and positive comportment at school are important, these are indirect outcomes of a sound yoga practice whose true goal is transformation and enlightenment. Other more qualitative data from our independent research showed that students' self esteem and body positivity improved as a result of our yoga classes. Students' sense of safety at school also increased. These results are what drive our organization to continue offering services to support students' inner and outer wellbeing.

However, with limited access to funding for more substantial qualitative research, improved test scores and reduced behavioral incidents are the data points that (1) are easily quantified and (2) catch the attention of potential funders. Locally, for instance, we have a significant focus on improving third grade reading scores, which are very low in many of the schools we work with. So, making a case of tying yoga to improved academic performance is a compelling argument to get our foot in the door, knowing that what we offer carries benefits far beyond test scores.

In the spirit of reimagining scholastic spaces with wellbeing at the center, I would like to share some best practices that we have learned over the years with Breathing Access. All of our classes take place during the school day and most of them occur during "specials" or non-core classes, during PE, or recess (which is not ideal because understandably many of the children prefer to play freely). We have also found that, not surprisingly, the classes run more smoothly when students are given the choice whether to participate in the class. Some of the teachers also get involved in the yoga classes which helps build camaraderie with their students.

We currently have seven amazing women yoga teachers on staff from diverse backgrounds and ethnicities. Personally, I situate myself within this context as Latinx and as a White woman. Although my cultural background and ethnicity are diverse, I fully recognize the privileges I receive because I am White presenting within a strict caste system of race in the United States (Wilkerson). We are always looking to work with more teachers of color because of how important it is for the students to work with teachers that look like them. All of our teachers have received training on trauma informed yoga and restorative justice circles, which seek to acknowledge and respect each person in the circle and also serve to neutralize what is often an adversarial teacher–student relationship. We emphasize a partnered approach to learning that Paulo Freire describes in that we are "coordinating" learning rather than imposing knowledge upon the students.

Funding is an ongoing challenge as we value long-term partnerships with our schools. This is because many of the students we work with face a lot of transition in their lives; whether it's changing schools, teachers, housing, or changes in their families. When we make a commitment to start working with a school, we do our best to keep the program funded so we don't become part of the problem, potentially causing more harm by becoming another attachment figure that failed to remain in their lives for any significant period of time.

We noted tremendous outcomes through a written survey of many of our elementary students at the beginning and end of one semester of yoga and mindfulness. Both teachers and students reported feeling more confident about their bodies and their intelligence. They also reported increased abilities to self-regulate emotions and fostered more positive feelings about school.

Dr. Essie McKoy, who is an author, entrepreneur, professor, and education leader, was the Principal of our inaugural partner school. She wanted us to start by focusing our work with the third grade students as that is when they begin standardized testing and often experience stress as a result. Dr. McKoy described her experience working with us as we piloted the program. She said she partnered with us because she believes in "educating the whole child."

Dr. McKoy also noted a drop in out-of-school suspensions, improved problem solving skills (in and outside of school), increased self-confidence, and improved physical health (according to some parents). Students also reportedly learned new skills and vocabulary. Dr. McKoy credited our whole child approach with also positively impacting academic performance saying, "Our school started with a -3.32 EVAAS [Education Value-Added Assessment System] growth index and in a short amount of time elevated to a +2.24 EVAAS growth index, exceeding expected growth and became a Piedmont Signature." A Piedmont Signature is an award given to a school in our region for significant academic achievement within one year.

Dr. McKoy went on to state that the yoga classes "brought the students closer together as they built trust amongst each other. They used their creativity and displayed enjoyment in being involved." She also described the sense of belonging that the students felt; being a part of something special and said they would always ask for the "yoga lady." The connection they felt is especially interesting because conversely, trauma is a disease of isolation. Talmy Givón describes in his 1971 essay titled "Linguistic Colonialism and De-Colonialisation: The School System as a Tool of Oppression," that colonialism succeeds by "instilling in the colonized people's consciousness the self-destructive and debilitating attitudes of cultural and personal alienation."

Similarly, Paulo Freire's book *Pedagogy of the Oppressed* describes how oppressors want marginalized people to feel like individual cases or like people living on the outskirts of society who yearn to be integrated. Freire theorized that, rather than looking at the structural problems that keep these people from fully being, the oppressors would like the marginalized to simply "adapt" to their current situation.

Yet, as author Miriam Greenspan describes in her book, *Healing Through the Dark Emotions*, healing happens in community. Our classes are an opportunity to facilitate this healing. School Counselors and Administrators have requested that we work with students that are having challenges at home. Unfortunately, many of our students observe traumatic incidents such as parents being arrested or violence in their homes and community.

During a luncheon we held for Breathing Access in 2019 to increase awareness and support for our programs, one of the elementary school principals we worked with broke down in tears. Tragically, one of the students in her school had taken their life and other students had observed this. While our classes are not equipped to address the comprehensive psychological needs of the surviving students, the Principal expressed gratitude in knowing that, because of our classes, the students had some skills to cope with such a terrible trauma.

While our instructors held healing space for our groups, they are also cautious never to overstep therapeutic boundaries, as they are not trained counselors. Rather, they work within the scope of their yoga training to address trauma and difficult emotions in an embodied way. Unfortunately, this is not an isolated incident, one researcher reports that, "Suicide is a leading cause of death in US elementary school-aged children, and the suicide rate in black school-aged children has increased in recent years" (Sheftall et al.). When I met with one of our school board members recently, one of her main concerns during COVID is increased suicide rates as a result of compromised mental health.

Survivors of trauma and abuse, "often experience extreme difficulty managing their own emotions and negotiating healthy and rewarding friendships and intimate relationships. They characteristically harbor persistent feelings of worthlessness and shame and grapple with intense personal scrutiny and self-blame" (Emerson and Hopper 15). For this reason, it is affirming to observe our students bonding and learning new skills to better manage their emotions. Our most experienced yoga teacher, Christine Bloomfeld observed:

> I have seen many of the students benefit from yoga and mindfulness in that our classes help them to improve focus, self-esteem and patience. We encourage them to express their feelings in a safe environment and give them tools to handle stress, anger and frustration. The girls I worked with last year often shared with me how they were using breathing techniques and calming methods I taught them in stressful situations in school and at home. When one girl told us that she had been bullied, the other girls showed compassion and empathy as we took turns saying something kind about each other. Yoga is much more than postures and relaxation. For these kids it gives them space to be safe to explore both physically and emotionally.

Yoga and arts 281

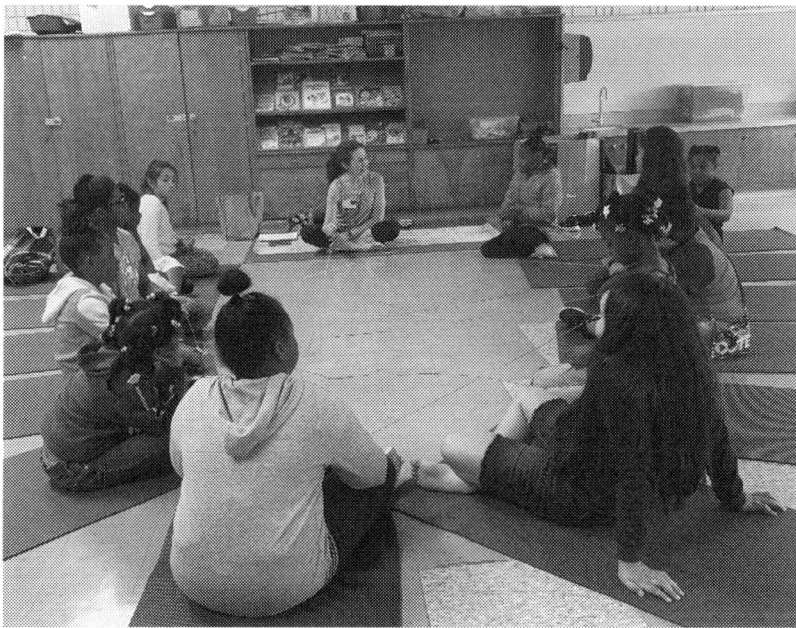

Figure 17.2 Photo by Christine Bloomfeld

In early March 2020, I was the substitute teacher for one of our fourth grade classes at one of our schools. I was new to the students, so when they walked in, I went down the line their teacher had asked them to form and shook their hands one by one, while learning their names and encouraging eye contact. One boy I noticed immediately had tons of energy; jumping up and down and asking if they could race in the gym. As a less experienced teacher, I might have viewed him as a potential threat to maintaining my control of the class. Fortunately, I had the wherewithal, the knowledge, and the wisdom to help guide and channel his energy towards his highest good and for the benefit of the entire class.

We use a talking piece (a small object) in our class from the Restorative Justice Circles method which allows for each person's voice to be acknowledged and heard. After we did our check in circle, I said I was looking for someone who is a leader in the class who could help to keep us focused. I told them I would leave the talking piece in front of that student's yoga mat and that I hoped to be able to leave it there for the entire class. I ceremoniously walked in front of several mats before stopping at this young man's mat where I gingerly placed the talking piece. He beamed with pride and rose to the challenge. I never even had to consider moving the piece because he was so intently focused throughout the session.

At the end of class he came to me and spelled his name proudly twice so I could remember him. He asked if he would see me again. My heart melted. Even though I was not scheduled to return for the remainder of that semester, I made a promise to myself to return. However, unfortunately due to the current COVID-19 crisis, I have not seen him since. But I find some comfort in knowing that I saw his potential and his strengths that day even if it was just for that class. I shudder to think of a different approach; one that might be harmful or shaming and ultimately adding to any trauma that this young man may have already suffered that an educator, administrator, or even a political leader might have taken to address the abundance of energy, intelligence, and potential that this child displayed.

I had the opportunity in February 2020 to talk with Michael Bloomberg before he gave a speech here in Winston Salem, NC. I asked him what he did to turn around the education system as Mayor of New York City." He said he gave high performing teachers a 43% raise over the course of five years so that the instructors that were talented, were motivated to continue teaching. Second, he "got rid of the kids that were disrupting the classroom". I said with a bit of surprise, "Where did they go?" There was a slight pause (he seemed less clear on his response), then responded, "Well I don't know, you'd have to talk to the teachers but we took them out because you can't have those kids ruining it for everyone."

Our conversation ended as he was rushed to the stage to deliver his campaign speech. And while I appreciate his concern about chaotic learning environments, I asked him where the children went because it matters. When a student is punished and sent to In School Suspension (ISS) or are expelled, they likely fall behind in their studies and are more likely to be arrested; creating a downward spiral (Blake and Marchbanks 7).

Recently we have been exploring a detention alternative yoga program with one of our Elementary and one of our High Schools. The Principals are interested in using the student's time in ISS to provide that student with rehabilitative programming to support their development. Yet, I think it's important that we not fall into the trap of students associating yoga with punishment, but rather as the opportunity for health and spiritual connection that it is. We are looking at offering yoga, mindfulness tools, and creative practices in this setting.

Another recent development in our programming and services was to expand our offerings to include African and Latin dance as well as visual art. We were also excited to add additional yoga classes for the middle school students we work with, because they were so popular. Most recently during the COVID pandemic, we offered online courses to support parents in managing stress, practicing self-care, and mindful parenting strategies.

We are currently working with one high school to offer virtual programming to support teachers and staff; equipping them with strategies to utilize in their online classes, as well as manage personal stress and provide tools for managing challenging situations. We will also offer interactive classes for students, including yoga, meditation, mindfulness, African dance and movement as well as visual arts. All classes are designed to help students learn in an embodied and engaging manner. We are also working with the county's school board to offer programming across the district.

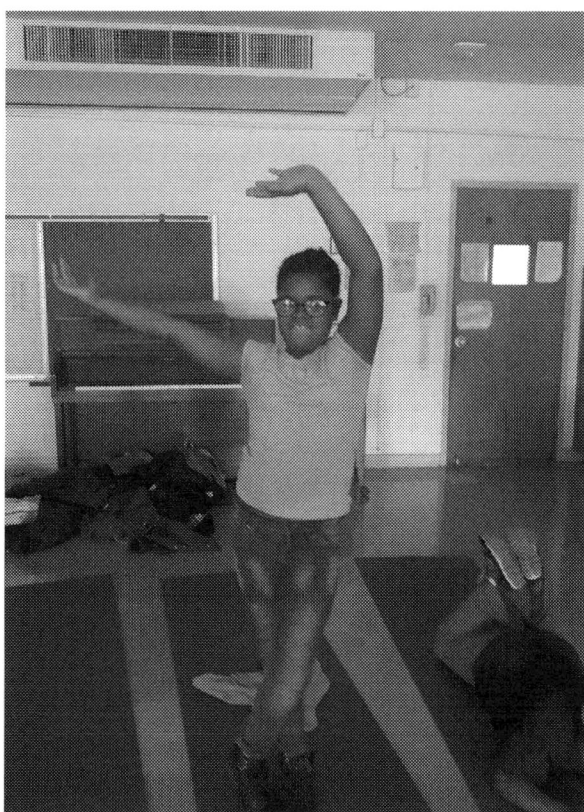

Figure 17.3 Rameka Warren, photo by Christine Bloomfeld

School and prison: Commonalities

In our work with both the schools and the prison, we found some surprising connections between the two systems. One similarity between schools and prisons is the poor nutrition they provide. While school lunches have improved nutritionally since congress passed stricter guidelines in 2010, they still offer "heavily processed foods, like corn dogs, tater tots, and cheese pizza" (Oberst). Similarly, food in prison is a highly processed product severely lacking in nutritional content and heavy in sodium ("Correcting Food").

Another similarity I noticed in the facilities we teach in, is the often gloomy appearance of many of the industrial style buildings, where grey and beige paint colors prevail. It's no surprise that many of the schools and prisons in the United States were designed by the same architects (Valencia). Also, most schools and certainly prisons are locked from the outside, literally providing a physical barrier to entry. Visitors (including parents and family members) must provide a driver's license or source of identification upon entering. One young person described the experience of entering school as, "Herded masses passing through the metal detectors" (Thorne). And Michelle Alexander, law professor, author, and civil rights advocate says students are "treated like potential criminals, even within their own schools and classrooms – doing time ends up seeming more like an inevitable stage of one's life" (qtd in. "Mutually Reinforcing").

Also, in both settings, law enforcement is present. And because the relationship with law enforcement is not equal for White people and people of color, their prevalence in the schools is an additional unequal stressor on students and families of color (Desilver et. al). Gene Demby, NPR co-host described this different experience in a recent interview, "for lots of white people the police are…public servants – they help out when something goes wrong…But for lots of communities of color, police are agents of chaos…they are omnipresent in many places. And there's almost constant contact with the police, and a lot of it is very tense contact" (Demby).

Then there is the history of industrialization in both systems – schools were designed to develop workers for manufacturing jobs and continue to follow the same inflexible models of education. Arne Duncan, former U.S. Secretary of Education and former CEO of the Chicago School system said, "Our K-12 system largely still adheres to the century-old, industrial-age factory model of education…But the factory model of education is the wrong model for the 21st century" (Duncan). Whereas industrialized prisons were designed to extract free manufacturing labor from their unpaid workforce and continue to receive either free or very cheap labor today – with 14 cents per hour as the national average (Moritz-Rabson).

But perhaps one of the most important connections between schools and prisons as it relates to the work we do, is how similar the philosophies on controlling bodies appear to be. In the schools, students are told where to stand, to follow single file lines, when to speak, who to sit next to, or even when to use the bathroom. In my experience as a parent, the more diverse the student body in terms of both economics and racial makeup, the more strict or discipline-oriented the school environment is.

This degree of control in the schools assumes that students are not trustworthy. After enough time of being treated as untrustworthy, it is surprising that more students do not act out this stereotype. Leaders in the school system seem to believe that if they can control students' bodies, then they can create safe learning environments. However, what they are perhaps inadvertently sacrificing is, in fact, true learning. Under this industrial model of education, teacher and student becomes an antagonistic relationship, characterized by dominance. It promotes what Freire calls an "ideology of oppression." True learning, he argues, is actually a process of openly questioning and wrestling with information rather than following oppressive rules that fail to respect the mind of the student.

Similarly, in the downtown detention center, inmates are under complete control. They are told where to stand, walk, whether they can attend our class, and must face the back of the elevator when changing floors. Clearly, these environments offer little freedom, autonomy, and choice. One student said, "There's no escape, just like in jail. There's no choice" (Thorne).

The tragedy is that many of the students in low income schools, as well as incarcerated individuals, are victims of trauma which is caused, in part, by removing choice. Judith Herman, a psychiatrist, author and one of the founding thought leaders of trauma treatment says, "trauma robs the victim of a sense of power and control; the guiding principle of recovery is to restore power and control" (Emerson and Hopper 23). Rather than building the autonomy that would support the recovery from trauma that many have endured, students and individuals living in incarceration have limited choices regarding their own bodies.

Our yoga classes aim to offer students an opportunity to reconnect with their own agency. While they are in our class, students can take up space, move freely, breathe and relax; a radical alternative to their day-to-day restrictions. We consciously cultivate this sense of choice in our trauma informed class curriculum. We offer modifications and remind students throughout sessions that they do not have to do anything they do not want to. One of our yoga teachers who is also a Licensed Clinical Therapist added, "I also use language that is an invitation not a mandate."

Our instruction often includes cues such as "listen to your body" and even "what your body is telling you is more important than what I am asking you to do." Students are encouraged to ask their body when it's time to come out of a pose, when to stay longer in a pose or whether to even practice the pose at all. Re-claiming this level of authority over one's own body and choices then becomes an integral part of reintegrating with one's inherent power and regaining trust in our own wisdom to choose.

The students, having followed someone else's rules all day, view their time in yoga as an opportunity to unwind, release, have fun, and play. Our instructors support these needs by providing a strong container to allow for their expression. And our most experienced instructors are masterful at allowing a balance between play and what may seem like rowdiness at times with the ability to bring them into a more calm and connected place. However, if the instructor does not have the training or capacity to give the students this psychic and physical space to explore and instead asks them to relax or to focus, the task seems nearly impossible.

Yet sometimes when we incorporate more freedom and flexibility into our classrooms, we receive pushback from school administrators. An administrator may enter a classroom during an important time of releasing pent up energy and misinterpret the students' behavior as being out of control or as disrespecting the instructor. I have seen well-meaning staff shut down a child, demanding that they "behave" when what they were doing was an important part of the process for them that day.

Another key aspect to trauma recovery is to reinstate a sense of safety. Herman states, "The first task of recovery is to establish the survivor's safety." We do this by offering meditations focused on cultivating a feeling of safety. We also invite students to keep their eyes open, if closing them doesn't feel safe. Even the way our mats are arranged in the room is designed to help students feel secure so that they can release, explore their bodies in space, and find true restoration.

Yoga in prison

We are fortunate in that the primary Corporal that we work with in the downtown detention center seems to grasp the notion that the women inmates need opportunities to let their guard down and be themselves. While she is new to this location and group of women, she has many years of experience working with women inmates. The Corporal said, they are still "feeling her out" because she is new to some of them, but she said to me, in confidence, that she was glad to see some of the women relaxing during our sessions enough to allow their personalities to begin to shine through.

Our partnership with the prison came about because our newly elected Sheriff had a personal connection to yoga, which he used to recover from an injury. When he first announced his desire to bring yoga into the prison, he said his staff was skeptical; as if doing so would somehow coddle the inmates – rewarding criminal behavior. But having witnessed the results, his staff is now asking for their own class! Also, the Sheriff has shared some of the early progress and results with Sheriffs from the surrounding seven counties in North Carolina and they have all expressed interest in starting a similar program in their own jails.

The response from the inmates has been overwhelmingly positive. The Corporal said some of the inmates started practicing yoga on their own in small groups outside of our sessions, which furthers healthy bonds amongst the participants and helps to deepen their yoga practice. Wardens have also reported less incidents of violent behavior and improved comportment overall.

In March 2020, I subbed for our weekly yoga class in our downtown detention center. It was my first time teaching at the prison and I was apprehensive; unsure of what to expect. The check in process can be fairly traumatic itself – our primary instructor for the detention center spoke to me about the rude treatment she received when she arrived to teach, like she was a criminal herself, until she explained who she was, which was my experience as well. I forgot my driver's license in my car (a requirement for entering the jail) and was treated harshly because of this error by the person checking me in. I had also attended a required training about how inmates can manipulate well-meaning outside visitors, complete with a display of weapons that were found fashioned of seemingly ordinary items, which contributed to my anxious feelings.

But when I met the students, my anxiety was relieved. They were warm and receptive. For many of them, our class is their first ever experience of yoga or mindfulness practice. The transformative results seem instant with many inmates who express such deep gratitude and interest in continuing to pursue the practice. The sense of relief from anxiety, stress, tension, and physical pain is palpable at the end of our classes. Our primary instructor and I also discussed a sense of community that is already present amongst the women. This cohesiveness or connection can be difficult to cultivate in a traditional yoga class yet it is already "built in" in this environment.

One of the students in class that day is a natural born leader. She had the attention of the group and held it with her humor. While I welcomed the laughter, I wondered at times during the class whether she was truly learning or whether she was distracting to the students next to her.

Yet she was the most vocal in her appreciation after the class. I discussed my experience with our primary instructor, who confirmed that this student has expressed a lot of interest in training to be a yoga teacher. The student had never taken a yoga class before but our instructor's consistent presence and teaching has presented her with a new role model and possibility for her own life. She says yoga helps her relax. It's one of the only opportunities the inmates have to feel safe enough to allow their guard down for a moment; allowing the body's nervous system to return to stasis where it can release stress, replenish, and recharge.

Part 4: Closing thoughts

The progress we see with our students is encouraging and gives us hope that much can be done and indeed is happening to bring yoga to both schools and prisons in an effort to bring true healing to these individuals who have suffered so much societal and personal trauma. Bringing mindfulness education to underserved communities in the United States is not new. In 1973, the Black Panther Party's Oakland Community School (OCS) opened in a poor East Oakland neighborhood where it served as the longest running community survival program until the party collapsed in 1982 and the school closed.

During its operation, the school "modeled innovative approaches to student learning: critical thinking skills, yoga, mindfulness, and restorative justice" states filmmaker Angela LeBlanc-Ernest. OCS also offered leadership opportunities and after school programming to their students and the community. Ericka Huggins, a former Panther Party leader and former director of OCS, says their innovative teaching "turned children from poor and marginalized communities who so often fall through the cracks in public school into eager scholars." Huggins, now a community college professor, called OCS "a model for education that was replicable anywhere." And one single mother whose children attended the school said, "My children grew up feeling proud of being black instead of feeling like it was a curse like a lot of children" (Drummond).

For young people, fulfilling their potential is an uphill battle when they are surrounded by environments and neighborhoods of denigration; an intentional result of oppression according to author and activist James Baldwin, which he describes as a "conspiracy to make Negroes believe they are less than human."

Baldwin argues that the role of educators is to educate the child as to a more accurate version of history that includes the truth about the contributions of Black people to the American economy and society. Teachers, according to Baldwin, have the responsibility to awaken students to the reasons behind the inequity with which they are surrounded in communities that are underserved economically. Yet, Baldwin describes the motivation of American society at large in keeping men and women of color uneducated as to their own value. This is because, "once he [the Negro child] suspects his own worth, once he starts believing that he is a man, has begun to attack the entire power structure."

Now is the time to educate students as to their own value. Yoga and the arts create opportunities to reconnect with one's true self; regaining control of our bodies, our worth, and uncovering our innate power. However, these services and tools are least available to poor Black and Brown students who need it most because they are the most vulnerable to the tragic effects of intergenerational poverty and institutional racism. Access to yoga education and trauma informed practices is an issue of equity. These tools must be made readily available to everyone who is interested in them regardless of color or economic status so that healing is available to all.

Bibliography

Andrade, Joaquim. "School Discipline and the 12 Learning Styles Theories". *Lulu.com*, 2018. https://books.google.com/books/about/School_Discipline_and_About_The_12_Learn.html?id=YYiCDwAAQBAJ Accessed 19 Aug. 2020.

Baldwin, James. "A Talk To Teachers". The Saturday Review, spps, December 21, 1963. https://www.spps.org/cms/lib010/MN01910242/Centricity/Domain/125/baldwin_atalktoteachers_1_2.pdf Transcript.

Blake, Jamilia J. and Miner P. Marchbanks III. "Assessing the Role of School Discipline in Disproportionate Minority Contact with the Juvenile Justice System: Final Technical Report". *National Criminal Justice Reference Service*. https://www.ncjrs.gov/pdffiles1/ojjdp/grants/252059.pdf Accessed 18 Aug. 2020.

Brown, Tony N. and Evelyn Patterson. "Wounds From Incarceration That Never Heal: Mass Incarceration is a Moral and Policy Failure". *New Republic*, June 28, 2016. https://newrepublic.com/article/134712/wounds-incarceration-never-heal Accessed 27 Aug. 2020.

"Correcting Food Policy in Washington Prisons How the DOC Makes Healthy Food Choices Impossible for Incarcerated People & What Can Be Done". *Prison Voice Washington*, 2016. http://prisonvoicewa.org/content/CorrectingFoodPolicy-2016-10-25.pdf Accessed 29 Aug. 2020.

Cruise, Shane Nash. *Reynoldstown: Race, Blight, Disease, Highway Construction and the Transformation of Winston-Salem, North Carolina*. MA History Thesis. North Carolina State University, 2011. https://www.scribd.com/document/401094810/Reynoldstown-Race-Blight-Disease-Highway-Construction-and-the-Transformation-of-Winston-Salem-North-Carolina Accessed 31 Aug. 2020.

Da Loba, Andre. "Devos Has Scuttled More Than 1200 Civil Rights Probes Inherited From Obama". *Propublica*. https://www.propublica.org/article/devos-has-scuttled-more-than-1-200-civil-rights-probes-inherited-from-obama Accessed 6 April 2020.

"Data Snapshot: School Discipline" Issue Brief No. 1. *U.S. Department of Education Office for Civil Rights*, March 2014. https://www2.ed.gov/about/offices/list/ocr/docs/crdc-discipline-snapshot.pdf Accessed 18 Aug. 2020.

Demby, Gene. Interview by David Greene. *For People Of Color, Relationships With Police Are Complicated*, 15 Aug. 2014. https://www.npr.org/2014/08/15/340562861/for-people-of-color-relationships-with-police-are-complicated. Accessed 31 Aug. 2020.

Desilver, Drew, Michael Lipka and Dalia Fahmy. "10 Things We Know About Race and Policing in the U.S". *Pew Research Center, FACT Tank*, June 2020. https://www.pewresearch.org/fact-tank/2020/06/03/10-things-we-know-about-race-and-policing-in-the-u-s/ Accessed 31 Aug. 2020.

Drummond, Tammerlin. "Black Panther School A Legend in Its Time". *East Bay Times*. http://www.eastbaytimes.com/2016/10/06/black-panther-school-ahead-of-its-time/. Accessed 2 April 2020.

Duncan, Arne. "The New Normal: Doing More with Less". *Qtd in U.S. Department of Education. Ed.gov. Remarks to American Enterprise Institute*, Nov. 2010. https://www.ed.gov/news/speeches/new-normal-doing-more-less-secretary-arne-duncans-remarks-american-enterprise-institute. Accessed 31 Aug. 2020.

Emerson, David and Elizabeth Hopper. *Overcoming Trauma Through Yoga: Reclaiming Your Body*. North Atlantic Books and The Trauma Center at Justice Resource Institute, Inc, 2011.

Herman, Judith. *Trauma and Recovery: The Aftermath of Violence - From Domestic Abuse to Political Terror*. Basic Books, 1992.

Huguley, James, et. al. "Just Discipline and the School to Prison Pipeline in Pittsburgh". *Heinz*. http://www.heinz.org/UserFiles/Library/Just_Discipline_and_the_School_to_Prison_Pipeline_in_Pittsburgh.pdf Accessed 3 April 2020.

Kamenetz, Anya. "Devos to Rescind Obama Era Guidance On School Discipline". *NPR*. https://www.npr.org/2018/12/18/675556455/devos-to-rescind-obama-era-guidance-on-school-discipline Accessed 3 April 2020.

Kauts, Amit and Neelam Sharma. "Effect of Yoga on Academic Performance in Relation to Stress". *International Journal of Yoga* 2(1) (2009): 39–43. doi:10.4103/0973-6131.53860. https://www.ncbi.nlm.nih.gov/pmc/articles/PMC3017967/ Accessed 31 Aug. 2020.

Moritz-Rabson, Daniel. "'Prison Slavery': Inmates Are Paid Cents While Manufacturing Products Sold to Government". *Newsweek*. Aug. 18. https://www.newsweek.com/prison-slavery-who-benefits-cheap-inmate-labor-1093729

"Mutually Reinforcing: Mass Incarceration and the School-to-Prison Pipeline". *The ACLU of Utah Activist*, 30 Nov. 2013, https://www.acluutah.org/blog/item/918-mutually-reinforcing-mass-incarceration-and-the-school-to-prison-pipeline#:~:text=Mass%20incarceration%20and%20the%20School%2Dto%2DPrison%20Pipeline%20(STPP,the%20STPP%2C%20creating%20a%20cycle. Accessed Aug. 25.

Najowski, C. and M. Noel. "When Parents Are Incarcerated, Their Children Are Punished, Too". *Monitor on Psychology* 50(8) (September, 2019). http://www.apa.org/monitor/2019/09/jn Accessed 28 Aug. 2020.

Nelson, Libby and Dara Lind. "The School to Prison Pipeline Explained". *Justice Policy Institute*. http://www.justicepolicy.org/news/8775 Accessed 4 April, 2020.

Oberst, Lindsay. "Why School Lunches in America Are Unhealthy and 10 Ways You Can Take Action to Improve Them" Food Revolution". *Network.com*, 2018. https://foodrevolution.org/blog/school-lunch-in-america/ Accessed 29 Aug. 2020.

Paybarah, Azi. "Sheriff Apologizes to Family of Inmate Who Died After Being Restrained". *New York Times*, 4 August 2020. https://www.nytimes.com/2020/08/04/us/john-neville-death-winston-salem-nc.html Accessed 20 Aug. 2020.

"School to Prison Pipeline". *ACLU*. https://www.aclu.org/issues/racial-justice/race-and-inequality-education/school-prison-pipeline Accessed 20 Aug. 2020.

Sheftall, Arielle H et al. "Suicide in Elementary School-Aged Children and Early Adolescents". *Pediatrics* 138(4) (2016): e20160436. doi:10.1542/peds.2016-0436

Thorne, Emily Rose. "Schools Are Like Prisons: How The School-to-Prison Pipeline Ruins Lives". *Medium.com*, 2019. https://medium.com/@emilyrosethorne6/schools-are-like-prisons-how-the-school-to-prison-pipeline-ruins-lives-b4c9c7d780d3#:~:text=%E2%80%9CSchools%20are%20like%20prisons%2C%20because,passing%20through%20the%20metal%20detectors. Accessed 31 Aug. 2020.

Valencia, Nicolas. "The Same People who Designed Prisons Also Designed Schools". *Architecture News*, May 2020. https://www.archdaily.com/905379/the-same-people-who-designed-prisons-also-designed-schools. Accessed 31 Aug. 2020.

Wilkerson, Isabel. *Caste: The Origins of our Discontents*. Random House, 2020.

"Youth Involved with the Juvenile Justice System". https://youth.gov/youth-topics/juvenile-justice/youth-involved-juvenile-justice-system Accessed 27 Aug. 2020.

"Zero Tolerance". *National Clearinghouse on Supportive School Discipline*. https://supportiveschooldiscipline.org/learn/reference-guides/zero-tolerance Accessed 27 Aug. 2020.

Chapter 18

Tending communities
Yoga as an integrative, collaborative, and transformative practice

Narin Hassan

In 2011, the year I was up for tenure in the School of Literature, Media, and Communication at Georgia Tech, I taught a seminar on "The Body and Cultural Representation." The course examined histories and politics of the body and focused closely on issues of gender and identity. We read material on racial science and Victorian medicine, discussed texts from the fields of literature, medical humanities, critical theory, and feminist criticism, and viewed films and visual images that addressed topics including histories of medicine, gender representation, and ethical, political, and legal issues surrounding the body. For the first time, I included texts that analyzed yoga as a cultural phenomenon and considered its migration to the West. Students read selections from Mark Singleton's *Yoga Body: The Origins of Modern Posture Practice* (Oxford, 2010) and Robert Love's *The Great Oom: The Improbable Birth of Yoga in America* (Viking, 2010). These books, both published the year before, explored the historical contexts of yoga and discussed its growing emergence within popular culture and as a subject of interdisciplinary scholarly study[1]. Along with excerpts from these texts, the class analyzed dominant narratives shaping our notions of gendered, healthy bodies, commodity culture, and communities of practice. We viewed popular images of the stereotypical "yoga body" in contemporary advertising as well as the YouTube "Yoga Girl" video which was circulating through social media at the time. 2011 seemed to be an important turning point for the emergence of yoga as a subject of intellectual inquiry as well as a darling attraction of popular culture.

During this segment of the semester, I was faced with a quandary about how much to share with students about my own longstanding relationship with yoga. I had been teaching at studios in Atlanta ever since being hired as a faculty member at Georgia Tech, but these two teaching experiences had resided in separate realms. Exposing this "side gig" could create a critical turn in our discussion and provide students with a different image of yoga culture, but could also impact and unsettle the classroom dynamic. Dominant images of yoga associate the practice with slick magazine images of slender figures performing what sometimes look like contortionist poses; individual bodies tend to be highlighted and sexualized while the mindful, thoughtful, collaborative side of yoga is often ignored, or simply harder to capture and convey in popular media. I feared the ways that the image of yoga teacher or "yoga girl" collided with that of a professor at a research institution where I had often been told that I "looked young" and "unlike a professor." I was also concerned that students could see me as, and primarily through, my body – popular images of yoga and the focus upon asana in Western contexts tend to present yoga solely as a physical pursuit of the body or a spiritual practice at odds with scientific and "objective" forms of thinking that my Georgia Tech students embrace. Further, in a class that addressed issues of bodies, race, and identity, students could read my South Asian background as a lens for my relationship with the practice and assume my interest in the subject simply because of my ethnicity. While it is important to critique the dominance of whiteness in yoga representation in the West and issues of appropriation, making authoritative claims about "authentic" yoga roots or one's own privileged cultural relationship to that history is equally problematic. Yoga as we know it is, and has been, a fusion of practices made possible through colonial histories and global interconnections. It currently tends to flow in privileged Westernized spaces, but is not always presented and practiced with its philosophical and historical roots in mind.

As feminist critics have long argued, the devaluing of women and their efforts has often been through the association of femininity to bodies and bodily processes[2] and in the same way, yoga's physical dominance can relegate it as a marginal and anti-intellectual practice. Sharing my experience with yoga could shift the dynamics of the classroom and impress claims to an identity often perceived in opposition to professorial authority. And then I did it. I told my wide-eyed and somewhat surprised students about my experience as a yoga teacher and practitioner highlighting how yoga did, indeed, benefit my scholarly thinking and teaching practices, and also how it trained me to think more deeply about what I was doing in the world. I shared some of my research on yoga and its relationship to globalization and feminism, placing some of my work outside of the academy more closely within it. At the time, the students had positive responses and seemed more engaged with the fact that they learned something about my life outside of Georgia Tech than with the details of yoga and my relationship to it.

In one of the final weeks of the semester, the class surprised me when a number of the students showed up to take my restorative yoga class at a local studio as part of an end of semester celebration that they organized. Suddenly, my worlds collided – as my college students mingled with the regulars in my yoga class (some of whom didn't know I was a college professor) and lined up on their mats we all shared a new experience as they witnessed a different side of my teaching outside of a traditional classroom setting. By reading their bodies and watching them move through poses, I perceived my college students in a new way and could better sense the burdens they carried in their bodies. The act of bundling students in blankets in savasana (our final relaxation pose) broke through the barriers that were held when we sat around a seminar table – so much of what we carry in our academic lives is held in the body, contained and restrained, and through yoga we can learn to release it and heal. This is why yoga had always been the perfect antidote to my work as a scholar. I had known that practicing yoga made me a better teacher to my academic students – more intuitive and aware of their needs, and conscious of the subtle forms of communication that can occur through the body. However, their inclusion in my studio class also highlighted the beneficial ways that principles and practices of yoga can be incorporated in academic settings. The act of touch, so often a practice we cautiously avoid in our classroom teaching, could be enacted in a careful way in the safe environment of a cozy studio and, further, the shared experience of focusing upon breath and quiet reflection served as an antidote to the active pace and potentially stressful space of a seminar. The experience decentered our classroom in a new way – I wished that students could have joined me in a yoga session at the beginning of the year because through acts of breathing deeply, meditating, and moving through poses together we could see that we all indeed were, and always are, embodied subjects in the process of learning.

We had two more final classes on campus after this experience, and the students who came to the yoga class connected with each other and with me in new ways in our classroom setting – the experience of being inside their bodies and having time for meditative reflection in a yoga class shifted the dynamics of the classroom. Students were more willing to share and confront their academic stress and connect themselves more deeply to material we were reading about bodies and our relationship to space. Since the course had dealt with issues that were sometimes divisive and tense – addressing topics that raised ethical questions in the areas of the reproductive technologies and the intersections of race and medicine, for example – awareness of our own embodiment and the living, breathing, interconnected qualities of our seminar environment gave students new ways to listen, analyze, and contribute within discussions.

The experience made me more aware of the ways to interpret and "hold" both of the teaching spaces I inhabit – the shared experience of yoga cultivated a more open and intuitive academic space on a college campus, and allowed me to interact with my students in a more productive way. And the nurturing qualities of my hands and a blanket – experiencing a sense of touch and comfort, created a new way to spark human connection with my students. Using props like bolsters, blankets, blocks, and belts to set my students up in gentle restorative postures allowed me to address the tension and convey the human need we have to be cared for. Through props and restful postures, students could discover new ways to support themselves and be more reflective and thoughtful. As a scholar in the humanities, that focus upon contemplation, feeling, and human contact could, and should, be central to the ways we think about our teaching – if the books we teach and the subjects we embrace ask our students to think about the world, the concerns and feelings of others, and the critical complexity of the quandaries we face, then we have to experience those issues head on – but not only with our heads and minds. We need to think beyond purely intellectual realms of the mind and also consider how we communicate with our bodies and how our embodiment and movement within communal spaces matters. We need to practice what Becky

Thompson proposes as a "pedagogy of tenderness," which "makes room for intimacy and vulnerability alongside deep study of guiding texts" (Thompson, 7).

The relationship of yoga with my academic life does not circulate only one way. The practice of being a yoga teacher and being a professor/scholar is becoming more deeply entwined – having an awareness of language and a capacity to read between the lines is as valuable and necessary when teaching yoga as it is to the critical practices of humanities scholarship. I can't always predict where a college classroom discussion will go and, in the same way, my yoga classes involve finding intuitive clues for what my students may need, what pose may align best after the other, and when to create the space for a more quiet or meditative practice. Yoga, like feminism, and like the collaborative classroom, is engaged with transformation and flux; it requires a process of confronting, balancing, and unearthing the complex questions, memories, thoughts embedded within us that don't easily come to the surface. Feminism and yoga are entwined – both encourage awareness, kindness, and compassion, and both work towards the recognition and balance of stillness and change – of remembering the potential to grow and evolve. Both also engage with issues of community and collaboration. Communication is central to my yoga classes as it is in the academic spaces I live in – and how we speak and how we listen to our students is critical to how we create spaces of learning in yoga classes as well as college campuses.

I share this personal story as a way to analyze yoga in contemporary culture and exemplify its potential for creating connection and supporting social justice within academic realms and within broader communities. My essay reflects upon the tensions of holding the dual role of yoga teacher and college professor and explores how social justice and community practices can be upheld and are critical to the spaces and institutions of yoga as well as the academy. Discussions of yoga, race, and social justice in the classroom open up the space of critical inquiry and shift the dynamics of the classroom, but they can also impact the culture and formation of other communities. Bringing together yoga and academic work can be a way to address social and cultural inequities and dismantle our assumptions about bodies and notions of the "individual" and the "collective." As Beth Berila notes:

> The merger of yoga and feminism, then, invites a turn toward not only the corporeal, but also toward embodied empowerment. Yoga is a critical site for embodiment, as it invites participants to sink into their felt sense and reflect upon emotional and physical sensations as well as cognitive ones. It also underscores the realization that feminists, yogis, and body practitioners have known, which is that we hold memory, wisdom, and trauma in our bodies. Since oppression creates deep trauma, it only makes sense that disrupting oppression and healing from it will require more than political and intellectual processes; it will also require embodied ones (Berila, *Yoga, The Body, and Embodied Social Change: An Intersectional Feminist Analysis*, 6).

I am particularly interested in examining how creating a "yoga space," whether it is within an academic classroom or a studio setting, can shift the dynamics of a community and foster new forms of collaboration and understanding as well as produce social change. As we do humanistic social justice work and make efforts to improve well-being around us, we need to consider issues of the body and touch – ways that yoga asks us to address knowing and understanding the body; issues of space and community – and how we connect with each other to build them; and finally, questions of identity – particularly how yoga can give us opportunities to reflect, challenge, and complicate narratives surrounding identity. Further, we need to reclaim and assert the presence of our bodies (and our yoga practices) within pedagogical spaces, spaces of the academy, and spaces within our communities.

In the example introduced above, sharing yoga with my students became the starting point for me to embrace my identity as a yoga teacher as well as an academic – it led me to recognize how acknowledging what is held in our bodies and working through the process of reclaiming the body (and its relationship to the mind and to the neural pathways we create) is a feminist act. For those of us who work in areas of social justice and gender equity (areas that ask us to consider and analyze the nature of embodiment), yoga can function as a critical component of self care and community care to restore and recharge us to do the work that desperately needs to be done in the world. Engaging with embodiment practices is critical to helping us recognize and address the impact of oppression and the various histories, traumas, and tensions we hold at a deeper level so that we can create individual and collective change. then continue with the next sentence which begins. Further, we can redefine how the body has been and continues to be represented in popular culture and challenge the dismissal of body work that so often dominates the culture of professional and academic spaces. Christy I. Wenger describes this kind of process as she explores contemplative pedagogies in the composition classroom. She writes: "As of yet, contemplative pedagogies are often unaware of the ways reclaiming the body in our classrooms is an overtly feminist act since women typically have been objectified as bodies and emptied as minds in Western culture and education" (35). While, as Elizabeth Grosz and others have shown, the body has been central to feminist theories as well, it resides most comfortably in the spaces of theory. Like Grosz, I'd like to encourage a dialogue of the body as a physical entity that needs to be visibly active in feminist spaces – we need to reclaim the role of the body and challenge assumptions that critique the body as lower on the hierarchical scales of culture. Further, we need to embrace the connections between our bodies and our mental, spiritual, emotional well-being – a process that yoga teaches us to do – and recognize the deep personal, ancestral histories and societal inequities and assumptions that shape our experiences and health.

Of course, these aspirational qualities of yoga also demand critique. Just as I find myself wanting to open up the worlds of yoga to my students and embrace it alongside my position as a scholar, teacher, and administrator, I feel slightly queasy about the increasingly weighted qualities of the term "yoga" and the varied practices that it embraces. As the broader cultures of yoga, mindfulness, and self-care become increasingly commodified, appropriated, and widely practiced, they also take on new forms and new ways of meaning. How can we hold on to the contemplative, collaborative qualities of yoga as a tool within the development of classroom and studio communities and also address the ways that it has become an increasingly popular practice that does not always address the needs and concerns of the communities it embraces? How does one embrace the role of yoga teacher at the same time as an academic and negotiate the often tense and toxic spaces of the academy? Yoga can be a tool for that process, but until it is integrated more fully into the spaces we inhabit, it can also uphold a position as a marginalized practice. And finally, how can we honor the multiple identities and spaces of yoga and its emphasis on touch as we introduce it within professional realms and various other aspects of our lives?

This, of course, needs to be negotiated as we consider ways that yoga in contemporary societies is evolving with an identity of its own – one that is often muddled by globalization and capitalism, and whitewashed as it seeps broadly within popular culture. Yoga, meditation, and mindful practices have their own cultures of inclusion and exclusion and can mirror and replicate cultures of oppression. Further, as yoga continues to boom as a billion-dollar industry and expand into various facets of society including corporate and educational spaces, it can re-inscribe ongoing societal inequities and injustices even as it manifests as a potential solution or "fix" for those very problems. Thus, we have to consider both the potentially liberating and oppressive tendencies of yoga as it expands in various realms and as we promote it as a possible antidote to our problems in this political and cultural moment. We can take an aspirational approach, and consider how our practices of yoga can seep into the rest of our lives in a positive way and impact our communities. For example, Be Scofield suggests that:

> For many contemporary yoga practitioners, there's a clear connection between cultivating inner states of peace on the mat and creating a harmonious and just world. In addition to documented health benefits, such as stress reduction, increased fitness, and emotional well-being, it's widely believed that spiritual practices such as yoga or meditation can provide grounding for more ethical and wise action. Compassion, kindness, and generosity are just a few of the qualities that many aspire to cultivate on the mat or cushion. In our fast-paced industrialized society, these methods offer opportunities to slow down and reconnect, while creating more space for discernment and contemplation of our actions. Through practicing yoga, one can hopefully gain a better understanding of the interconnectedness of all things. Many believe, or at least hope, that this renewed sense of awareness will inspire us to take action against injustice in the world" (Scofield, 134).

As the popularity of yoga increases and takes on new forms and functions within mainstream culture, it can be infused with the existing problems and in turn serve injustice and coercion. Thus, our aspiration work needs to acknowledge the ongoing tensions and inequities that impact students and seep into the spaces of yoga just as they do within our culture. As Beth Berila notes, in her introduction to the collection *Yoga, The Body, and Embodied Social Change*: "mainstream yoga in the West is often infused with discrimination, becoming yet another tool for oppression. It can be difficult if not impossible to do deep self-study and reach some level of liberation through a yoga practice when the practice itself has been inscribed with oppression…In the face of what some have classed the yoga industrial complex, many yogis have reasserted the spiritual roots of yoga, calling out Western emphasis on *asana*" (3).

My thoughts on this subject are informed by my longstanding relationship to yoga as both a student and a teacher, as well as the valuable critical material that has been emerging on the subject within the last decade or so. As I note early in this essay, I am in the process of shifting the space of yoga from being "outside" of my academic life, to a more integrated process within. Of course, my yoga practice informs my work and how I live my life – and in this way, it has always impacted how I organize a classroom and the other aspects of my academic work. But more recently, I find the need for it to be more central in all aspects of my life – as an intentional, radical, and necessary act. Since that first moment of introducing my college students to it theoretically and practically, various shifts have brought yoga into my tiny corner of academic life. Colleagues and friends have increasingly attended my classes, and I have approached my own research through the lens of yoga – tracing its complex histories and writing a manuscript on the global intersections of gender, travel, and yoga in the 19th century My academic thinking has, in turn, informed my courses, as I am able to share the research of this new project, and of extended trainings and workshops, with my community of yoga students. The dominance of social media in our culture – as a space in which the personal and public become more intertwined – has made it so my yoga teaching has become more public in the past few years. When you teach at yoga studios that need to market classes and share activities, it is hard to avoid being "tagged" in photos or highlighted in studio news. Thus, I've begun to develop my own social media presence (and create more reflective and diverse kinds of social media images) in terms of how my yoga teaching is a critical part of my life that helps me organize my academic work and productivity and also encourages me to think more critically and inclusively. And students in recent years have been much more open to learning about and incorporating practices of yoga and meditation in their own lives. In a course last semester, one of my male students, an aspiring yoga teacher himself, began a presentation by asking the class to take three deep breaths and then do some simple movements in the classroom. This initiated what became a more regular process of starting many of our classes with breath-work and gentle stress-releasing movement which the students themselves requested.

I decided in 2018 to take a bigger leap by working collaboratively to create a community space for yoga – I call our space a "community space" because the role of "studio owner," in the traditional sense, has taken a while to embrace, and, in the formation of our space we have intentionally created a nontraditional business model. Our "Little Yoga Co-op" is organized as a shared space between two teachers with independent businesses engaged in the development of a community based, affordable place for practice. My shift towards taking the leap of building and supporting a yoga space was largely based upon the need to connect with and build community and more fully integrate yoga in my own life and the lives of others. I wanted to create a living, breathing, open yoga space, make decisions of my own with careful thought and integrity, and in turn to host and tend to a space in a whole new way – as a collaboratively defined, slowly evolving, healing environment to hold a community of learners and teachers – nonacademic and academic alike.

The style of yoga I study and teach Purna Yoga – with a lineage that roots back to Sri Auribindo, an Indian freedom fighter who claimed "all life is yoga" and believed the practice should be integrated into our everyday lives, as a way for us to pursue social justice – and the careful asana of B.K.S. Iyengar, who, through his brilliant use of props and therapeutic sequencing and alignment, helped to make yoga accessible and beneficial for everyone. The creators of Purna Yoga, Aadil Palkhivala and Savitri, integrate yoga asana with Heartfull Meditation, as well as the study of yoga philosophy, nutrition, and pranayama, making all of these aspects of life critical to the practice. As I share and practice, I recognize the lineage of the practice as well as its potential to inspire others through its expansive and integrative approach. The style considers yoga as a path for transformation and evolution and for living and for impacting the world. Purna Yoga trainings and workshops also have a strong emphasis on the power of communication and the importance of language in the practice of teaching – part of why I was attracted to this style is because its attention to alignment, detail, refinement, and rigor along with its emphasis on clear language naturally aligned with the work I was already doing as a professor and writer. It is a naturally "intellectual" style of yoga with a strong emphasis on studying a philosophical lineage and refining various aspects and roots of yoga practice; it is intersectional in the ways that it addresses yoga as a complete lifestyle method and attempts to balance and reveal the interconnectedness of our thoughts, daily routines, and mental and physical practices. It closely supports my work in the classroom with its strong focus on pedagogy, communication, and clarity in language as well as its emphasis on yoga as a critical path to finding ones dharma or purpose. As I continue to study in this tradition, I find myself wondering how I can integrate the various parts of my teaching and my life. What would it be like to host a classroom in a studio? Or to have students see the building of a community from the ground up? And how can I incorporate some of the critical aspects of Purna Yoga – a focus upon transformation, evolution, and light to a classroom space and a broader community within an academic institution?

The development of the Little Yoga Co-op, shared with Lynn Brandli, a Certified Iyengar yoga teacher, came about in a grassroots and community-based way. Lynn and I have known each other for almost 15 years, and have lived in the same close-knit neighborhood of Grant Park in Atlanta in that period. When we made the decision to share a studio, we both felt that the space needed to be one with a history and strong roots in community – and much of our collaboration and planning initially took place as we were in the midst of tasks like painting, cleaning, and refinishing old floors. We discovered stories about how the space was a center for activities surrounding justice and community organizing. Living in a neighborhood that is increasingly gentrified and full of shiny new spaces, we took the task of honoring and caring for an older space and embracing its energy and history. We also decided that instead of following a typical studio model, we would create a space for collaboration – where two women's businesses could thrive together through cross-promotion, and where our neighbors could also embrace the space for cultural activities and social justice events. Within our first month of opening, we received requests for opening the space up for a social justice event and also for a poetry book launch. We also opened the space for girl scout meetings, which has given young girls the opportunity to see yoga as inclusive, active, educational, and collaborative. A recently formed women's leadership and entrepreneurial group – the Southeast Lady MOB (MOB stands for My Own Boss) – which I have been a part of, used the space for meetings and social events. Through these gatherings, the space has become a grassroots center for women to support each other in the development of new initiatives – as writers, business owners, artists, and women working in the nonprofit sector – and for more social interaction and collaboration between women. I have offered free yoga sessions for various groups, led classes on health, yoga, and self care for teens, and organized workshops related to yoga and its connection to dharma and well-being. This is just the beginning of imagining a yoga space as expansive – the work that happens in the space addresses all forms of wellness and also supports growth of various forms within our community. In the future, I imagine the space could function in ways that Matthew Remski recommends in his proposals for practitioners and yoga studios (123–125) and with the flexibility and openness of a space built not only for yoga practice, but also for conversation and community collaboration[3].

Much of the work of building our co-op took place over a summer – during a time when I was teaching at Georgia Tech, but with fewer campus responsibilities outside of that one class. Now that our co-op has been a reality for more than two years, the process of thinking through how the space integrates with my academic life has become more of a priority. I still find myself being tentative about sharing these aspects of "my other life" in academic realms, although as I do so, I am reminded that the men in my department run marathons, take long walking tours, and embark on all kinds of physical and intellectual activities outside of campus without any sense of concern. And some of them engage in entrepreneurial activities outside of campus in other realms. As my husband recently claimed – our little co-op can be envisioned as my "lab" – the equivalent of the many research and teaching spaces that academics create for themselves that also exist as communities of learning and growing. And this is where I realize that the act of teaching is a feminist act, and also an act of social justice that is deeply embedded in my work and demands continued integration in my research and teaching. In the same way that I, as a junior faculty member, sometimes had to show up to faculty meetings with my baby in a sling – or attend a conference with a toddler in tow, I feel like yoga and my connection to it needs to be more integrated and embraced with the intellectual contours of my life. It may be a risk to integrate yoga more fully into my academic classes, but would also be a chance to have students connect with each other and with me in new ways. But the classroom space is not the only space where yoga has the potential for empowerment and for forging more meaningful and tender ties – creating communities of faculty who can be in their bodies and more aware of their own potential and living in their dharma can create powerful shifts in the academic spaces we inhabit and create more cohesive and supportive work environments. A collaboration with Anneliese Singh, a fellow Purna Yoga teacher and academic, has resulted in "mini-retreat" experiences combining restorative yoga with yoga nidra in sessions where we focus upon creating nurturing, collaborative spaces for people to focus upon their "sankalpa" (intention) and take the time for reflective and meditative practice. Our goal is to bring this to various communities, including academic spaces – our upcoming workshops for academics include topics addressing yoga as a path to creativity and productivity, yoga for the eyes and vision, and sessions focused upon academic issues such as finding balance between research and teaching integrating yoga as a means of balancing and organizing your life.

I've been a studio owner for two years, and the work of maintaining an active academic career with studio ownership has been a whirlwind of exciting and also sometimes exhausting work. The task has been incredibly rewarding, especially as the process has led to some incredible collaborations – with my partner Lynn, and also with other local and small businesses owned by women. This has also been a period of deep thinking and strategizing for academic writing – the more yoga I practice and teach, the more I find myself thinking about the connections between yoga and writing, and the importance of the practice for my academic sanity and productivity, as well as my pedagogical efforts. There is also a very healthy shift in the dynamic of my relationships – especially in the process of clearing space for new friendships and partnerships. Because I don't rely solely upon yoga for financial support, I can take some leaps and risks with that business, and focus closely upon building relationships with other women and truly building a powerful collaborative community. The space itself has also attracted new students from the neighborhood as well as former students who attended my classes at other locations. From its inception our space has functioned as more than just a yoga studio. Along with donating the space for workshops on topics related to race and social justice, and meetings for various community groups, we have also held an annual holiday market representing the creative work and wellness-based products and services of over 20 local women artists and entrepreneurs. With my own classes I have felt a deeper sense of "ownership" in terms of my role as a yoga teacher – I always strived to build community in my classes, but this year I could schedule my own activities before and after classes and this has included hosting events like a baby shower for a student who attended class throughout her pregnancy and pop-up events focused upon attracting particular groups such as teenage girls and their mothers. The process of converging my "yoga life" with my academic one has fostered new relationships and shaped my academic work in meaningful ways. For the first time last year, I had a group of faculty from my department come to class, and the experience, once again, allowed us to engage with each other in ways that promoted self-care as well as community care – we all recognized the need for more grounded, healing spaces and opportunities for deeper connection.

The process of owning and running a studio also brings up important questions about the importance of honoring our environments and building nurturing spaces within them. One of my biggest reflections in the past month has had to do with thinking about the energetics and spiritual responsibility towards the space itself. Our building is historic – it was built in 1905 and has an enduring presence in our neighborhood, serving as a church for many years and also as an event space. It was a church in the critical years of the civil rights movement, and, from what we have heard from passers-by and from our landlord, it was a beacon in Atlanta – not just as a church but also as a space of convergence for activists within the civil rights movement. We are trying to gather and learn more about the history of that space, but it seems to carry the energy of that vital period in our history. As current renters, we try to honor that lineage, and also present the space as a reminder of the long history of the city. While the neighborhood is rapidly gentrifying, and is now surrounded by new buildings and condos attracting young professionals in Atlanta, we value the old, uneven floors and wooden walls along with a stage which used to function as a sacred and ceremonial space in the years when the building served as a church and shelter for the community. Now, in 2020, we find ourselves thinking not only about how we are providing yoga as a sacred and healing practice but also about how we are honoring and continuing the lineage of the space. In the same way that Sri Aurobindo argues for a yoga that focuses upon evolution, transformation, and action in the world, I see the development of the space and its evolution as critical to serving the needs of our community and the unifying practices of yoga and meditation at this time. And the theoretical and practical application of that process relies upon me critically thinking about the space and yoga itself – aligning academic work on social justice and community building with the work of teaching and building a diverse, kind, and welcoming yoga community.

Our newest challenge has emerged in 2020 as a result of the global health situation surrounding the coronavirus. I write this "addendum" or revision of my essay while sheltering at home and embarking on the process of a whole new virtual model of teaching. It has now been ten months of temporarily closing the studio and teaching through Zoom and Facebook live. This has felt like creating a whole new business, and each day the forced online "experiment" has brought new challenges and new ways to learn – my teaching has been enriched by the presence of colleagues in classes from around the world – I thought of calling a recent class the "Victorian yoga salon" because so many 19th-century academics I know were in it. I've become a better teacher because online teaching means being painfully aware of how your words and expressions translate on camera, and I've learned to eliminate the various "tics" or filler words you use to explain things. This period has been the most isolated in many ways, but also the richest as I've taken classes with all my teachers who are also teaching online, and completed the last phase of an advanced 500 hour training graduating online instead of in person. While the screen has shifted the way we do things, it has also enriched this time at home and connected many of us even more deeply. It also has allowed us to think about how to evolve, progress, and think carefully about priorities, what we value, and what kind of life we want to create for ourselves when the pandemic begins to subside. I cannot imagine getting through this phase without my yoga and meditation practice, and without the lifestyle and philosophical support that my yoga experience brings to my life. While it has been a struggle to do the work of writing a new book (on gender, colonial travel, and the global expansion of yoga) at this time, practicing and thinking about yoga has been a crucial part of each day. We face so many unknowns now, and the pandemic brings many things into question – when we may return to our studios, how long we can afford to sustain them, and how this phase will change the way we teach in more permanent ways. Many of my students are becoming accustomed to yoga on screen, and the convenience of practicing from home. Others desperately miss the community and chatter after class. Some have been more out of touch and dealing with the stress and upheaval of work at home, or uncomfortable with the idea of practicing with technology. As I grapple with the different shifts of the online experience, I wonder how my teaching will have to evolve – and how long it will take before I can give adjustments, give students big hugs, or wrap them up in studio blankets for savasana. While the pandemic has created limits to yoga studio teaching, the practice of yoga is now much more integrated in my remote teaching experience on campus. Unlike my first timid foray into sharing "my yoga life" with college students ten years ago, now my fall class (on Literature and Medicine – a timely, and sometimes stressful topic for the times) has material on yoga more fully integrated – not only as a theoretical aspect of the class but also as a practice students can experience for their own well being. I'm collaborating on an initiative in my department that offers students and the faculty/staff community free access to my studio classes, and I have made my academic responsibilities include frequent check-ins with students to address how we are taking care of ourselves and prioritizing our health and wellness at this time. The tragic lack of leadership from institutions and political structures surrounding the pandemic has opened up ways for all of us to address and strategize care amongst ourselves, and given us more of a sense of urgency to show how yoga and its vast practices and benefits are strikingly necessary at this time. We can no longer think of our work as yoga practitioners as being a band-aid or cozy supplement to the work we do in classrooms, workspaces, and communities we inhabit – the pandemic, racial tensions in the United States and around the globe, political upheavals, and uncertain and vulnerable environmental and health situations have shown us that yoga is and must be integrated and prioritized to support and strengthen our own well-being and improve the various structures and communities that surround us.

Bringing together yoga and academic thinking is an integrative and intersectional process. Just as feminists and theorists of race, sexuality, and class have argued for the value of considering the intersectional aspects of our identities and relationships, I suggest that we need to consider yoga as an intersectional bridge or web that we can integrate within our lives to create more harmonious linkages between our various identities, spaces, and communities. This can be a process of reclamation – where we can define and promote the thoughtful and rigorous practices of yoga that come from various lineages. While yoga is a flexible practice – one that can mean many things to many people and take many forms, we need to honor its roots and varied lineages and recognize its current forms and often hybridized fusions of cultures and practices. However we honor and practice, we can explore its potential transformative and collaborative value in the various spaces we inhabit and also integrate it as part of who we are. As yoga practitioners and teachers in other spaces, we need to recognize the value of bringing our varied knowledge into all the spaces we create and build. We then can be part of the process of redefining and reclaiming yoga, but this time not in the flashy corporate and fast-paced images we so often see, but instead in the space of intentional, tender, tending communities shielded with the protection and grounding of a blanket.

Notes

1 Critical work on yoga and its relationship to Western culture expanded in the 1990s with seminal work by Joseph Alter, Elizabeth De Michelis, and others, with much of this work produced by scholars in the fields of anthropology and religious studies. More recent texts have begun to analyze yoga in its contemporary and popular culture contexts. The publication of *21st Century Yoga* (Horton and Harvey eds.) in 2012 and works such as *Yoga, The Body, and Embodied Social Change* (Berila et al eds.) reveal the ways in which yoga is emerging as an important interdisciplinary and intersectional subject of study. These recent texts also focus upon analyzing the potential of yoga as a means of social justice.

2 See the long tradition of work in feminist theory that grapples with Cartesian models of a mind-body divide and addresses ways that women and bodily processes are devalued. This tradition begins with the work of figures such as Simone de Beavoir and continues with critics including Denise Riley, Susan Bordo, Elizabeth Grosz, Judith Butler, and many others. Mary Douglas has shown how the body can be powerful symbolically, and Michel Foucault has theorized how it can be regulated and monitored in our daily lives. Following Foucault, Bordo has explored how disciplining the female body endures as a strategy of social control. As we acknowledge our bodies in classrooms and spaces we inhabit, we need to recognize and challenge the

ongoing regulatory qualities of the body and its cultural representation. Acknowledging the importance of "self-care" also requires transforming dominant ways of thinking about physical practices of the body as frivolous or unproductive acts. Further, we can theorize the value of yoga as a "transformative practice" that challenges the ongoing binaries of our culture and the devaluation of the body and its relationship to the mind as a vital collaboration.

3 In his essay, "Modern Yoga will Not Form and Real Culture," from *21st Century Yoga* (Horton and Harvey eds.), Remski argues that yoga studios need to function as foundational spaces for communities – for example, he proposes that kitchens can function as soup kitchens (122) and also recommends a list of ideas for studio owners and practitioners to make yoga more accessible, inviting, and supportive. These include ideas like classes that have a fluid beginning time (122), creating family programming and affirmations for relationships (126) and sliding scale fees (125). These are just a few of the many suggestions he makes to create more welcoming community based yoga spaces.

Bibliography

Barbezat, Daniel and Mirabel Bush. *Contemplative Practices in Higher Education*. San Francisco: John Wiley and Sons, 2014.

Berilla, Beth. *Integrating Mindfulness into Anti-Oppression Pedagogy*. Social Justice in Higher Education. Routledge, 2015.

Berilla, Beth et al. (eds). *Yoga, The Body, and Embodied Social Change: An Intersectional Feminist Analysis*. Lanham, Maryland: Lexington Books, 2016.

Grosz, Elizabreth. *Volatile Bodies. Toward a Corporeal Feminism*. Bloomington: Indiana University Press, 1994.

Horton, Carol and Roseanne Harvey. *21st Century Yoga. Culture, Politics, and Practice*. Chicago: Kleio Books, 2012.

Jagger, Alison M. and Susan Bordo. *Gender/Body/Knowledge. Feminist Reconstructions of Being and Knowing*. Rutgers: Rutgers University Press, 1989.

Love, Robert. *The Great Oom. The Improbable Birth of Yoga in America*. Viking Books, 2010.

Price, Janet and Margaret Shildrick, *Feminist Theory and the Body. A Reader*. Edinburgh: Edinburgh University Press, 1999.

Singleton, Mark. *Yoga Body: The Origins of Modern Postural Practice*. Oxford: Oxford University Press, 2011.

Wenger, Christy I. *Yoga Minds, Writing Bodies: Contemplative Writing Pedagogy*. Anderson, SC: Parlor Press, 2015.

Index

2004 International Association of Black Yoga Teachers 256
2016 presidential election 4

abolition 128
Abu-Jamal, Mumia 53–54, 63n5
Adams, Erin 220–221
Afghanistan, refugees 184–185
Africa, John 53–54
Africa, Pam 54
Africa, Ramona 53–54, 56
Africa Jr., Mike 54
Ahimsa 31–32, 246, 247, 249, 251
Alexander, Michelle 284
Allen, Maryrose 163–164
American Dance Festival Studios 13–14
Americanized yoga 230
amygdala 72
An, Sohyun 222
antiracism 17–20; interconnection 21–22
Antony, M. 85
Apple, Michael 233
apprenticeship of observation 233
Arbery, Ahmaud 131n8
Ardhanarishvara 169–171
Argenal, Amy 39
asana 9, 12, 27, 29, 35, 59, 118, 123, 129, 131n3, 136, 137, 166, 168, 172, 178–181, 203, 205–206, 210, 215–216, 226, 241, 297
Ashton, Catherine 182
asylum seekers 176–179
Aurobindo, Sri 204, 301

Bajaj, Monisha 39–40
Baldwin, James 287–288
banking system of education 86
Barkataki, Susanna 29, 246, 251
Bautista, Claudia 205–211
Beaujeu, J.A. 160
Beaujeu-Hawley, Madame 160
becoming 215–216
Berila, Beth 294, 297
Bhagavad Gita 245
Bhajan, Yogi 259
Biswas, P. 85
Black girls 257–258
Black liberation 63n6
Black Lives Matter 128, 167, 244
Black Lotus Collective 30–34
Black Panther Party 53; Oakland Community School (OCS) 287
Black Power era, Philadelphia 54–55
Black women, female slaves 161
Blackhorse, Amanda 143
Blackness 124, 126, 161
Blake 243–244
Bloomberg, Michael 282
Bloomfeld, Christine 280
bodies, reclaiming 295
body-based neurological functions 73
Boone Universalist Unitarian Church 10
Bourne, J. 85
Braden, Anne 18
Braden, Carl 18
brahmacharya 33
brain breaks 229–230
Brandli, Lynn 298
breastfeeding 188
breath 79; survival responses 70–73
Breathing Access 277–283
Breathing Room 275–276; yoga in schools 277–283
Brett, Emily 88
Brillo advertisement (1968) *113*

Bring it to the Mat: Yoga, Mindfulness and Racial Justice 9
Broca's area 72
Brooks, Louise 110
brown, adrienne maree 22, 77
Brown yogis 42
Bryan, William "Roddie" 131n8
Buckle, Jennifer L. 182, 185
Budh (Mercury) 169
Burton, Jazmyn 57

California Department of Corrections and Rehabilitation (CDCR) 180–181
Campaign to Bring Mumia Home 57
Caplan, Marianna 194
Cartesian dualism 136–137
caste-privileged 41
Castile, Philando 118, 130n1
CDCR (California Department of Corrections and Rehabilitation) 180–181
Chandra (Lunar God) 169
Chandra, Shefali 111
Chaudhury, Aadita 57
Chauvin, Derek 131n7
Chris 243–244
Circle of Hope 182, 186, 196–197
class observations, Ourmala and OMPowerment Project case study 94–95
coconspiratorship 76–77
Cognitive Behavioural Therapy 85
Cole, Elizabeth 269
Cole, Teju 86
collective energy 33
collective fear 9
collective liberation 7
collective visibility 30
College of Education 219
colonialism, settler colonialism 124–126
commercialization of yoga 29
community 296; Black Lotus Collective 30–34; niyamas (observances) 33–34; refugees 185–188; yamas (social restraints) 31–33
community building 275–276
community space 297–300
complementary and alternative health 256
Consider This: A Read-In for 21st Century Literacies 11
contemplative practices 51
corn, Diné (Navajo) 145
COVID-19 129; asylum seekers 178
Craven, Christa 162–163

Crawford, Joan 110
Creative Social Stewardship 5
Crenshaw, Kimberlé 86, 115, 258
critical literacy 40
crown of the head, Diné (Navajo) 147
CRT (critical race theory) 86, 102
CTZNWell Summit 14
cultural appropriation 28–29
cultural healing 34–36
cultural trauma 28, 183

Dadosky, John 137
Dance studies 137–138
Dancer's Pose, Diné (Navajo) 149–150
Darya 240–241
DASS-21 (Depression Anxiety Stress Scale-21) 261,265–267
data collection, Ourmala and OMPowerment Project case study 87–88
decolonization 30, 41, 126, 154n7
decolonizing methodologies 154n6
Demby, Gene 284
demographics, K-12 yoga research 258–259
Depression Anxiety Stress Scale-21 (DASS-21) 261,265–267
DERS-SF (Difficulties in Emotion Regulation Scale-Short Forms) 261,264–265
detention alternative yoga programs 282
Difficulties in Emotion Regulation Scale-Short Form (DERS-SF) 261,264–265
Diné (Navajo) 133; Laughter, Haley 138–150
Diné philosophies 136
Dream Defenders 59
Dunbar-Nelson, Alice 161
Duncan, Arne 284
Dwyer, Sonya Corbin 182, 185

eagles, Diné (Navajo) 134
Eat, Pray, Love (Gilbert) 111–112
education: becoming 215–216; mindfulness in teachers 228–232; neoliberalism 226; purpose of 205–207; teacher education 226–227; theory/practice divide 232–234; Year of India *see* Year of India
eight limbs for radical healing 29–30
El Centro de Estudiantes High School 59
Elegy (Girmay) 130
Embodied Learning Summit 10, 12

embodied self-reflection 215–216
embodiment 73–77, 294
energy 33
engaged pedagogy 206
engaging yoga critically 40–42
epigenetics 68–69, 79–80
eugenics 158
Europe, refugees 177–178
Everett, Rupert 165
exercise 158–160

Fabletics 166
Facing History and Ourselves 205
fall events, Year of India 224–225
families, asylum seekers 179
family yoga class (Oakland, CA) 42–44; instructor's perspectives 44–45; kids/parents' perspectives 45–47
fear, collective fear 9
female slaves 161
feminism 294, 295
Fernandez, Johanna 53
fertility 168–169
Fight, Flight, Freeze, Submit, Fawn (FFFSF) 69–71, 73, 75–76, 78–79
Fine, Michelle 269
Five Essential Questions 9, 13, 14
Florence 213–214
Flowerthief 29
Floyd, George 127, 131n7, 167
FMI (Freiberg Mindfulness Inventory) 88
focus 231
folx 77
Fonda, Jane 110
Ford, Jillian 222
Foster, Susan 152
Free Your Mind, Free Mumia, Free Them All 57
Freedom Square Encampment 131n4
Freiberg Mindfulness Inventory (FMI) 88
Freire, P. 85–86, 99, 100, 204, 206, 215, 279, 284
future of YBL (Yoga for Black Lives) 126–130

gabriel, jean-jacques 57, 58
Gay, Ross 123
gender, expanded definitions of 168–172
gender expression 169–170
gender-fluidity 168
generational trauma 49
"Get Free Fest" 57
"Get Free Manifesto" 57

Gilmore, Ruth Wilson 129
Ginwright, Shawn A. 49–51
Girls Justice League 59
girls of color, K-12 yoga research 257–258, 269
Girmay, Aracelis 130
Givón, Talmy 279
Global Learning and Mindfulness through the Study of India 222–223
Goode, Wilson 52
Goop 109
Gottschild, Brenda Dixon 148
gratitude journals 240–241
Greece, refugees 176–178
Greenspan, Miriam 280
Grosz, Elizabeth 295
guru-śiṣya relationship 84–85
gymnastics 160

Haines, Staci K. 179
hair, Diné (Navajo) 143
Harshman, J. 229
Hartsfield, Denise 274
Harvard Trauma (HT) Questionnaire 88
Hatha yoga 181
Headstand, Diné (Navajo) 148–149
healing 78; cultural healing 34–36; eight limbs for radical healing 29–30; politicized healing, Philadelphia 56–59; radical healing 49–51, 56; Yusra 193–194
healing circle 182; Javad 191–193; Neda 194–195; Zahra 188–191
healing justice 50–51
health 115–116
HEALTHY ACTIVE NATIVES!!!! 134
Heartfull Meditation 298
Henry 246–249
Hepatitis C 54
Herman, Judith 284–285
Hindu Nationalist legacy 246
Hindu nationalists 57
Hinduism 41
history of yoga in US 158–164
Hogan 136, 142, 151
Home (Shire) 179
Hot Hooghan Yoga 136, 150–153
hot yoga 221
Hozho Total Wellness 133, 136, 143
Hozho Yoga (2017) 133–136, 138–150
Hudson, Kate 166
Huggins, Erica 171, 287
Human Rights Watch 178

identity mask activity 208
ideology of oppression 284
imperial trauma 28
incarcerated people 180
India 28, 244–246
insider-outsider roles 182–183, 185
insula 72, 74
integrative health 256
integrative medicine 256
interconnectedness 243, 296
interconnection 17; antiracism 21–22
internalized oppression 31–32
interoception 73–75
interpersonal relationships 80
intersectional balancing 75
intersectionality 86
intrapersonal relationships 80
Iran: migrants 183–184; refugees 242
Iyengar, B.K.S. 85, 136, 242, 249, 298

Jackson 246–250
Javad, healing circle 191–193
Joines, Allen 277
Jois, Pattabhi 85
Jones, Grant 35
Jubilee School, Philadelphia 54–55
Juntos 55

K-12 yoga research 257–258, 268–269; DASS-21 (Depression Anxiety Stress Scale-21) 265–267; demographics 258–259; DERS-SF (Difficulties in Emotion Regulation Scale-Short Forms) 264–265; MAAS-S (Mindful Attention Awareness Scale-Adolescent) 261–263; study procedures 260; Y4Y (Y.O.G.A. for Youth) 259–260
Kahn-John, Michelle 136
Kannaki 170–171
Karma yoga 182, 245
Karpovich, Peter V. 163
Kaushik-Brown, Roopa 235
Kelley, Robin D.G. 50
Kensington CAPA, Philadelphia 54–55
Khalsa, Keval Kaur 257
Khomeini, Ayatollah 183
Khour 185
Kindred Healing Justice Collective 51
Koithan, Mary 136
Krishnamurti, J. 205, 206
Kruse-Peeples, Melissa 145, 146
Kueng, J. Alexander 131n7
Kumanyika, Chenjerai 115

Kumar, Rebecca 166
Kundalini yoga 180; Y4Y (Y.O.G.A. for Youth) 259–260
Kyleah, Ms. 49, 61–62

Lajja Gauri 172n5
Lakota people 135
Lane, Thomas K. 131n7
Laughter, Haley 133–137, 151–152, 154n7; *Hozho Yoga* (2017) 138–150
Lauren 214–215
Laxman, family yoga class (Oakland, CA) 44–45
learning 284
LeBlanc-Ernest, Angela 287
Lee, Cynthia Ling 247
leisure-wellness 112
Leonard, Thomas 116
Leonardo, Z. 233
liberation 19; collective liberation 7
Lighthouse Reports 177
"Little Yoga Co-op" 298
lordosis 15n2
Lortie, D. C. 233
Love, Robert 291
Lululemon 56, 112, 171

M&E (Monitoring and Evaluation) 83
MAAS-S (Mindful Attention Awareness Scale-Adolescent) 261–263
MacDonald, Laquan 129, 131n9
Macy, Joanna 17
Madonna 112, 164–166
Mahabarata 168
mainstreaming of yoga 56–59
Majumder, Sarasij 225
Malakasa camp 185
Manigault-Bryant, James 39
Manuel, Zenju Earthlyn 17, 21–22
Mattingly, Kate 137
McDowell, Carol 241
McKoy, Essie 279
McMichael, Gregory 131n8
McMichael, Travis 131n8
men, yoga and 192
Menakem, Resmaa 188
Midland, Julia 88
migrants 82–83
Miller, Amara 38
Mindful Attention Awareness Scale-Adolescent (MAAS-A) 261–263
mindfulness, teachers 226
Mindfulness and Resistance 5

Mindfulness and Resistance: The Body as Chronicle workshop 11–12
moccasins 133, 153n1
Modi, Prime Minister 246
Monáe, Janelle 166
Monitoring and Evaluation (M&E) 83
Monroe, Marilyn 110–111
Moore, Laura Jane 153n1
Morales-Williams, Mari 18, 58
MOVE 52–55
MOVE 9 54, 63n7
movement 79
Mun, Roksana 55
Muscular Christianity 163
Musial, Jennifer 154n7
music 33; YBL (Yoga for Black Lives) 122; "Yoga for Spirit" 60

Naim 177
Nair, Lakshmi 228
"Naked Athena" 167
Native peoples 134–135; settler colonialism 135–136
Neda, healing circle 194–195
negative eugenics 158
neoliberalism 225
nervous systems 72
neuroception 73
neurological intersectionality 76
neuroplasticity of survival 76, 78
Neville, John 276
The Next Best Thing (2000) 165
Nicole 212–213
"Night Owl" 133–134
niyamas (observances), community 33–34
non-binary entity 169
nonviolence 19
Norman, M. 231

Oakland Community School (OCS) 287
Off The Mat, Into The World 181
OMPowerment Project 83, 86–87, 102, 175, 196–197; analysis of study 100–101; class observations 94–95; participant demographics 91; participant feedback 97–98; teacher surveys 98–99; teacher-training module observations 92–94
online teaching 302
oppression 3, 7–8, 10, 49; internalized oppression 31–32
oppressors 100
orientalism 84

orthoexia nervosa 114
Ourmala 83, 86–87; analysis of study 99–102; class observations 94–95; participant feedback 95–97; teacher surveys 98–99; teacher-training module observations 92–94
Owens, Rod 34–35

Page, Cara 51
Pahlavi, Mohammad Reza 183
PAL (Police Athletic League) 60
Palkhivala, Aadil 298
Paltrow, Gwyneth 109–110
parent industrial complex 38
participant feedback: OMPowerment Project 97–98; Ourmala 95–97
participant observation 83
Parvati 170
Patanjali's Yoga Sutras 19, 29, 204, 249
Patankar, Prachi 41, 57
peace 3
pedagogy of tenderness 294
Pedro 210–212
Pegacornasana 166
Philadelphia: Black Panther Party 53; MOVE 53–55; politicized healing 56–59; radical healing and healing justice 50–51; state-sanctioned trauma 51–52; "Yoga for Spirit" 59–62; youth 54–55
Philadelphia Student Union (PSU) 54–55
physical education 159–160
Piepzna-Samarasinha, Leah Lakshmi 50
Police Athletic League (PAL) 60
politicized healing, Philadelphia 56–59
positive eugenics 158
Pratipaksha Bhavanam 240–241, 252
pratyahara 190, 194
prefrontal cortex 72
prisons 286–287; schools and 283–286
problem-posing education 215
proprioception 73, 75
psoas 15n2
PSU (Philadelphia Student Union) 54–55
Pummel, Brittany 175
Purkiss, Ava 161
Purna Yoga 298
pushbacks 176–177

Queer and Trans yoga 59

racism 22
racists, White people 18

radical healing 30, 49–51, 56
Railey, Janelle 275
Rathbone, Josephine 163
refugee camps 185
refugees 175; Afghanistan 184–185; experiences in 2020 176–180; Iran 242; yoga and 185–188
Refugym 175
"Re-Invention" (2004), Madonna 164–165
relationships 80; teacher/student relationship 84–85
Remski, Matthew 299
resilience 179
resistance 9
restorative justice 247, 249
Restorative Justice Circles method 281
Reynolds, Diamond 118, 130n1
Rizzo, Frank 52
Rodriguez, Sanjuana 222–223
Rosebud Reservation 135, 153n3
Roth, Sammy 139, 141, 142, 143, 144, 153n2, 154nn9–11
Rousseau, Jean Jacques 158
Royster, Jordan 83
Rumi 275

Sabik, Natalie 269
Sadequee, Sonali 224
safety 286
Sailers, Akilah 122
SAMA (Small and Mighty Acts) 5–6
sampling, Ourmala and OMPowerment Project case study 88–90
samskaras 180
SAND (Strategy and Network Development) 59
Santoyo, Juliana 30
satya (truthfulness) 32
saucha 34
savasana 243–244
school justice partnership 274
School Resource Officers (SRO) 273
school to prison pipeline (STPP) 273–274
schools 227, 277–283; prisons and 283–286
Scofield, Be 296
Segall, A. 233
self-awareness 187, 206
self-care 110–113
self-compassion 32
self-liberation 206
self-reflection 215–216
self-regulation, OMPowerment Project 93

settler colonialism 84, 124–126, 135–136
Shilappatikaram 170
Shire, Warsan 179
Shiva 170
silence 74
Silverfox, Robin 133
Singh, Anneliese 300
Singh, Roopa 224
Singleton, Mark 291
slaves 161
Small and Mighty Acts (SAMA) 5–6
A Small Needful Fat (Gay) 123
Smith, Linda Tuhiwai Smith 154n6
Social Darwinism 158–159
social justice 206
social media 297
Somers, Suzanne 110
songs, Laughter, Haley 141
Sood, Sheena 18, 41–42, 57, 58, 239
Spencer, Herbet 158
Spiegel International 177
spiritual bypassing 20–21
spirituality 84
Sri Vidya Tantra tradition 19
SRO (School Resource Officers) 273
St. Denis, Ruth 110, 112
St. Onge, Patricia 17
state-sanctioned trauma, Philadelphia 51–52
Sterling, Alton 118, 131n2
STPP (school to prison pipeline) 273–274
Strategy and Network Development (SAND) 59
students: Blake 243–244; Chris 243–244; Darya 240–241; Florence 213–214; Henry 246–249; Jackson 246–250; Lauren 214–215; Nicole 212–213; Pedro 210–212; Thomas 210; Vanessa 213–214
study procedures, K-12 yoga research 260
Sudbery, Imogen 178
suicide 280
Summerville, Amelia 160
survival responses 69–70; breath 70–73
survival systems 69–70
survivance 153n5
suspension rates 257–258
"Sustaining Organizers through Self/Collective Care" 58
Svadhyaya 9, 180, 242
Swift, Taylor 166
systems 80

Taliban 184
Tantra Hatha asana practice 19
Tantra yoga 19–20
tapas 34
Tara 169
Taylor, Alan 184
Taylor, Breonna 131n8
teacher education 226–227
teacher surveys, Ourmala and OMPowerment Project case study 98–99
teacher/student relationship 84–85, 101
teacher-training module observations, Ourmala 92–94
"Thick Girl Yoga Full Embodied Expression" 253
thinness 160
Thomas 210
Thompson, Becky 293–294
Thompson, Kerry Frances 146, 227
Three Leagues Deep exercise 7–8
Three Sisters Garden 145–146
Tigunait, Pandit Rajmani 19
Todd, Jan 159, 160
trauma 49, 179, 275,280; cultural trauma 28, 183; generational trauma 49; imperial trauma 28; state-sanctioned trauma, Philadelphia 51–52
trauma recovery, safety 286
trauma-informed yoga training 181
The Tree 181
true womanhood 161
Trump, Donald 21
truthfulness (satya) 32
tsiiyéé 143
Turn Up for Freedom (T.U.F.F.) Girls 59

Ujjayi Pranayama (Victorioius breath) 250
United Nations High Commissioner for Refugees (UNHCR) 175, 176
US, history of yoga 158–164

vagus nerve 69
Van Dyke, Jason 129, 131n9
Vanessa 213–214
velvet ghetto 115
Verbrugge, Martha H. 164
violence 250
Vitaly 243–244
Vizenor, Gerald 153n5
Vonne, Vidya 204

"Waging Wellness" yoga series 58
Walker, Adrian 131n8
Warren, Rameka 283
Washington, Harriet 116
wellness 110–111; whiteness and 113–115
Wenger, Christy I. 295
West LA College 239
Western yoga 28–29
Wherry, Christina S. 253
White antiracism 18–19
White hygiene 115–116; White womanhood and 110–111
White people, racists 18
White privilege 19–21, 84
white supremacists, Hindu nationalists and 57
White supremacy 20, 115
White womanhood, White hygiene 110–111
whiteness 18–19, 21, 22, 29, 84, 125; wellness and 113–115
White-saviour industrial complex (WSIC) 86
Winston Salem, North Carolina 277
Wollstonecraft, Mary 159
WSIC (White-saviour industrial complex) 86, 102

Y4Y (Y.O.G.A. for Youth) 259–260
yamas (social restraints), community 31–33
Yanez, Jeronimo 118, 130n1
YASP (Youth Art & Self-Empowerment Project) 55
YBL (Yoga for Black Lives) 118–122; class structure 122–124; future of 126–130; settler colonialism 124–126
Year of India 219, 222–224; events 224–225; mindfulness in teachers 228–232
Year Of program 219–220
Yellow Bird, Michael 30
Yeye Devi Collective 57–58, 63n12
YMCAs 163
Yoga (2015) 166
yoga fashion industry 171
Yoga for Black Lives (YBL) 118–122; class structure 122–124; future of 126–130; settler colonialism 124–126
"Yoga for Spirit" 49, 59–62
Y.O.G.A. for Youth (Y4Y) 259–260
yoga industrial complex 38

yoga interventions 102, 209
yoga pedagogy 85
yoga porn 171
yoga space 295
yoga studies 84
Yoga Sutra 33, *Pratipaksha Bhavanam* 240
Yoga to Transform Trauma 182
"Yogini Sistahs for Liberation" 58
youth, Philadelphia 54–55

Youth Art & Self-Empowerment Project (YASP) 55
Youth United for Change (YUC) 55
yuj 251
Yusra, healing circle 193–194

Zahra, healing circle 188–191
Zehr, Howard 249
zero-tolerance 274
Zong, G. 226

Printed in the United States
By Bookmasters